Experimental Hematology Today—1987

Experimental Hematology Today—1987

S.J. Baum G.W. Santos F. Takaku
Editors

Recent Advances and Future Directions in Bone Marrow Transplantation

Proceedings of a Symposium Held in Conjunction with the 16th Annual Meeting of the International Society for Experimental Hematology, August 23–28, 1987, Tokyo, Japan

With 36 Illustrations

Springer-Verlag
New York Berlin Heidelberg
London Paris Tokyo

S.J. Baum
Department of Physiology
Uniformed Services University of the Health Sciences
Bethesda, MD 20817, USA

G.W. Santos
Department of Oncology
The John Hopkins Hospital
Baltimore, MD 21205, USA

F. Takaku
Third Department of Internal Medicine
Faculty of Medicine
University of Tokyo
Tokyo, Japan

Library of Congress Cataloging-in-Publication Data
Recent advances and future directions in bone marrow transplantation.
(Experimental hematology today ; 1987)
Includes bibliographies.
1. Bone marrow—Transplantation—Congresses.
I. Baum, Siegmund J. II. Santos, G. W. (George W.)
III. Takaku, Fumimaro. IV. International Society for Experimental Hematology. Meeting (16th : 1987 : Tokyo, Japan) V. Series. [DNLM: 1. Bone Marrow—transplantation—congresses. W1 EX504P 1987 / WH 380 R2945 1987]
RB145.E97 1987 612'.11s 87-28771
[RD123.5] [617'.44]
ISBN-13: 978-1-4612-8339-3 e-ISBN-13; 978-1-4612-3762-4
DOI: 10.1007/978-1-4612-3762-4

Camera-ready copy provided by the editors.

9 8 7 6 5 4 3 2 1

Acknowledgments

The organizers of the symposium and the International Society for Experimental Hematology wish to acknowledge the generous assistance and grants provided by the following organizations of the United States Government:

National Heart, Lung, and Blood Institute, National Institutes of Health, Department of Health and Human Services, Public Health Service, Bethesda, Maryland 20892.

Fleet Health Care Systems, Code 405, Naval Medical Research and Development Command, Naval Medical Center National Capital Region, Bethesda, Maryland 20814-5044.

The generous assistance provided by the following persons was also greatly appreciated:

Dr. Alan S. Levine, National Heart, Lung, and Blood Institute, National Institutes of Health, Public Health Service, Bethesda, Maryland 20892.

Commander Thomas J. Contreras, Technology Area Manager, Biomedical/CBR, ONT-223, Office of Naval Technology, 800 North Quincy Street, Arlington, Virginia 22217-5000.

Furthermore, the generous grant provided by the following organization was greatly appreciated:

Leukemia Society of America, Inc., 733 Third Avenue, New York, New York 10017.

The Editors

Contents

Contributors

Massimo Aglietta, M.D., Associate Professor, University of Torino, School of Medicine, Torino, Italy

Fabrizio Agostinelli, Biologist, Assistant in Hematology, Divisione di Ematologia, Ospedale Civile, Pesaro, Italy

Richard F. Ambinder, M.D., Instructor of Oncology, The Johns Hopkins Hospital, Baltimore, Maryland, USA

Claudio Anasetti, M.D., Assistant Member, Fred Hutchinson Cancer Research Center, Seattle, Washington, USA

Hans Kerzel Andersen, D.V.M., Associate Professor, Institute of Medical Microbiology, University of Aarhus, Aarhus, Denmark

Emanuele Angelucci, M.D., Assistant in Hematology, Divisione di Ematologia, Ospedale Civile, Pesaro, Italy

Frederick R. Appelbaum, M.D., Associate Professor of Medicine, University of Washington, and Associate Member, Fred Hutchinson Cancer Research Center, Seattle, Washington, USA

Shigetaku Asano, M.D., University of Tokyo, Institute of Medical Science, Tokyo, Japan

Jens Henrik Badsberg, Ph.D., Assistant Professor and Statistician, Statistical Research Unit, University of Copenhagen, Copenhagen, Denmark

Donatella Baronciani, M.D., Assistant in Hematology, Divisione di Ematologia, Ospedale Civile, Pesaro, Italy

A.J. Barrett, M.D., F.R.C. Path., Department of Hematology, Westminster Hospital, London, United Kingdom

Siegmund J. Baum, Ph.D., Department of Physiology, Uniformed Services University of the Health Sciences, School of Medicine, Bethesda, Maryland, USA

Patrick Beatty, M.D., Assistant Member, Fred Hutchinson Cancer Research Center, and Assistant Professor of Medicine, University of Washington, School of Medicine, Seattle, Washington, USA

William Bensinger, M.D., Assistant Member, Fred Hutchinson Cancer Research Center, and Assistant Professor of Medicine, University of Washington, School of Medicine, Seattle, Washington, USA

William E. Beschorner, M.D., Associate Professor of Pathology and Oncology, The Johns Hopkins Hospital, Baltimore, Maryland, USA

Carolyn Bigelow, M.D., Associate in Clinical Research, Fred Hutchinson Cancer Research Center, Seattle, Washington, USA

Alessandro Bocconcelli, M.D., Fellow, Divisione di Ematologia, Ospedale Civile, Pesaro, Italy

Mortimer M. Bortin, M.D., Professor of Medicine, Department of Medicine, The Medical College of Wisconsin, Milwaukee, Wisconsin, USA

Raleigh A. Bowden, M.D., Acting Assistant Professor of Pediatrics, Department of Pediatrics, University of Washington, and Assistant Member, Program in Infectious Diseases, Fred Hutchinson Cancer Research Center, Seattle, Washington, USA

Susan Brennan, M.S., Senior Research Technician, The Johns Hopkins Oncology Center, Baltimore, Maryland, USA

Paul A. Brown, Research Technician, Fred Hutchinson Cancer Research Center, Seattle, Washington, USA

C. Dean Buckner, M.D., Program Head, Chemotherapy and Supportive Care, Fred Hutchinson Cancer Research Center, and Professor of Medicine, University of Washington, School of Medicine, Seattle, Washington, USA

Mary J. Buffo, B.S., Cancer Research Laboratories, Allegheny-Singer Research Institute, Allegheny General Hospital, Pittsburgh, Pennsylvania, USA

William H. Burns, M.D., Associate Professor of Oncology and Medicine, Department of Oncology and Medicine, The John Hopkins University School of Medicine, The Johns Hopkins Oncology Center, Baltimore, Maryland, USA

Anna Butturini, M.D., Assistant Professor, University of Parma, Parma, Italy

A. Michele Carella, A.M., M.D., Associate Professor of Hematology, Department of Hematology, San Martino Hospital, Genova, Italy

Filippo Centis, M.Sc., Fellow in Research, Divisione di Ematologia, Ospedale di Pesaro, Pesaro, Italy

Josette Champagne, M.D., Childrens Hospital of Los Angeles, Department of Research Immunology/BMT, Los Angeles, California, USA

Richard E. Champlin, M.D., Associate Professor of Medicine, Department of Medicine, Division of Hematology/Oncology, UCLA Medical Center, Los Angeles, California, USA

James Chang, M.R.C. Path, Hematology Department, Christie Hospital and Holt Radium Institute, Manchester, United Kingdom

Martin Cheever, M.D., Associate Member, Fred Hutchinson Cancer Research Center, and Associate Professor, University of Washington, School of Medicine, Seattle, Washington, USA

Reginald A. Clift, F.I.M.L.S., Associate Staff Scientist, Fred Hutchinson Cancer Research Center, Seattle, Washington, USA

Paolo Coleselli, M.D., Associate Professor, Pediatrics Department, University of Padova, School of Medicine, Padova, Italy

Maxwell Cooper, Childrens Hospital of Los Angeles, Department of Research Immunology/BMT, Los Angeles, California, USA

Edward A. Copelan, M.D., Assistant Professor of Medicine and Assistant Director, The Ohio State University, Bone Marrow Transplantation Program, Columbus, Ohio, USA

George W. Counts, M.D., Professor of Medicine, Department of Medicine, University of Washington, School of Medicine, and Member, Microbiology/Infectious Diseases, Fred Hutchinson Cancer Research Center, Seattle, Washington, USA

L.H. Coutinho, M.D., Paterson Institute for Cancer Research, Christie Hospital and Holt Radium Institute, Manchester, England

Yves DeClerck, M.D., Assistant Professor of Pediatrics, University of Southern California School of Medicine, Los Angeles, California, USA

H. Joachim Deeg, M.D., Professor of Medicine, Lombardi Cancer Research Center, Georgetown University, Washington, D.C., USA

T.M. Dexter, Ph.D., D.Sc., M.R.C. Path., Professor and Head of Department, Experimental Hematology, Paterson Institute for Cancer Research, Christie Hospital, Manchester, United Kingdom

Karel A. Dicke, M.D., Ph.D., Professor of Medicine, Internist, Department of Hematology, Bone Marrow Transplantation Section, UT–M.D. Anderson Hospital and Tumor Institute, Houston, Texas, USA

Meris Donati, Biologist, Assistant in Hematology, Divisione di Ematologia, Ospedale Civile, Pesaro, Italy

Kris Doney, M.D., Associate Member, Fred Hutchinson Cancer Research Center, and Associate Professor of Medicine, University of Washington, School of Medicine, Seattle, Washington, USA

Albert D. Donnenberg, Ph.D., Assistant Professor of Oncology, Immunology, and Infectious Diseases, The Johns Hopkins Hospital, Baltimore, Maryland, USA

Veronica Draper, Childrens Hospital of Los Angeles, Department of Research Immunology/BMT, Los Angeles, California, USA

Evan Farmer, M.D., Associate Professor, Dermatology, The Johns Hopkins Hospital, Baltimore, Maryland, USA

Joseph W. Fay, M.D., Director, Bone Marrow Transplant Program, Charles Sammons Cancer Center, Baylor University Medical Center, Dallas, Texas, USA

Alexander Fefer, M.D., Member, Fred Hutchinson Cancer Research Center, and Professor of Medicine, University of Washington, School of Medicine, Seattle, Washington, USA

Ann C. Fischer, Laboratory Technician, The Johns Hopkins Hospital, Baltimore, Maryland, USA

Debra Frei-Lahr, M.D., Instructor, Department of Medicine, Barnard Cancer Center, Washington University, School of Medicine, St. Louis, Missouri, USA

Kenneth Friedman, M.D., Research Postdoctoral Fellow, The Johns Hopkins Hospital, Baltimore, Maryland, USA

Gösta Gahrton, M.D., Professor, Department of Medicine, Huddinge Hospital, Huddinge, and Karolinska Institute, Stockholm, Sweden

Robert Peter Gale, M.D., Ph.D., Associate Professor of Medicine, Department of Medicine, Division of Hematology/Oncology, University of California, Los Angeles School of Medicine, and President, The Armand Hammer Center for Advanced Studies in Nuclear Energy and Health, Los Angeles, California, USA

Maria Galimberti, M.D., Assistant in Hematology, Divisione di Ematologia, Ospedale Civile, Pesaro, Italy

Claudio Giardini, M.D., Assistant in Hematology, Divisione di Ematologia, Ospedale Civile, Pesaro, Italy

Clizia Giorgi, Biologist, Assistant in Hematology, Divisione di Ematologia, Ospedale Civile, Pesaro, Italy

John Goldman, D.M., F.R.C.P., F.R.C.Path., Senior Lecturer, Royal Postgraduate Medical School, London, United Kingdom

E.C. Gordon-Smith, M.D., Department of Hematology, St. George's Hospital Medical School, London, United Kingdom

Theodore C. Graham, Animal Laboratory Supervisor, Fred Hutchinson Cancer Research Center, Seattle, Washington, USA

Alois Gratwohl, M.D., Division of Hematology, Department of Internal Medicine, Kantonsspital, University of Basel, Basel, Switzerland

Philip Greenberg, M.D., Associate Member, Fred Hutchinson Cancer Research Center, and Associate Professor of Medicine, University of Washington, School of Medicine, Seattle, Washington, USA

John Hansen, M.D., Member, Fred Hutchinson Cancer Research Center, and Professor of Medicine, University of Washington, School of Medicine, Seattle, Washington, USA

Geoffrey P. Herzig, M.D., Associate Professor of Medicine, Department of Medicine, Barnard Cancer Center, Washington University, School of Medicine, St. Louis, Missouri, USA

Roger H. Herzig, M.D., Director, Bone Marrow Transplantation Program, Cleveland Clinic Cancer Center, Department of Hematology and Medical Oncology, Cleveland Clinic Foundation, Cleveland, Ohio, USA

Allan D. Hess, Ph.D., Associate Professor of Oncology, Immunology, and Infectious Diseases, Department of Oncology, The Johns Hopkins Hospital, Baltimore, Maryland, USA

Roger Hill, M.B., Ch.B., M.R.A.C.P., F.R.A.C.P., F.R.C.P.A., Assistant Professor of Medicine, University of Washington, School of Medicine, and Assistant Member, Fred Hutchinson Cancer Research Center, Seattle, Washington, USA

Winston G. Ho, M.D., Associate Professor of Medicine, Department of Medicine, Division of Hematology/Oncology, UCLA Medical Center, Los Angeles, California, USA

Mary M. Horowitz, M.D., Assistant Professor of Medicine, Department of Medicine, The Medical College of Wisconsin, Milwaukee, Wisconsin, USA

Leonard J. Horwitz, M.D., Assistant Internist, Instructor in Medicine, Department of Hematology, Bone Marrow Transplantation Section, UT-M.D. Anderson Hospital and Tumor Institute, Houston, Texas, USA

Takao Ichioka, M.D., Postdoctoral Fellow in Neurology, The Johns Hopkins University School of Medicine, and The Kennedy Institute, Baltimore, Maryland, USA

Tadaatsu Ito, M.D., Assistant Professor, Department of Pediatrics, Teikyo University School of Medicine, Tokyo, Japan

Niels Jacobsen, M.D., Ph.D., Bone Marrow Transplantation Unit, Department of Infectious Diseases, Copenhagen University Hospital, Copenhagen, Denmark

Sundar Jagannath, M.D., Assistant Professor and Assistant Internist, Department of Hematology, Bone Marrow Transplantation Section, UT-M.D. Anderson Hospital and Tumor Institute, Houston, Texas, USA

Richard Jones, M.D., Clinical Fellow, Department of Oncology, The John Hopkins Hospital, Baltimore, Maryland, USA

Akihisa Kanamaru, M.D., Ph.D., Lecturer, Second Department of Internal Medicine, Hyogo College of Medicine, Nishinomiya, Hyogo, Japan

Niels Keiding, Ph.D., Research Professor, Statistical Research Unit, University of Copenhagen, Copenhagen, Denmark

John H. Kersey, M.D., Professor, Department of Laboratory Medicine and Pathology and Pediatrics, University of Minnesota, Minneapolis School of Medicine, Minneapolis, Minnesota, USA

Yasuo Kishimoto, Ph.D., Professor of Neurology, The Johns Hopkins University School of Medicine, and The Kennedy Institute, Baltimore, Maryland, USA

Deborah L. Kociban, B.S., Cancer Research Laboratories, Allegheny-Singer Research Institute, Allegheny General Hospital, Pittsburgh, Pennsylvania, USA

Yoshihisa Kodera, M.D., Division Head of Hematology, The Japanese Red Cross Nagoya First Hospital, Nagoya, Japan

William Krivit, M.D., Ph.D., Professor of Pediatrics, Unversity of Minnesota Medical School, Minneapolis, Minnesota, USA

C. Frederick LeMaistre, M.D., Assistant Professor of Medicine, University of Texas Health Science Center, Department of Medicine, Division of Hematology, San Antonio, Texas, USA

Berit Lönnqvist, M.D., Associate Professor, Department of Medicine, Huddinge Hospital, Huddinge, Sweden

James N. Lowder, M.D., Cleveland Clinic Cancer Center, Departments of Immunology and Cancer Research and Hematology-Medical Oncology, Cleveland Clinic Foundation, Cleveland, Ohio, USA

Guido Lucarelli, M.D., Chief of Hematology, Divisione di Ematologia, Ospedale Civile, Pesaro, Italy

Gunnar Lund, M.D., Associate Professor, Department of Radiology, University of Nebraska, Omaha, Nebraska, USA

Enrico Madon, M.D., Director, Clinica Pediatrica, Università di Torino, Torino, Italy

Flavia Manenti, M.D., Assistant in Hematology, Divisione di Ematologia, Ospedale Civile, Pesaro, Italy

Lina Mangoni, M.D., Associate Professor, Hematology Unit, University of Parma, School of Medicine, Parma, Italy

Annunziata Manna, M.D., Fellow, Divisione di Ematologia, Ospedale Civile, Pesaro, Italy

Marisa Manna, Biologist, Assistant in Hematology, Divisione di Ematologia, Ospedale Civile, Pesaro, Italy

Maria Teresa Marchetti-Rossi, M.Sc., Fellow in Research, Divisione di Ematologia, Ospedale di Pesaro, Pesaro, Italy

Donatella Marchionni, Biologist, Assistant in Hematology, Divisione di Ematologia, Ospedale Civile, Pesaro, Italy

Paul Martin, Ph.D., Associate Member, Fred Hutchinson Cancer Research Center, and Associate Professor of Medicine, University of Washington, School of Medicine, Seattle, Washington, USA

Tohru Masaoka, M.D., Director, Fifth Internal Medicine Center for Adult Diseases, Osaka, Japan

Dana Matthews, M.D., Acting Instructor, University of Washington, School of Medicine, Seattle, Washington, USA

William Stratford May, M.D., Assistant Professor of Oncology, The Johns Hopkins Hospital, Baltimore, Maryland, USA

Richard F. Mayer, M.D., Professor of Neurology, The University of Maryland, School of Medicine, Baltimore, Maryland, USA

George McDonald, M.D., Associate Member, Fred Hutchinson Cancer Research Center, and Associate Professor, University of Washington, School of Medicine, Seattle, Washington, USA

Robert McGuffin, M.D., Associate Member, Program Head, Infectious Diseases and Clinical Virology, Fred Hutchinson Cancer Research Center, and Assistant Professor of Medicine, University of Washington, School of Medicine, Seattle, Washington, USA

Joel Meyers, M.D., Associate Professor of Medicine, Department of Medicine, University of Washington, School of Medicine, and Associate Member and Head, Program in Infectious Diseases, Fred Hutchinson Cancer Research Center, Seattle, Washington, USA

H. Mizoguchi, M.D., Department of Medicine//Hematology, Tokyo Women's Medical College, Tokyo, Japan

Takao Mori, M.D., Associate Professor, Third Department of Internal Medicine, Kanazawa University Medical School, Kanazawa, Japan

Yasuo Morishima, M.D., First Department of Internal Medicine, Nagoya University School of Medicine, Nagoya, Japan

Yoshiaki Moriyama, M.D., Associate Professor, First Department of Internal Medicine, Niigata University School of Medicine, Niigata, Japan

Hugo W. Moser, M.D., Professor of Neurology and Pediatrics, The Johns Hopkins University School of Medicine, and President, The Kennedy Institute, Baltimore, Maryland, USA

Ruggero Mozzana, M.D., Associate Professor, University of Milano, School of Medicine, Milano, Italy

Hideo Mugishima, M.D., Instructor, Department of Pediatrics, Nihon University School of Medicine, Tokyo, Japan

Jukka Nikoskelainen, M.D., Ph.D., Associate Professor, Department of Medicine, University of Turku, Turku, Finland

Catherine Nissen, M.D., Division of Hematology, Department of Internal Medicine, Kantonsspital, University of Basel, Basel, Switzerland

James P. OKunewick, Ph.D., Senior Scientist, Director of Experimental Hematology and Flow Cytometry Facility, Cancer Research Laboratories, Allegheny-Singer Research Institute, Allegheny General Hospital, Pittsburgh, Pennsylvania, USA

Mariangela Palazzi, M.D., Fellow, Divisione di Ematologia, Ospedale Civile, Pesaro, Italy

Ortensia Paradisi, Biologist, Assistant in Hematology, Divisione di Ematologia, Ospedale Civile, Pesaro, Italy

Robertson Parkman, M.D., Professor of Pediatrics and Microbiology, University of Southern California, School of Medicine, Los Angeles, California, USA

Carlo Pazzaglia, M.D., Fellow, Divisione di Ematologia, Ospedale Civile, Pesaro, Italy

Finn Bo Petersen, M.D., Assistant Member, Fred Hutchinson Cancer Research Center, Seattle, Washington, USA

Gordon L. Phillips, M.D., Associate Professor of Medicine, University of British Columbia, and Director of Leukemia and Bone Marrow Transplant Program of British Columbia, Vancouver, British Columbia, Canada

D.H. Pluznik, Ph.D., National Institute of Dental Research, National Institutes of Health, Bethesda, Maryland, USA

Paola Polchi, M.D., Assistant in Hematology, Divisione di Ematologia, Ospedale Civile, Pesaro, Italy

Patrizia Politi, M.D., Assistant in Hematology, Divisione di Ematologia, Ospedale Civile, Pesaro, Italy

Adolfo Porcellini, M.D., Director, Division of Hematology and Bone Marrow Transplantation Center, and Associate Professor of Hematology, Department of Hematology, Ospedale Civile, Pesaro, Italy

Jukka Rajantie, M.D., Assistant Professor, Childrens Hospital, University of Helsinki, Helsinki, Finland

Norma K.C. Ramsay, M.D., Professor, Department of Pediatrics, and Director, Pediatric Bone Marrow Transplantation, University of Minnesota Hospital and Clinics, Minneapolis, Minnesota, USA

Donna E. Reece, M.D., Clinical Assistant Professor of Medicine, University of British Columbia, Vancouver, British Columbia, Canada

Elizabeth C. Reed, M.D., Senior Fellow in Medicine, University of Washington, School of Medicine, and Fred Hutchinson Cancer Research Center, Seattle, Washington, USA

Luigi Resegotti, M.D., Chief of Internal Medicine, Divisione di Medicina Interna, Ospedale di Torino, Torino, Italy

Alfred A. Rimm, Ph.D., Professor, Biostatistics/Epidemiology, and Head, Division of Biostatistics/Clinical Epidemiology, Department of Medicine, The Medical College of Wisconsin, Milwaukee, Wisconsin, USA

Olle Ringdén, M.D., Ph.D., Professor, Department of Clinical Immunology, Huddinge Hospital, Huddinge, Sweden

Vittorio Rizzoli, M.D., Professor of Hematology, Hematology Unit, University of Parma, School of Medicine, Parma, Italy

Scott D. Rowley, M.D., Assistant Professor of Oncology, The Johns Hopkins Hosptial, Baltimore, Maryland, USA

Tapani Ruutu, M.D., Head, Division of Hematology, Department of Medicine, University of Helsinki, Helsinki, Finland

Jean E. Sanders, M.D., Associate Professor of Pediatrics, University of Washington, School of Medicine, and Associate Member, Fred Hutchinson Cancer Research Center, Seattle, Washington, USA

Brenda M. Sandmaier, M.D., Oncology Fellow, Fred Hutchinson Center Research Center, Seattle, Washington, USA

George W. Santos, M.D., Professor of Oncology and Medicine, Department of Oncology, The Johns Hopkins Hospital, Baltimore, Maryland, USA

Rein Saral, M.D., Associate Professor of Oncology and Medicine, The Johns Hopkins Hospital, Baltimore, Maryland, USA

Friedrich W. Schuening, M.D., Associate in Clinical Research, Fred Hutchinson Cancer Research Center, Seattle, Washington, USA

Kenji Shinohara, M.D., Assistant Professor, Third Department of Internal Medicine, Yamaguchi University Medical School, Ube, Japan

Howard Shulman, M.D., Associate Member, Fred Hutchinson Cancer Research Center, and Associate Professor of Pathology, University of Washington, School of Medicine, Seattle, Washington, USA

Martti A. Siimes, M.D., Associate Professor, Childrens Hospital, University of Helsinki, Helsinki, Finland

Mary Silanskis, Laboratory Technician, The Johns Hopkins Hospital, Baltimore, Maryland, USA

Jack Singer, M.D., Assistant Member, Fred Hutchinson Cancer Research Center, and Professor of Medicine, University of Washington, School of Medicine, Seattle, Washington, USA

Shawn J. Skerrett, M.D., Acting Instructor, Department of Medicine, University of Washington, School of Medicine, and Associate Investigator, Seattle Veterans Administration Medical Center, Seattle, Washington, USA

Sherrill J. Slichter, M.D., Scientific Director, Puget Sound Blood Center, Seattle, Washington, USA

Giovanni Sparaventi, M.D., Fellow, Divisione di Ematologia, Ospedale Civile, Pesaro, Italy

Bruno Speck, M.D., Professor of Medicine, Division of Hematology, Department of Internal Medicine, Kantonsspital, University of Basel, Basel, Switzerland

Gary Spitzer, M.D., Professor of Medicine, Internist, Department of Hematology, Bone Marrow Transplantation Section, UT–M.D. Anderson Hosptial and Tumor Institute, Houston, Texas, USA

Patricia Stewart, M.D., Associate Member, Fred Hutchinson Cancer Research Center, and Associate Professor of Medicine, University of Washington, School of Medicine, Seattle, Washington, USA

Rainer Storb, M.D., Head of the Program in Transplantation Biology, Fred Hutchinson Cancer Research Center, and Professor of Medicine, University of Washington, School of Medicine, Seattle, Washington, USA

Keith Sullivan, M.D., Associate Member, Fred Hutchinson Cancer Research Center, and Associate Professor of Medicine, University of Washington, School of Medicine, Seattle, Washington, USA

Fumimaro Takaku, M.D., Professor, Third Department of Internal Medicine, Faculty of Medicine, University of Tokyo, Tokyo, Japan

Nadia Talevi, M.Sc., Fellow in Research, Divisione di Ematologia, Ospedale Civile, Pesaro, Italy

Nydia G. Testa, M.D., Ph.D., Paterson Institute for Cancer Research, Christie Hospital and Holt Radium Institute, Manchester, United Kingdom

E. Donnall Thomas, M.D., Associate Director for Clinical Research, Fred Hutchinson Cancer Research Center, and Professor of Medicine, University of Washington, School of Medicine, Seattle, Washington, USA

André Tichelli, M.D., Division of Hematology, Department of Internal Medicine, Kantonsspital, University of Basel, Basel, Switzerland

Auli Toivanen, M.D., Ph.D., Associate Professor, Department of Medicine, University of Turku, Turku, Finland

Glauco Torlontano, M.D., Professor of Hematology, Hematology Unit, School of Medicine, Pescara, Italy

Eitoku Toyoshima, M.D., Postdoctoral Fellow, Department of Neurology, The University of Maryland School of Medicine, Baltimore, Maryland, USA

Peter J. Tutschka, M.D., Professor of Medicine, The Ohio State University, and Director, The Ohio State University Bone Marrow Transplantation Program, Columbus, Ohio, USA

Georgia B. Vogelsang, M.D., Assistant Professor of Oncology, The Johns Hopkins Hospital, Baltimore, Maryland, USA

Liisa Volin, M.D., Research Fellow, Department of Medicine, University of Helsinki, Helsinki, Finland

John E. Wagner, Jr., M.D., Postdoctoral Fellow, The Johns Hopkins Hospital, Baltimore, Maryland, USA

Sharyn Walker, Ph.D., Associate Professor of Pediatrics and Microbiology, University of Southern California, School of Medicine, Los Angeles, California, USA

Chester B. Whitley, Ph.D., M.D., Assistant Professor, Department of Pediatrics, University of Minnesota, Minneapolis, Minnesota, USA

Andrew Will, M.B.C.H.B., M.R.C.P., Pendlebury Childrens Hospital, Manchester, United Kingdom

John R. Wingard, M.D., Assistant Professor of Oncology and Medicine, Departments of Oncology and Medicine, The Johns Hopkins University School of Medicine, and The Johns Hopkins Oncology Center, Baltimore, Maryland, USA

Drew J. Winston, M.D., UCLA Medical Center, Los Angeles, California, USA

Robert Witherspoon, M.D., Associate Member, Fred Hutchinson Cancer Research Center, and Associate Professor, University of Washington, School of Medicine, Seattle, Washington, USA

Steven N. Wolff, M.D., Associate Professor of Medicine, Vanderbilt University, Nashville, Tennessee, USA

Andrew M. Yeager, M.D., Associate Professor of Oncology and Pediatrics, The Johns Hopkins University School of Medicine, Baltimore, Maryland, USA

Christine K. Young, B.S., Cancer Research Laboratories, Allegheny-Singer Research Institute, Allegheny General Hospital, Pittsburgh, Pennsylvania, USA

Introduction

Siegmund J. Baum

It has become a tradition to commence important meetings of this society with reminiscence and nostalgia. Bone marrow transplantation, which has a history of only 30 to 40 years, permits this process, since some of the early investigators are still with us. For example, over the past 15 years, we have had three symposia in honor of Egon Lorenz. As we all know, the team of Lorenz, Uphoff and Congdon was involved in the first successful transplantation of syngeneic and allogeneic bone marrow into irradiated mice (1). Subsequently, these investigators theorized that a humoral factor probably was responsible for the radiation protection, as documented by the injection of rat bone marrow into irradiated mice (2). This created interesting debates between the humoral factor people (as represented by Lorenz) and the cellular replacement groups (vociferously advocated by Leonard Cole) (3).

At about the same time, Alpen and Baum (4), using a larger mammal, the dog, demonstrated that injecting autologous marrow post irradiation would protect lethally irradiated animals (see Table). Certainly, protection was obtained from the cellular constituents of the bone marrow.

We undertook to test on dogs the hypothesis of Gengozian and Makinodum (5) that increasing the radiation dose will increase immunologic tolerance for allogeneic implants. They found increased effectiveness at well over LD_{50} in mice. For this reason, we chose 600 R--a dose equivalent to twice the LD_{50} in dogs--for the test dose. We found that infusion of allogeneic marrow into these dogs was not protective. Later, it was found that higher doses of radiation were needed to achieve immunologic tolerance.

Table: Survival Time and Mortality in Dogs Exposed to 400R Whole Body Irradiation*

Treatment	Dead/Total	Survival (%)	Mean Survival Time (days)
Autologous Bone Marrow	0/8	100	----
Homologous Bone Marrow	6/7	14.3	12.5
Saline	4/4	0	12.3
Controls	7/8	12.5	13.4

* Reprinted with permission from Alpen and Baum, 1958, (Ref. 4).

Since it was assumed that human beings would be similarly affected, discussions were held concerning what procedure to follow when animals or humans received a lethal radiation dose which has not yet eliminated immune responses. Should one subject humans to additional doses of radiation?

Three decades have passed since these early experiments. A considerable number of investigators have been intrigued with the problems of bone marrow transplantation not only for postirradiation protection, but certainly also as a treatment modality for a variety of blood cell diseases and metabolic or genetic disorders. We have come here as a convocation to relate what we have learned since those early days, to present our achievements and indeed also our failures, and to discuss what we can predict for the future. We have received great support and recognition for this effort. And, as our presentations and discussions take place over the next three days, I anticipate that this support and recognition will prove to be well deserved.

Finally, one of our sponsors has asked why we have not considered ethical and socioeconomical issues in our presentations. A session on these topics probably should be considered for our next annual meeting. I was involved in this type of discussion once, 15 years ago, when the National Academy of Sciences counseled the Naval Medical Hospital on the advisability of permitting bone marrow transplantation in humans previously exposed to supralethal gamma irradiation. The Navy had some personnel in the terminal stages of leukemia and some staff members desired to make a final attempt at saving lives.

After lengthy debate, the overwhelming majority of committee members voted in favor of transplantation as a final effort in the fight against this dreadful disease. One member sincerely dissented. He asked what assurance of success we had: Would it aggravate the condition of the patient? What quality of life would exist even after successful therapy? He thoughtfully added what he understood to be the position of the British medical community at that time: Why can we not let terminal patients die in dignity? Considering all the options, the Navy hospital proceeded with the treatment of ten patients, one of whom lived for one year post treatment. I am certain that we all are looking forward to the report from Mortimer Bortin at this symposium, in the hopes of hearing the extent to which recent efforts have yielded greater improvements and promise.

I started this introduction relating how bone marrow transplantation began as a consideration for the rescue of radiation victims. In the last presentation of this symposium, Robert Gale--who nobly volunteered to help the victims of Chernobyl--will discuss the results of this accident. Was the present state of the art helpful? To what extent can we do better in the future?

In the anticipation of good tidings, it gives me great pleasure to open this symposium Recent Advances and Future Directions in Bone Marrow Transplantation.

REFERENCES

1. Lorenz E, Uphoff D, Reid TR, Shelton E: Modification of irradiation injury in mice and guinea pigs by bone marrow injections. J Natl Cancer Inst 12:197, 1951.

2. Congdon CC, Lorenz E: Humoral factor in irradiation protection: Modification of lethal irradiation injury in mice by injection of rat bone marrow. Am J Physiol 176:297, 1954.

3. Cole LJ, Habermeyer JG, Bond VP: Recovery from acute radiation injury in mice following administration of rat bone marrow. J Natl Cancer Inst 16:1, 1955.

4. Alpen EL, Baum SJ: Modification of X-radiation lethality by autologous marrow infusion in dogs. Blood 13:1168, 1958.

5. Gengozian N, Makinodan T: Mortality of mice as affected by variation of the X-ray dose and number of nucleated rat bone marrow cells injected. Cancer Res 17:970, 1957.

I. Experimental Bone Marrow Transplantation: S.J. Baum and F. Takaku, Chairpersons

1: Graft-versus-Host Disease and Graft-versus-Leukemia in Experimental Systems

James P. OKunewick, Deborah L. Kociban, Mary J. Buffo, and Christine K. Young

INTRODUCTION:

The development of monoclonal antibodies (MABs) has provided us with valuable new tools for studying the mechanisms of immune response. In our laboratories, we have been employing them in particular in the study of the role of T-cells in graft-vs-host (GvH) disease and in graft-vs-leukemia (GvL).

The original identification of T-cells as a prime mediator of GvH response, however, very much pre-dated the development of MABs, and stemmed from the observation that in rodents transplanted unmatched allogeneic marrow was often a poor inducer of GvHR (1-3). By contrast, in humans transplanted marrow from unmatched donors yields a nearly one hundred percent incidence of GvHR (4). The observed reason for this difference was that rodent marrow was comparatively poor in lymphocytes (3). Therefore, in order to duplicate the level of the human response in rodent systems it was necessary to supplement the transplanted marrow with cells taken from the spleen, thymus or lymph nodes (2, 3).

In an early classic study, Vos et al. (2) demonstrated that the addition of lymph node (LN) cells to the donor marrow not only could increase the overall incidence of acute fatal GvHR, but that the relative incidence was also proportional to the number of LN cells added. We later confirmed this observation with spleen and marrow cells in a separate mouse model (5), and found that both the incidence of fatal GvHR and the median survival times of the transplant recipients were exponential functions of the percentage of spleen cells in the cell mixtures engrafted. At the same time, we observed that those recipient mice which did not fatally succumb to GvHR within 60 days post-transplant had a better than ninety percent probability of surviving indefinitely, even though a few of them might continue to show protracted evidence of chronic GvHR (5). Since the proportion of marrow cells decreased as the spleen cells were increased, these findings were consistent with the theory which proposed that the ultimate source of effector cells for acute GvHR was not among the pluripotent hematopoietic stem cells, but among already differentiated lymphoid cells or lymphoid committed precursors.

The above being the case, it was obvious that it might be practical to prevent or reduce GvHR by selectively removing the lymphoid cells prior to transplantation. Studies done by several workers using antilymphocyte serum or antilymphocyte globulin proved this to be true (6-8), particularly with mouse models, although the initial results with clinical application of the technique in humans were less encouraging (9). Retrospectively, those clinical difficulties were probably due to a low strength and lack of specificity of the material available at the time. Nevertheless, the necessary direct proof that the active lymphoid cells involved in GvHR were indeed T-cells came from animal studies in which the donor cells were exposed to polyclonal antithymocyte globulin prior to engraftment, which in turn resulted in a reduction in fatal GvHR (10). Subsequently, similar results were obtained in several laboratories with the use of a monoclonal antibody directed specifically against the Thy-1 marker of mouse T-cells (11-13).

Along with the introduction of MAB technology, additional facets to the problem of understanding GvHR have begun to manifest themselves. Among these have been the possibility that the expression of GvHR in experimental systems may be influenced by the particular distribution and proportions of T-cell subsets within the tissue used as the source of T-cells (e.g. LN versus spleen versus thymus). Likewise, there appear to be differences between the nature of the GvHR induced when the donor and recipient are mismatched for both their major and minor histocompatibility determinants, as opposed to being mismatched in their minor histocompatibility determinants alone. Also, certain studies have indicated that which strain is the donor and which is the recipient can affect the probability of GvHR induction, with reciprocal and equal two-way intensity definitely not always being the case (14). Finally, independent of major histocompatibility (MHC) influences, the particular nature and extent

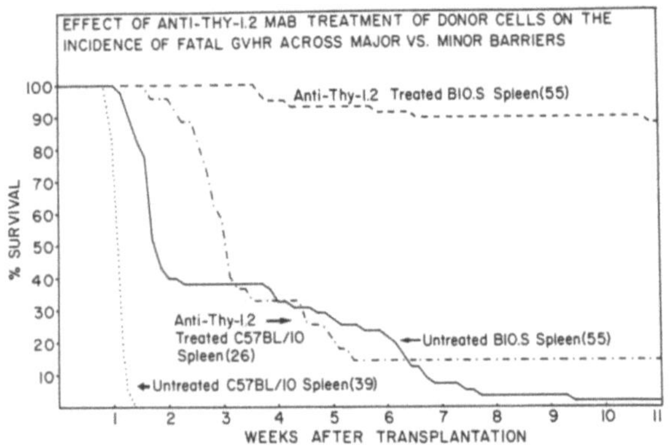

Figure 1. Effect of ex-vivo treatment of the donor cells with anti-Thy-1 MAB on GvHR induced in SJL/J recipients by 10^7 engrafted spleen cells from major barrier (C57BL/10) and minor barrier (B10.S) mismatched donors. Number in parenthesis indicates number of recipients.

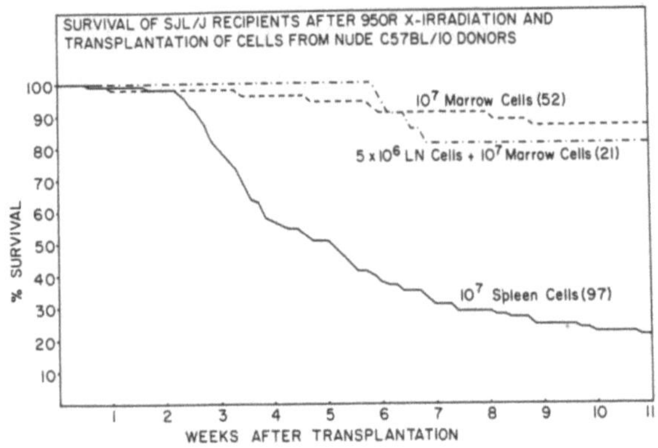

Figure 2. Survival of SJL/J recipients engrafted with spleen, marrow, or marrow plus lymph node cells from MHC-mismatched nude (athymic) C57BL/10 donors. Number in parenthesis indicates number of recipients.

of donor-recipient disparities at the minor histocompatibility loci (MiHL) may by itself alone critically influence the GvH reaction mechanisms to a degree greater than has been previously appreciated (15, 16).

The current armamentarium of MABs directed against T-cells and T-cell subsets provide us with some very powerful tools for investigating these problems and the mechanisms of GvHR. Those that have been applied chiefly to date in the mouse include anti-Thy-1 (a pan-T-cell MAB which reacts with virtually all T-cells); anti-L3/T4 (a recently developed anti-helper MAB equivalent to Leu-3 or T-4 in man); anti-Lyt-1 (previously thought to be an anti-helper MAB, but now known to recognize other immature T-cells in addition to the mature helper cells); and anti-Lyt-2 (an anti-cytolytic/suppressor cell MAB equivalent to human T-8).

EXPERIMENTAL TECHNIQUE:

Our basic model for studying GvHR has used the SJL/J mouse as the recipient, with the C57BL/10 and the B10.S as donors. The SJL/J has the MHC type of H-2^s, while the C57BL/10 is H-2^b. The B10.S is a congenic derivative of the C57BL/10, bred to yield a mouse with the same MHC type of H-2^s held by the SJL/J, but retaining the MiHL configuration of the C57BL/10 (12, 15). Thus, with this model we can study the combined influences of MHC plus MiHL disparities together as well as separate out the influence of the MiHL disparities alone. In addition, as part of our studies into MHC-GvHR we have used the nude (athymic) C57BL/10 as a donor congenitally free of mature T-cells.

The technique for T-cell depletion by the MABs has been previously described by us (12, 17). Briefly, donor cells obtained from the spleen, lymph nodes and/or femoral marrow are rendered into a single cell suspension in Ca and Mg-free Hank's solution, adjusted to the desired concentrations, and divided into equal aliquots, one of which is used as the non-MAB-treated control. To the other aliquots the appropriate MABs are added in a quantity at least 10^3 higher than that necessary to achieve complete lysis and the cells are incubated at 4°C for 15 minutes; complement is then added and incubation is continued for another 45 minutes at 37°C. Simultaneously, the non-MAB-treated cells to be used in the control animals are handled in the same manner, but with only the addition of complement. To check for completeness of ablation by the particular MAB, a sample is taken for flow-cytometry analysis. At the completion of the above ex-vivo treatment the cells are injected into 12-week-old female SJL/J mice prepared for transplant two hours previously by total body irradiation (9.5 Gy X-ray). Following transplant the recipients are housed 2 per cage under sterile conditions, and observed for 11 weeks for signs of GvHR and for survival. All mice dying are autopsied to confirm whether GvHR was the probable cause of death.

EFFECTS OF ANTI-Thy-1 MAB ON SPLEEN CELL INDUCED GvHR ACROSS MAJOR AND MINOR BARRIERS:

Figure 1 compares our findings for the influence of MHC plus MiHL factors (C57BL/10 donors) versus MiHL factors alone (B10.S donors) on acute GvH response, with the survival curves plotted according to Kaplan-Meier statistics (12). Clear differences can be seen in the survival patterns, both with and without ex-vivo treatment of the cells with anti-Thy-1.2. Fatal GvHR developed quite rapidly in the recipients of MHC-mismatched C57BL/10 spleen cells and all the animals were dead before the end of the second week. In contrast, fatal GvHR developed more slowly when the MHC-matched B10.S were used as donors. Also, the survival curve assumed a biphasic shape, with an early incidence of deaths peaking between the first and second weeks and a delayed incidence between fourth and eighth weeks. Ex-vivo treatment of the donor cells was successful in preventing fatal GvHR in 90 percent of the recipients of spleen cells from the MHC-matched, but MiHL-disparate, B10.S donors. However, with the MHC-mismatched totally allogeneic C57BL/10 donors only a small fraction of the fatal response was eliminated, with the main effect being to shift the survival curve to the left, and to delay death until the second to sixth week. There were also distinct differences between the survivors of

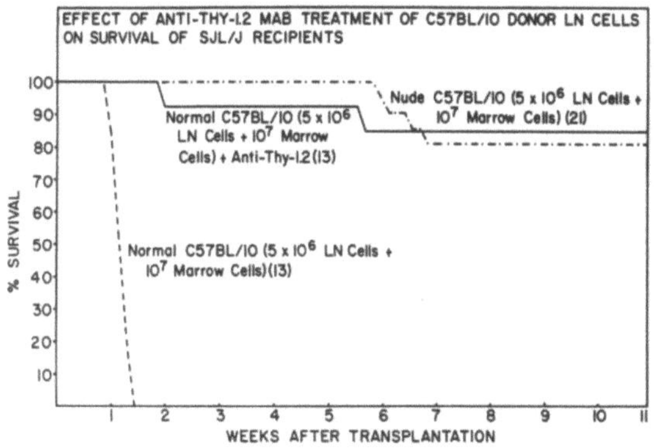

Figure 3. Effect of ex-vivo anti-Thy-1-MAB treatment of normal C57BL/10 donor lymph node plus marrow cells on survival of SJL/J recipients; comparison with the survival response to nude C57BL/10 lymph node plus marrow cells. Number in parenthesis indicates number of recipients.

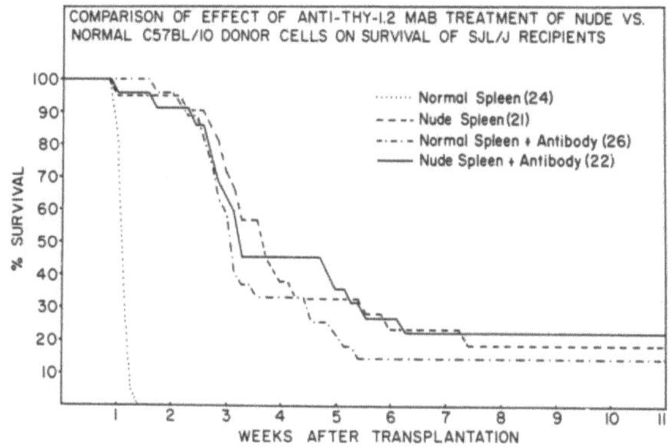

Figure 4. Effect of ex-vivo anti-Thy-1 MAB treatment of the donor cells on SJL/J recipients of 10^7 spleen cells from normal C57BL/10 donors or nude (athymic) C57BL/10 donors. Number in parenthesis indicates number of recipients.

the two sets, in that all of the surviving recipients of anti-Thy-MAB treated C57BL/10 spleen cells developed persistent chronic GvHR, while virtually none of the recipients of anti-Thy-MAB treated B10.S spleen cells showed any evidence of chronic GvHR.

To further investigate this comparatively poor response of the MHC-mismatched transplant to ex vivo treatment with anti-Thy-1.2 MAB we conducted a set of studies using the congenitally T-cell deficient nude mouse as a donor; the hypothesis being that since these mice do not possess mature T-cells, then their tissues should not induce GvHR. Figure 2 illustrates the results obtained when spleen cells, marrow cells or LN cells mixed with marrow were transplanted into SJL/J recipients. The resultant was a survival curve for the spleen cell recipients that was strikingly similar to that of Figure 1 for the recipients of anti-Thy-1 treated spleen cells from normal donors. By contrast, the recipients of nude mouse marrow or LN cells showed the expected response of no GvHR and of few deaths.

We then turned to an examination of the effect of using ex vivo anti-Thy-1.2 treatment on LN cells (mixed with marrow) from normal C57BL/10 donors instead of spleen cells. The results as shown in Figure 3 indicated that, in contrast to the effect of spleen cell transplant, treatment of the normal C57BL/10 LN cells with the anti-Thy-Mab effectively eliminated most of the GvHR fatalities and produced a survival curve similar to that of Figure 2 for the nude mouse LN cells.

Carrying the studies a step further, we then treated spleen cells from the nude (athymic) mouse donors with anti-Thy-MAB and compared the survival response to that of spleen cells from normal C57BL/10 donors, also treated with anti-Thy-MAB. The results, shown in Figure 4, indicated that there was no effect of the MAB on survival of the nude spleen recipients, and that the resultant survival remained essentially the same as that seen with normal C57BL/10 spleen cells treated with MAB and as that seen with nude speen cells not treated with MAB. To confirm that these recipients of nude mouse spleen cells were indeed dying of GvHR, samples of the tissues from the mice receiving nude spleen cells were sent to Wm. Beschorner at Johns Hopkins for independent histopathology evaluation, and the findings were positive (18).

These results, as we have described them above, have pointed out several things of importance to the understanding of the nature of GvHR. First, there may be fundamental differences in the mechanisms of acute GvHR when it is induced across major plus minor histocompatibility barriers as opposed to only the minor barriers. Clearly, the reaction induced by the H-2 matched B10.S spleen cells was less intense than that induced by the related fully allogeneic C57BL/10 donor. Second, although anti-Thy-MAB depletion of the T-cells nearly completely obliterated the MiHL-GvHR induced by B10.S spleen cells, it only slightly affected the MHC-GvHR induced by normal C57BL/10 spleen cells and had no effect whatsoever on the MHC-GvHR induced by nude C57BL/10 spleen cells. This in turn raises the possibility that in MHC-GvHR there may be an additional inducer that is either not a T-cell or is still too primitive to be displaying T-cell markers at the time of transplant. Thirdly, the tissue source of GvH inducer cells can critically affect both the expression of experimental GvHR and the interpretation of the results. This is evidenced by the observations that nearly all of the GvHR induced by C57BL/10 LN cells could be prevented by ex vivo treatment of the cells by anti-Thy-1, but that when C57BL/10 spleen cells were so treated a substantial anti-Thy-MAB resistant element of the response remained.

ROLE OF T-CELL SUBSETS IN MINOR HISTOCOMPATIBILITY GvHR INDUCED BY SPLEEN OR LYMPH NODE CELLS:

Having explored the effects of anti-Thy-1 MAB on GvHR, we next focused our attention on the effects of MABs directed at the subsets of T-cells. For this we chose to use the MiHL-GvHR model involving the B10.S donors as being the more clinically relevant one. For our initial MABs we chose anti-Lyt-1 and anti-Lyt-2. The former was chosen because the

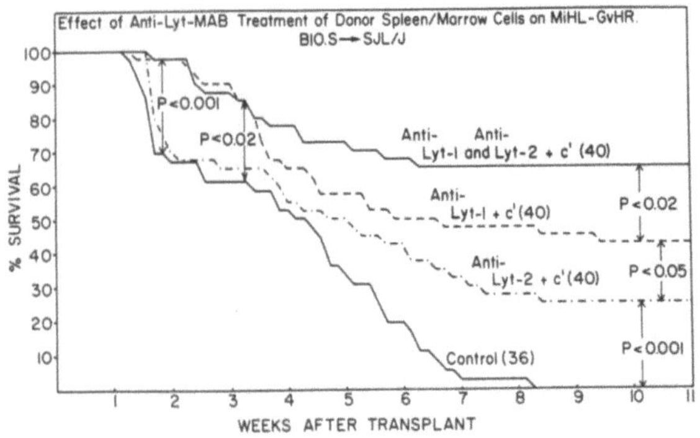

Figure 5. Effect of ex-vivo anti-Lyt-1 and/or anti-Lyt-2 MAB treatment of donor spleen/marrow cells in minor barrier acute GvHR; 5 x 10^6 spleen cells plus 5 x 10^6 marrow cells (as measured before MAB treatment) engrafted into SJL/J recipients. Number in parenthesis indicates number of recipients. P-values calculated using Kaplan-Meier statistics.

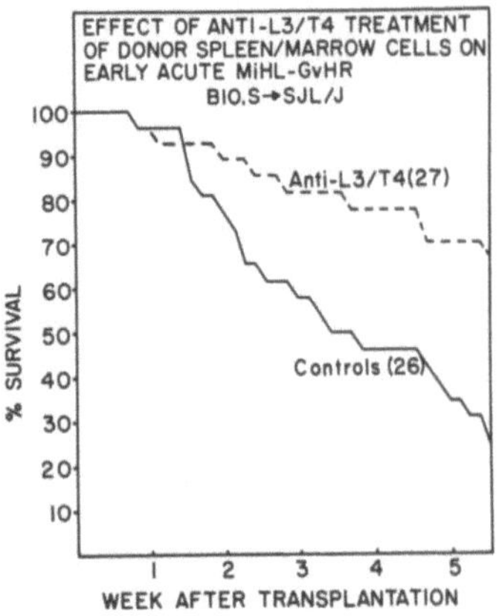

Figure 6. Effect of ex-vivo anti-L3/T4 MAB treatment of donor spleen/marrow cells on the early phase of minor barrier acute GvHR; 5 x 10^6 spleen plus 5 x 10^6 marrow cells (as measured before MAB treatment) engrafted into SJL/J recipients. Number in parenthesis indicates number of recipients.

Lyt-1 marker is found on both immature T-cells and on mature T-helpers. In more recent studies, currently still underway, we are also employing the helper-cell specific anti-L3/T4 MAB. The anti-Lyt-2 MAB was chosen because that marker is specific for mouse T-cytolytic/suppressor cells. Although there is some overlap between the two Lyt MABs among the immature cytolytic cells, especially in that subset which strongly expresses both Lyt-1 and Lyt-2 (i.e. the Lyt-1^+2^+ cells), the more mature of the cytolytic/suppressor cells do not express enough Lyt-1 antigen to be lysed by that MAB, whereas all of the mature helper cells do (19). Also, in our hands none of the Lyt-2^+ cytolytic cells express L3/T4, but all of the Lyt-1^+ helper cells do express it. Therefore, for experimental purposes, a reasonable separation of the T-cell subclasses can be achieved with the above MABs. These subclasses are: Lyt-1^+L3/T4^+ helper cells; Lyt-1^-2^+ cytolytic cells; and Lyt-1^+2^+ immature cells.

Also, since we were interested in comparing the response elicited by the LN cells as well as spleen cells, we chose in both cases to use those cells mixed with marrow. This was necessary because, in contrast to the mouse spleen, mouse LN cells do not contain enough pluripotent hematopoietic stem cells to allow for reconstitution of the non-lymphoid elements. Using flow-cytometry data to estimate the relative numbers of T-cells, the spleen-marrow and LN-marrow mixtures were adjusted to contain the same number of Thy-1 positive cells and approximately equivalent ratios of pluripotent stem cells.

Figure 5 illustrates the effect of the anti-Lyt-1 and anti-Lyt-2 MABs on MiHL-GvHR induced by B10.S spleen-marrow cell transplant. The lower (control) curve is again a biphasic similar to that seen in Figure 1, with the exception that there were fewer early deaths. Ex vivo treatment of the cells with anti-Lyt-2 MAB significantly increased survival, but the effect of the anti-Lyt-1 MAB was still more significantly greater. Further, while anti-Lyt-1 protected against the early phase of deaths, anti-Lyt-2 did not. Since the anti-Lyt-2 MAB eliminated all Lyt-2 positive cells (i.e. Lyt-1^+2^+ as well as Lyt-1^-2^+) and since the effect of the anti-Lyt-1 MAB was greater than that of the anti-Lyt-2, it must be concluded that there was a contribution of Lyt-1 positive cells to the GvHR over and above that which can be attributed to any Lyt-1^+2^+ cells alone. This was further confirmed by the results obtained when the cells were treated simultaneously ex vivo with both antibodies. As the data show, the resultant survival following the double MAB treatment was significantly greater than that seen using either Lyt-MAB alone. Curiously, however, it did not achieve the level of effect that was seen when spleen cells were treated with anti-Thy MAB. This might suggest that there may be a contribution to the response by some primitive T-cells in which the Lyt markers are not yet sufficiently defined or expressed to achieve lysis of the cells by the anti-Lyt-MABs.

To confirm that T-helper cells may be contributing to the effect of the Lyt-1 cells, we have been conducting a parallel set of studies using the anti-L3/T4 MAB. The results of these studies to date have shown that ex vivo treatment of B10.S spleen-marrow cells with that MAB also protects against the early deaths (Figure 6), thus confirming a probable influence of T-helper cells on the early element of acute MiHL-GvHR. Supportive of this, Atkinson et al. (20) have recently reported a decrease in GvHR in their clinical studies of patients receiving marrow treated with anti-T-4 MAB, the antibody for human T-helper cells.

In Figure 7, we have examined the effects when B10.S lymph nodes were used as the source of T-cells for inducing GvHR. From this several differences can be seen in the LN-induced GvHR as opposed to spleen-induced GvHR. To begin with, even though the numbers of Thy-1 positive cells injected were equivalent in both cases

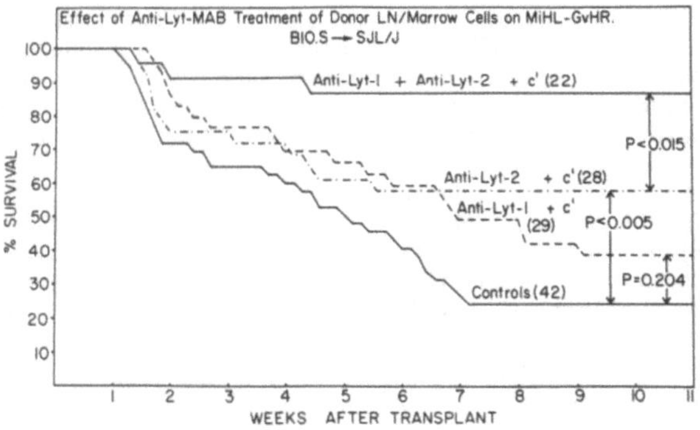

Figure 7. Effect of ex-vivo anti-Lyt-1 and/or anti-Lyt-2 MAB treatment of donor LN/marrow cells in minor barrier acute GvHR; 2 x 10^6 LN cells plus 1 x 10^7 marrow cells (as measured before MAB treatment) engrafted into SJL/J recipients. Number in parenthesis indicates number of recipients. P-values calculated using Kaplan-Meier statistics.

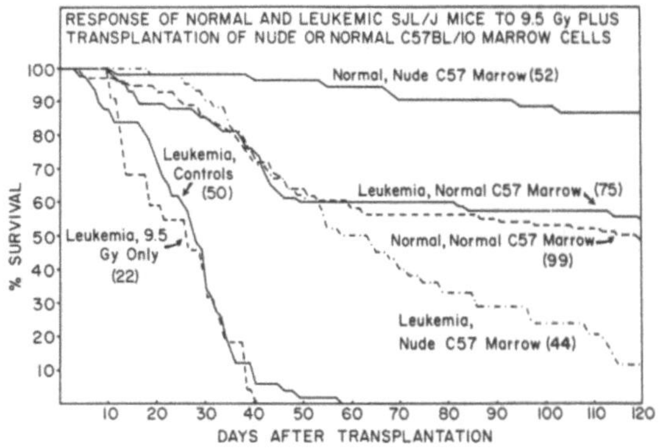

Figure 8. Contrast in GvL and GvH response induced across major barriers following transplant of 10^7 marrow cells from normal C57BL/10 donors versus T-cell deficient nude C57BL/10 donors into normal or Rauscher leukemic SJL/J recipients. Number in parenthesis indicates number of recipients. Leukemia controls and irradiated leukemia controls received no cell transplant.

(17), the number of surviving mice in the LN control group did not drop to zero. Nevertheless, the control curve did exhibit a biphasic behavior. Still greater differences can be found in the response to treatment of the cells with the individual anti-Lyt-MABs. In this case when anti-Lyt-1 was used alone, although it had some marginal effect on early lethality, whatever other protection it provided did not exceed that of the anti-Lyt-2 and by the end of 11 weeks was no longer significant. On the other hand, anti-Lyt-2 treatment did protect, although again that protection was only against the delayed fatalities and not the early ones. By contrast, when the LN-marrow cell mixtures were exposed to both anti-Lyt-MABs together, the protection achieved was highly significant for the entire period, approaching that seen using anti-Thy-1 and B10.S spleen cells. These results, comparing the single MAB treatment with the simultaneous exposure to both MABs, are quite similar to the classic studies of Cantor and Boyse (21) obtained in their in vitro demonstration of the interactions of T-helper cells with cytolytic T-cells to enhance the activity of the latter.

Added to the above, the lack of significant effect of the anti-Lyt-1 MAB when applied by itself in the LN studies suggests that the LN may differ from the spleen in the spectra of mature and immature Lyt-1^+ cells they possess. Consistent with this, the near complete effect of the combined MAB exposure in eliminating fatal GvHR suggests that, again in contrast to the spleen, nearly all of the LN cells active in GvHR probably have their Thy-1, Lyt-1, and Lyt-2 markers well defined.

THE ROLE OF T-CELLS IN GRAFT-VS-LEUKEMIA:

In earlier studies using Rauscher viral leukemia we established that transplanted marrow cells from B10.S donors could exert a graft-vs-leukemia effect in SJL/J recipients without at the same time inducing GvHR (22). Spleen cells on the other hand, induced a level of GvHR that all but obscured any beneficial GvL effect (23). Slavin et al. (24) in a separate study obtained similar results with the murine BCL_1 leukemia in (BALB/c x C57BL/6)F_1 hybrids treated with C57BL/6 marrow. In addition, we also observed that the MiHL determinants appeared to exert a greater influence on GvL than did the MHC determinants (22), and this was supported by a concurrent study done in rats by Westcott et al. (25). These results suggested that the GvL effect may, in fact, be separable from GvHR. On the other hand, clinical efforts to reduce GvHR by T-cell depletion of the donor marrow have frequently resulted in an increase in leukemic relapse, leading to the inference that there must be some commonalities between GvHR and GvL. This presents a basic question, which is whether or not the same T-cells responsible for inducing GvHR are also the functional T-cells for GvL.

To address this question, we have initiated two sets of studies; one using nude mice as donors, the other using B10.S donors along with anti-Lyt MABs to delete specific T-cell subsets. Figure 8 contrasts the effects of using marrow from normal and nude C57BL/10 donors on Rauscher leukemic SJL/J mice. As the control data show, both irradiated and unirradiated leukemic control SJL/J mice exhibited very poor survival. By contrast, when the leukemic recipients were irradiated and given normal C57BL/10 marrow cells, they showed a good survival of up to 50% at 4 months after treatment. When normal SJL/J control mice were given the identical treatment, they also showed the same survival at 4 months, with the bulk of the deaths due to GvHR. Hence, the data would seem to suggest that the GvH reaction might be one of the governing factors in eliciting the GvL effect. On the other hand, when marrow from nude C57BL/10 donors was engrafted there was no GvHR, but there was still a strong GvL effect which, although it was lesser than that obtained using normal marrow, yielded a significantly better survival ($p < 0.0001$) than that of the controls. Therefore, the GvL effect must be also at least

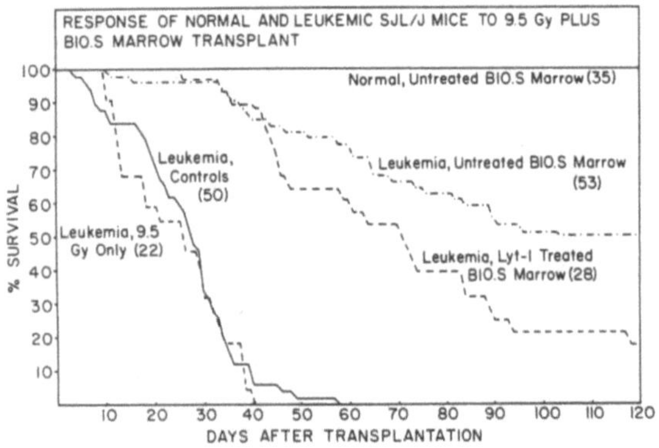

Figure 9. Effect of anti-Lyt-1 MAB ex-vivo treatment of B10.S donor marrow cells on GvL and GvHR induced across minor barriers following transplant of 10^7 cells (as measured before MAB treatment) into normal and Rauscher leukemic SJL/J mice. Number in parenthesis indicates number of recipients.

in part independent of the T-cells which induce GvHR.

Figure 9 illustrates the response observed using B10.S donor marrow and anti-Lyt-1 MAB T-cell depletion. As the upper curve indicates, B10.S marrow induced no fatal GvHR in SJL/J recipients. When irradiated leukemic mice were given these marrow cells, an excellent GvL response was seen, resulting in 50% survival at 4 months. In contrast, when the donor marrow cells were treated with anti-Lyt-1 MAB, a portion of the GvL effect was lost, just as had been observed with the nude mouse transplants.

Although marrow from B10.S donors does not induce GvHR, it does contain a small number of Lyt-1^+ T-cells, most of which are L3/T4 positive T-helper cells. Therefore, our preliminary interpretation of these results is that GvL may be in part a T-cell dependent reaction, and that T-helper cells may contribute to this reaction. However, these T-helper cells are not necessarily the same ones involved in GvHR. Moreover, both the nude mouse data and the B10.S data suggest that a significant element of the GvL response may not be T-cell dependent. Thus, while T-cell depletion may negatively affect a portion of the GvL response (consistent with what has also been observed in the clinic) there may also be other non-T-cell mechanisms operative in GvL.

DISCUSSION:

The data described in this paper indicate some of the complexities involved attempting to illucidate the mechanisms of GvHR. Among them it can be seen that the interpretation of the results can be strongly influenced not only by whether the donor and recipient are matched versus unmatched at the MHC, but also by the tissues chosen as the source of T-cells to induce GvHR. This is most clearly demonstrated with the use of spleen cells versus LN cells to induce MHC-GvHR.

The failure of anti-Thy-MAB treatment to completely ablate the GvHR induced by normal C57BL/10 spleen cells, and its confirmation using nude C57BL/10 donors, strongly suggests that the spleen may contain some cell type not found in the lymph nodes. Gillis et al. (26) have reported that the spleens of nude mice possess primitive Thy-1-negative T-cell precursors that can be induced to mature in vitro into Thy-1^+ cells. We have observed the same thing with T-cell cultures in our own laboratory. Consistent with that, old (>6 mo) nude mice do exhibit a small but measurable number of Thy-1^+ cells in their spleens and lymph nodes (27). However, the nude donors used in our studies were much younger than that age, and flow cytometry analysis of their tissues showed no significant number of T-cells. Substantiating this were the results indicating that anti-Thy-MAB treatment of the nude C57BL/10 spleen cells had absolutely no effect on the level of GvHR induced, and that when normal C57BL/10 spleen cells were treated with the anti-Thy-MAB they produced the same pattern of GvHR fatalities as the transplanted nude spleen cells. Therefore, the conclusion is strongly forced upon us that the mouse spleen contains some Thy-1-negative element that is not found in lymph nodes but which nonetheless is capable of eliciting a strong GvH response across MHC barriers.

The nature of this mediating element remains unknown. However, two obvious possibilities are that it might be a primitive T-cell progenitor which matures within the host to induce GvHR, or it may be an NK-cell. Previous studies done by us and using thymectomized recipients suggest that the former may be somewhat the case (28), but with regard to any NK-cell influence our data to date have been inconclusive. It is also evident from the work of Vallera et al. (13), as well as being consistent with our earlier studies using combinations of spleen and marrow in varying percentages (5), that the effects of the GvHR mediators in the spleen can be diluted down by the addition of marrow cells to the cells being engrafted. This dilution of effect may be a passive resultant due simply to the reduction in T-cell numbers or it may reflect some active mechanism; and that raises another question which we have not specifically dealt with in this paper, which is the possible induction of suppressor cell activity in GvHR (29, 30) when spleen and marrow cells are mixed.

From the clinical standpoint one can argue as to whether or not the presence of a Thy-1-negative GvHR inducer cell in the spleen is of relevance, because one does not transplant spleen cells with human marrow transplant. However, the fact that the observed response is there, and that it renders anti-Thy-MAB treatment less effective in preventing fatal MHC-GvHR as compared to MiHL-GvHR, should cause the transplant physician to be aware of the possibility that unexpected difficulties may be encountered if transplants using depleted T-cell cells from unrelated HLA-mismatched donors are attempted. By contrast, and as it has already been observed in the clinic, the use of T-cell depletion with matched or partially matched sibling donors offers better hope.

Turning to the matter of minor-barrier GvHR, the results described in this paper suggest that the mechanisms of acute MiHL-GvHR are equally complex as those of MHC-GvHR. In addition, it should be emphasized that although the data indicated a biphasic response, both phases were indeed elements of the acute GvH response. Chronic MiHL-GvHR, which we have observed among the long-term survivors in the control groups that received untreated cells from the MHC-matched donors, exhibits different overt and histopathological signs, the most obvious being the skin reaction and alopecia.

The existence of a biphasic response in itself suggests that there may be separable components to the mechanism of acute MiHL-GvHR (12, 17, 28). Of these two components, our results, obtained with the anti-Lyt-1 and anti-L3/T4 MABs, suggest that the early phase may be directed by helper-cells. These results are in good agreement with the earlier work of Mason (31) done in rats and are supported by the clinical findings of Atkinson et al. (20). With respect to the second component of the biphasic response, the results obtained with the Lyt-2 MAB suggest that the delayed phase may reflect a more slowly developing expression of acute GvHR which may be brought about by cytloytic T-cells acting without the aid of T-helper cells. Thus, the basic reaction appears to follow that of a classic immune response mechanism where the cytolytic T-cells are capable of acting on their own, but in which helper-cells contribute by accelerating the reaction and increasing its intensity.

Based on work done by Pietryga et al. (32) and of Cobbold et al. (33), there is no doubt that helper-cells also play a similar critical role in MHC-GvHR. In fact, the data obtained by Pietryga et al. (32) using spleen-marrow transplants to induce MHC-GvHR, are virtually identical with our own MiHL-GvHR data of Figure 5.

It must be emphasized, however, that there are two important considerations that can affect the interpretation of the results when one is dealing with experimental acute MiHL-GvHR in the laboratory. The first of these (as has also been noted for MHC-GvHR) is the tissue used as the source of T-cells. The second is the particular type of MiHL disparity that exists between the donor and recipient (15). With respect to the influence of the source tissue, in comparing Figure 6 with Figure 5 it can be seen that, if one used only the LNs as the sole T-cell source and only examined the effect of anti-Lyt-1 or of anti-Lyt-2 alone, it would appear that helper-cells play no part in LN-induced MiHL-GvHR and that the response is entirely and exclusively dependent on Lyt-2$^+$ cytolytic cells. Indeed, it was on data such as this that Korngold and Sprent (34, 35) based their earlier premise that MiHL-GvHR was exclusively a helper-independent Lyt-2$^+$ mediated reaction. However, more recently they too have now found evidence for helper-cell (L3/T4$^+$ cell) involvement in MiHL-GvHR (36). The reasons for the differing influences of spleen versus LN cells in the induction of MiHL are not yet totally clear. However, they may relate to the relative degree of maturity of the T-cells found in each tissue. As already mentioned, the data suggest that the splenic T-cells may be less mature in that there appears to be an element of splenic Thy-1$^+$ cells which are not strongly expressing either Lyt-1 or Lyt-2 but which can still induce GvHR. Conversely, the results obtained with the exposure of LN cells to the combined Lyt-MABs suggest that both Lyt-1$^+$ helper cells and Lyt-2$^+$ cytolytic cells do contribute to the LN induced GvH response and also that nearly all of the LN Thy-1$^+$ cells must be expressing one of the other of these two antigens. The fact that we observed fewer deaths in the control animals receiving LN cells, as contrasted to spleen cells, even though equivalent numbers of Thy-1$^+$ cells were engrafted is also consistent with the possibility that the LN T-cells are more mature than splenic T-cells. To be specific, given the accepted premises of immunology, among any population of <u>fully</u> mature helper-T-cells or cytolytic-T-cells there would be a significant segment which would already be irreversibly committed to a response against other specific antigens not involved in the GvH response. Those cells, though present and counted among the Thy-1$^+$ cells, would most likely not contribute to the GvHR.

The second consideration, that of MiHL disparity, is equally important to the interpretation of the experimental data, as it definitely affects the expression of the early phase of acute MiHL-GvHR and may govern whether helper-cells may or may not influence and contribute to the reaction in certain donor-recipient combinations. As Cantrell and Hildemann (15) have observed, MiHL-GvH reactions can be divided into "strong, moderate and weak." The weaker the histocompatibility, the later the time of onset and the greater the number of cells required to induce GvHR. The B10S. spleen cell GvHR induced in SJL/J is an example of a strong MiHL reaction with a well defined helper-cell input. However, we have also observed in our laboratory that the transplant of B10.D2 spleen cells into BALB/c recipients induces a very weak reaction in which no significant helper-cell activity could be found, and against which only the Lyt-2 MAB was effective. By contrast, the same B10.D2 spleen cells injected into DBA/2J recipients induced a moderate reaction in which helper-cell activity was clearly evident, though less pronounced than that of the B10.S plus SJL/J combination.

Therefore, the results of these minor histocompatibility studies suggest that in interpreting the laboratory data as well as the clinical data for MiHL-GvHR, reasonable caution should be used; in that the source tissue of the T-cells, the degree of MiHL disparity, and probably also the relative maturity of the T-cells when engrafted can all affect the experimental observations. Those factors being considered, however, the results clearly indicate that MiHL-GvHR is dependent on the presence of cytolytic-T-cells in the graft and, depending on the above conditons, can be accelerated and intensified by the action of helper-T-cells engrafted with the cytolytic-T-cells.

With respect to the role of T-cells in the Graft-vs-leukemia (GvL) effect, the data from our laboratory (22, 23) and those of the others (24, 25, 39) who have examined the question in mouse models are all in agreement. The GvL effect is at least in part separable from GvHR. On the other hand, at least a segment of it is mediated by T-cells, with the resultant that elimination of T-cells or the use of marrow from congenitally T-deficient donors reduces the level of GvL activity. In particular, among the T-cells active in GvL in the mouse are those of the Lyt-1^{+} subset, which is the component that includes mature and immature helpers along with immature cytolytic T-cells. The reduction of GvL activity when these cells are eliminated from the donor marrow corresponds well with the clinical experience that the use of T-depleted marrow to prevent GvHR results in a higher incidence of leukemic relapse as compared with the more standard clinical approach (37). Nonetheless, our experimental evidence indicates that not all of the GvL effect is eliminated with the elimination of T-cells from the transplant; and this suggests that other mechanisms may also play a role in GvL (38). Moreover, while a portion of the GvL effect can be attributed to donor T-cell activity, the particular T-cells involved are not necessarily the same as those mediating GvHR. Nevertheless, they may still fall within the same subclasses, such that separating them from the effector cells for GvHR may not be practical at present. At the same time, however, if T-cells are not the only mediators of GvL, a potential for exploiting the mechanisms to increase the GvL effect may still exist.

SUMMARY:

In summary, the data from mouse models studied by our laboratory and others indicate that acute GvHR across either major or minor barriers involves both helper-T-cells and cytolytic-T-cells. In addition, suppressor-T-cells may influence the response in ways that are not yet fully understood. Helper-cell activity is probably an omnipresent element to all MHC-GvHR. However, with MiHL-GvHR the presence or absence of helper-cell activity is decidedly dependent on the nature of the minor histocompatibility disparities between the donor and recipient. MiHL-GvH reactions may be divided into three categories: strong, moderate and weak. Helper-cell activity in MiHL-GvHR is most evident when the MiHL disparities result in a strong reaction, and least evident when the GvH reaction is weak. Cytolytic-T-cells are a component to the weak as well as the strong reactions and apparently can induce GvHR by themselves without significant helper-cell input, but the reaction is slower in developing and less intense in its expression as compared to helper-cell assisted GvHR. It should also be noted with caution that the expression of GvHR, as it is induced in the laboratory, can be strongly influenced by factors inherent to the tissue used as the T-cell source, to the extent that seemingly (although not actually) conflicting results may be observed when the T-cells used to induce GvH reaction are obtained from the spleen as compared to the lymph nodes. The data suggest that the spleen in particular may contain T-cells that are more primitive than those found in the lymph nodes, which in the case of MHC-GvHR may in fact be too primitive to be expressing T-cell antigen. With respect to GvL, the mouse data suggest that T-cells do play a role in the effect, such that their elimination will reduce the extent of the GvL activity. However, the data also suggest that there may be other mechanisms involved as well. In addition, it is evident that GvHR and GvL may be separable effects and that those T-cells participating in the GvL effect may not necessarily be the same ones mediating GvHR.

REFERENCES:

1. van Bekkum DW, de Vries MJ (1967) Radiation Chimaeras. New York, Academic Press.
2. Vos O., de Vries MJ, Collenteur JC, van Bekkum DW (1959) Transplantation of hemologous and heterologous lymphoid cells in X-irradiated and non-irradiated mice. J Nat Cancer Inst 23:53-73.
3. van Bekkum DW, Wagemaker G, Vriesendorp HM (1979) Mechanisms and avoidance of graft-vs-host disease. Transplant Proc 11:189-195.
4. Thomas ED, Storb R, Clift RA, Fefer A, Johnson FL, Neiman PE, Lerner KG, Glucksberg H, Buckner CB (1975) bone marrow transplantation. N Eng J Med 832-843, 895-902.
5. OKunewick JP, Meredith RF, Brozovich BJ, Seeman PR, Magliere K (1980) Exponential relationship between spleen cell concentration and fatal GvH response following transplantation of allogeneic spleen/marrow mixtures. Transplantation 29:507-510.
6. Suvatte V, Githem J, Colofiare J (1968) Modification of graft-vs-host reaction by antilymphocyte serum. Transplantation 6:826-832.
7. Bau J, Thierfelder S (1973) Antilymphocyte antibodies and marrow transplantation I. The effect of antilymphocytic serum on xenogeneic engraftment. Transplantation 15:564-567.
8. Rodt H, Thierfelder S, Eulitz M (1974) Anti-lymphocytic antibodies and marrow transplantation III. Effect of heterologous anti-brain antibodies on acute secondary disease in mice. Eur J Immunol 4:24-29.
9. Weiden PL, Doney K, Storb R, Thomas ED (1979). Antithymocyte globulin for prophylaxis of graft-vs-host disease. Transplantation 27:227-230.
10. Thierfelder S, Hoffmann-Fezer G, Rodt H, Kummer U (1982) Cell manipulation with antibodies: Differential effects of anti-T and ATG. In: Baum SJ, Ledney GD, Thierfelder S (eds) Experimental Hematology Today 1982. New York, Karger pp 103-110.
11. Korngold R, Sprent J (1978) Lethal graft-vs-host disease after bone marrow transplantation across minor histocompatibility barriers in mice. Prevention by removing mature T cells from marrow. J Exp Med 148:1687-1698.
12. OKunewick JP, Meredith RF, Raikow RB, Buffo MJ, Jones DL (1982) Possibility of three distinct and separable components to fatal graft-vs-host reaction. Exp Hemat 10:277-289.
13. Vallera DA, Soderling CCB, Carlson GJ, Kersey JH (1981) Bone marrow transplantation across major histocompatibility barriers in mice. Transplantation 31:218-222.
14. Hamilton BL (1984) Absence of correlation between cytolytic T lymphocytes and lethal murine graft-vs-host disease in response to minor histocompatibility antigens. Transplantation 38:357-360.

15. Cantrell JL, Hildemann WH (1972) Characteristics of disparate histocompatibility barriers in congenic strains of mice I. Graft-vs-host reactions. Transplantation 14:761-770.
16. OKunewick JP (1985) Review of the effects of anti-T-cell monoclonal antibodies on major and minor GvHR in the mouse In: Baum SJ, Pluznik DH, Rozenszajn LA (eds) Experimental Hematology Today - 1985, New York, Springer-Verlag pp 133-143.
17. OKunewick JP, Buffo MJ, Kociban DL (1987) Evidence for two distinct mechanisms in acute fatal graft-vs-host reaction across minor histocompatibility barriers. Exp Hemat 15:365-372.
18. OKunewick JP, Beschorner WE, Buffo MJ, Kociban DL (1985) Histopathology of a possible graft-vs host reaction induced by nude mouse spleen cells. Transplantation 39:447-449.
19. Ledbetter JP, Rouse RV, Micklem HS, Herzenberg LA (1980) T-cell subsets defined by expression of Lyt-1,2,3 and Thy-1 antigens. J Exp Med 152:280-295.
20. Atkinson K, Cooley M, Farrelly H, O'Flaherty E., Concannon A, Dodds A, Biggs JC (1986) $T-4^{+}$ cells can initiate graft-vs-host disease in a dose dependent fashion: a comparative study of T-depleted and non-depleted human marrow transplants. Exp Hemat 14:447.
21. Cantor H, Boyse EA (1975) Functional subclasses of T lymphocytes bearing different Ly antigens. J Exp Med 141:1390-1399.
22. Meredith RF, OKunewick JP (1983) Possibility of graft-vs-leukemia determinants independent of the major histocompatibility complex in allogeneic marrow transplantation. Transplantation 35:378-385.
23. OKunewick JP, Meredith RF (1978) Adoptive immunotherapy of viral leukemic mice I. Comparison of spleen and marrow transplantation from allogeneic, hybrid and immunized syngeneic donors in inducing remission and survival. Exp Hemat 6 (Suppl 3):17.
24. Slavin S, Vitetta E, Morecki S, Weiss L (1982) Antileukemic effects of allogeneic bone marrow allografts in mice. In: B and T Cell Tumors, New York, Academic Press, pp 513-517.
25. Westcott O, Dorsch S, Roser B (1979) Adoptive immunotherapy of leukemia in the rat, without graft-vs-host complications. J Immunol 123:1478-1483.
26. Gillis S, Union NA, Baker PE, Smith KA (1979) The in vitro generation and sustained culture of nude mouse cytolytic T-lymphocytes. J Exp Med 149:1460-1476.
27. MacDonald HR, Lees RK, Sordat B, Zaech P, Maryonski JL, Bron B (1980) Age-associated increase in expression of the T-cell surface markers Thy-1, Lyt-1 and Lyt-2 in congentially athymic mice. J Immunol 126:865-870.
28. OKunewick JP, Meredith RF, Braunschweiger PG, Buffo MJ, James DL, Beschorner WE (1982) Definition and prevention of graft-vs-host disease with the use of monoclonal antibodies. Exp Hemat 10 (suppl 12):12-22.
29. van Bekkum DW, Knaan-Shanzer S (1983) Identity of suppressor cells of graft-vs-host disease. Transplant Proc 15:1451-1453.
30. Pickel K, Hoffman MK (1977) The Ly phenotype of suppressor T-cells arising in mice subjected to a graft-vs-host reaction. J Exp Med 145:1169-1175.
31. Mason DW (1981) Subsets of T-cells in the rat mediating lethal graft-vs-host disease. Transplantation 32:222-226.
32. Pietryga DW, Blazar BR, Soderling CCB, Vallera DA (1987) The effect of T-subset depletion on the incidence of lethal graft-vs-host disease in a murine MHC-mismatched transplantation system. Transplantation 43:442-444.
33. Cobbold S, Martin G, Waldmann H (1986) Monoclonal antibodies for the prevention of graft-vs-host disease and marrow graft rejection. Transplantation 42:239-247.
34. Korngold R, Sprent J (1982) Features of T-cells causing H-2-restricted lethal graft-vs-host disease across minor histocompatibility barriers. J Exp Med 155:872-883.
35. Korngold R, Sprent J (1983) Lethal GvHD across minor histocompatibility: Nature of the effector cells and role of the H-2 complex. Immunol Rev 71:5-29.
36. Korngold R, Sprent J (1987) Variable capacity of L3T4 cells to cause lethal graft-vs-host disease across minor histocompatibility barriers in mice. J Exp Med 165:1552-1564.
37. Mitsuyasu RT, Champlin RE, Ho WG, Winston D, Feig S, Wells J, Terasaki P, Billing P, Weaver M, Gale RP (1985) Prospective randomized controlled trial of ex vivo treatment of donor bone marrow with monoclonal anti-T-cell antibody and complement for prevention of graft-vs-host disease. Transplant Proc 17:482-485.
38. Lotzova E, McCredie KB, Dicke KA, Friereich EJ (1978) Natural killer cells in man: Their possible involvement in leukemia and bone marrow transplantation. Exp Hemat 6 (Suppl 10):38.
39. Truitt RL, LeFever AV, Shih CC (1987). Graft-vs-leukemia Reactions: Experimental models and clinical trials. In: Gale RP, Champlin R (eds) Progress in Bone Marrow Transplantation, New York, Alan R. Liss, pp 219-232.

2: Syngeneic Graft-versus-Host Disease: Failure of Self: Non-Self Discrimination

A.D. Hess, A.C. Fischer, G.B. Vogelsang,
W.E. Beschnorner, and G.W. Santos

Graft-versus-host disease (GVHD) occurs after allogeneic bone marrow transplantation (BMT) and is primarily thought to be the response of donor lymphocytes to foreign histocompatibility antigens of the recipient (1). However, the recent description of GVHD after autologous and/or syngeneic BMT has raised critical questions with regard to our understanding of the immunobiology of GVHD, the antigens which induce this reaction and the mechanisms accounting for the development of donor to host tolerance in the lymphohematopoietic chimera (2,3). The occurrence of syngeneic GVHD implicates that histocompatibility differences are not an absolute requirement for GVHD as once postulated by Billingham (4) but may include a dysregulation of self:non-self discrimination. (1)

An animal model of syngeneic GVHD has recently been described which may allow some insight into the complex immunological mechanisms associated with GVHD and autoaggression (5,6). Severe autoimmunity occurs after syngeneic and/or autologous BMT in rats and treatment with cyclosporine (CsA). This autoaggression syndrome results after cessation of CsA therapy and has been termed syngeneic GVHD because of its similarity to GVHD (acute and chronic) occurring after allogeneic BMT with respect to the histological damage and target organs (6). This disease can be adoptively transferred with splenic T lymphocytes into naive rats that have been irradiated and reconstituted with normal marrow. Associated with syngeneic GVHD is the development of cytotoxic cells (CD8+) reactive to public class II major histocompatibility determinants (7). Similar class II recognition by (CD4+) helper T cells has been reported in a more chronic form of this autoimmune syndrome (8). The relationship of the effector cells in syngeneic GVHD and in the chronic form of this autoimmune syndrome remains unclear.

The mechanisms accounting for syngeneic GVHD remain unknown but the thymus appears to play a central role since thymic shielding during irradiation prevents the development of this syndrome. Similarly, the failure to adoptively transfer this syndrome into non-irradiated animals has implicated the presence of an autoregulatory cell controlling the development of syngeneic GVHD. (6) The present studies were undertaken to sequentially characterize syngeneic GVHD histologically and identify the infiltrating lymphocytes phenotypically. Furthermore, the role of autoregulatory cells in controlling the development of this syndrome were assessed in adoptive transfer experiments.

MATERIALS AND METHODS

Animals. Lew (RT11) female rats (Corona virus-free), 6-8 weeks old were purchased from Harlan Sprague Dawley, Inc., Indianapolis, IN.

Radiation. Lewis rats were irradiated (1050 rad) at 120 rads/min from a dual-source 137Cs small animal irradiator (Atomic Energy of Canada Ltd., Kanata, Ontario, Canada).

Marrow Transplantation. Donor animals were killed by CO2 asphyxiation. Marrow from femurs, tibias, and humeri was collected in Hank's solution supplemented with 50 U/ml penicillin and 50 ug/ml streptomycin. The marrow cells were adjusted to a concentration of 6×10^7 nucleated cells/ml and 1 ml was infused into recipient animals by intravenous injection through the tail vein 1 day after irradiation.

Antibiotics Rats received medicated drinking water supplemented with bactrim, neomycin, and polymixin B, and were given 1 mg/d gentamycin subcutaneously for 10 days as previously described (7).

Cyclosporine. CsA was the generous gift of Sandoz, Ltd., Basel, Switzerland. The powdered CsA was dissolved in 95% ethanol and added to a 4% Tween-20 solution in deionized H20. Rats were weighed daily and received 1 ml/100 g/d subcutaneously from the day of marrow infusion for 40 consecutive days. The total dose of CsA per day per rat was 15 mg/kg. Control animals received the identical quantities of the drug diluent (ethanol, 4% Tween-20, H20) without CsA.

Adoptive transfer experiments. Spleen cells (3×10^7) from animals with active syngeneic GVHD were harvested and infused together with marrow (6×10^7) from normal Lewis rats into recipients prepared with irradiation, busulfan (30 mg/kg, suspended in 3% methylcellulose injected intraperitoneally) or cyclophosphamide (100 mg/kg:suspended in saline injected intraperitoneally) as previously described (9).

Assessment of GVHD. Rats were examined daily for signs of clinical GVHD, such as red ears, dermatitis, or diarrhea. Skin biopsies were taken at frequent intervals. Previously described criteria were used for the histological documentation of GVHD (10).

Immunoperoxidase. The relative number and location of lymphocytes expressing various membrane antigens was determined with the avidin-biotin complex method of immunoperoxidase. (11) Primary antibodies included OX8 (cytotoxic/suppressor cells), and/or W3/25 (helper/inducer cells), (Sera Laboratories, distributed by Accurate Chemical and Scientific Corp., Westbury, NY).

Sections of skin and tongue were frozen in cold isopentane (-105 C). Five-micron sections were cut, air-dried, and fixed in cold acetone, Endogenous avidin and biotin receptors were blocked, and endogenous peroxidase was inactivated with methanol and hydrogen peroxide. The slides were incubated with optimal dilutions of primary mouse monoclonal antibodies (1:200 to 1:800) for 30 minutes at room temperature and washed with phosphate-buffered saline (PBS) with 0.2% bovine serum albumin (BSA). This was followed by affinity-purified goat anti-mouse IgG (heavy and light chain, 1:800) absorbed to remove cross-reactivity with rat immunoglobulins. After washing, the slides were then incubated with biotinylated horse anti-goat IgG (1:800, Vector Laboratories, Burlingame, California). The bound antibodies were revealed with a complex of avidin and biotinylated horseradish peroxidase (Vector Laboratories) and a substrate containing diaminobenzidine (0.06%) in hydrogen peroxide (0.01%). The color was enhanced with 0.5% copper sulfate. The slides were counter-stained with Giemsa stain, dehydrated, and cover-slipped.

RESULTS

Sequential Histological Characterization of Syngeneic GVHD. Initial studies were undertaken to histologically characterize syngeneic GVHD sequentially following the initial onset of this syndrome. Tongue, skin, liver and gastrointestinal tract were evaluated for the presence of acute and/or chronic GVHD. The criteria used for acute GVHD included lymphocytic infiltration, dyskeratosis, vacuolar degeneration and epidermolysis (severe): the histological criteria for chronic GVHD were collagen deposition hyperkeratosis and fibrosis as previously described (10). Results shown in Table 1 revealed that at the onset of clinical syngeneic GVHD (erythema and dermatitis), 4 of 6 animals had histological evidence of acute GVHD while 2 where primarily diagnosed as chronic GVHD. Thereafter, the majority of animals exhibited histological evidence of chronic GVHD after the initial onset of this autoaggression syndrome suggesting a maturation from an acute disorder into a more chronic form of this autoimmune disease.

The lymphoid cells infiltrating the epidermis and submucosa of the tongue were also phenotypically evaluated by immunoperoxidase in this sequential analysis. The results shown in Table 2 demonstrate the presence of equal numbers of cells bearing the CD4 (W3/25; helper T cell subset) and/or the CD8 (OX8; cytotoxic/suppressor subset) determinants at the initial onset of syngeneic GVHD. At present we cannot exclude cells expressing both determinants especially in the epidermis. As the autoaggression syndrome develops (days 3-4 and 6-8 after the initial onset of syngeneic GVHD) mononuclear cells bearing the CD4 determinant appear to dominate the epidermal and submucosal infiltrate with a CD4/CD8 ratio of 3.6.

Demonstration of Autoregulatory Cell Controlling Syngeneic GVHD. Recent studies have demonstrated that syngeneic GVHD can be adoptively transferred into irradiated recipients but not into unmodified animals (6) suggesting the presence of autoregulatory cells controlling the development of syngeneic GVHD. To test this hypothesis, spleen cells ($3x10^7$) from animals with active syngeneic GVHD (early onset) were adoptively transferred along with fresh Lewis marrow cells into secondary Lewis recipients. In order to perturb an autoregulatory system, the recipients were treated with total or hemibody irradiation (1000R), low dose irradiation (500R) busulfan (30 mg/kg) or cyclophosphamide (100 mg/kg). The results are summarized in Table 3. Successful transfer of syngeneic GVHD only occurred if the secondary Lewis recipients were total and upper body irradiated with 1000R, or treated with cyclophosphamide. Secondary syngeneic GVHD routinely was observed 10-20 days after adoptive transfer. In contrast syngeneic GVHD could not be transferred into secondary recipients either left untreated or prepared with low dose total body irradiation (500R), lower body irradiation with 1000R or treatment with busulfan. These results suggest that an autoregulatory system can be detected and is sensitive to irradiation (1000R) and cyclophosphamide but resistant to lower doses of irradiation (500R) and busulfan. The finding that upper body irradiation but not lower body irradiation allowed for successful transfer of syngeneic GVHD suggests that this autoregulatory system may be thymic dependent.

Another approach to demonstrate an autoregulatory system was utilized. Normal spleen cells ($6x10^7$) were adoptively transferred with spleen cells ($3x10^7$) from animals with active syngeneic GVHD (and normal Lewis marrow cells) into secondary Lewis recipients prepared with total body irradiation (1000R). The results in Table 4 show that normal spleen cells successfully prevented the adoptive transfer of syngeneic GVHD.

In contrast, animals only receiving spleen cells from rats with syngeneic GVHD but not normal spleen cells developed this autoaggression syndrome. The identity of the autoregulatory of the cell remains unknown but appears to be thymic dependent.

DISCUSSION

Tolerance to self major histocompatibility (MHC) antigens is one of the fundamental tenets of immunology (12). Implicit in this concept of tolerance is the ability of the immune system to discern and discriminate between self and non-self. To account for tolerance to self MHC antigens, Burnet put forth the concept of clonal selection whereby self reactive clones are deleted during the ontogeny of the immune system in the neonate (12). However, autoregulatory T cells in the control of self tolerance has received strong experimental support (13, 14). Acquisition of tolerance to self MHC antigens is not limited to the developing immune system in the neonate, but must also occur after autologous, and/or syngeneic BMT (1). Reconstitution of the immune system after autologous and/or syngeneic BMT with effective self:non-self discrimination occurs quite rapidly with apparent normal T cell function. Perturbation of the developing immune system could lead to severe autoaggression. Recent studies have shown that treatment of animals with CsA following syngeneic and/or autologous BMT leads to severe autoaggression resembling allogeneic GVHD with the development of CD4+ and CD8+ effector cells recognizing class II MHC antigens including self (5,6,7,8); the immunologic homeostasis accounting for self:non-self discrimination was perturbed by CsA treatment during immunologic recovery.

The mechanism by which CsA leads to syngeneic GVHD and allows for the development of class II MHC-reactive T cells after syngeneic and/or autologous BMT remains unknown. Two criteria appear to be essential for the induction of syngeneic GVHD: 1) thymic and/or total-body irradiation and 2) CsA treatment. (5,6,15) Studies by Glazier et al have shown that thymic shielding during irradiation prevents the development of syngeneic GVHD. (6) On the other hand, Cheney and Sprent have demonstrated that the transfer of spleen cells from a CsA-treated , non-irradiated host into an irradiated recipient resulted in the development of syngeneic GVHD. (15) These data indicate that thymic irradiation is not essential to generate the autoreactive cell but suggest that irradiation may abrogate a host regulatory mechanism.

The present studies provide strong experimental support for the existence of such an autoregulatory system in unmodified animals which controls the development of syngeneic GVHD. This autoregulatory system is sensitive to irradiation (1000R) and cyclophosphamide treatment but resistant to busulfan, and to low dose irradiation. This regulatory system appears to be thymic dependent. These findings are remarkably similar to the regulatory system controlling donor to host tolerance after allogeneic BMT. (9) Further support of such an autoregulatory system is the ability of normal spleen cells to suppress the adoptive transfer of syngeneic GVHD. However, the ratio of normal spleen cells to syngeneic GVHD effector cells appears to be important in suppression of this syndrome. (8) It will be of interest to fully characterize and phenotype this autoregulatory cell and compare it with the regulatory cells controlling the development of donor to host tolerance after allogeneic BMT.

Although the abrogation of the autoregulatory system is essential for induction of syngeneic GVHD, the role of CsA therapy appears to be important for the generation of the effector mechanisms leading to altered self recognition. This effect seems to be related to the affect of CsA on thymic function. Previous studies have shown that CsA treatment leads to a rapid depletion of medullary thymocytes (6), altered T cell differentiation with an apparent release of immature thymocytes into the peripheral blood (16) and a reduction of class II MHC expression in the thymic medulla (15). This pronounced effect on the thymic medulla and on class II MHC antigen expression appears to play a central role in the generation of the effector cells of syngeneic GVHD. One possible explanation to account for the generation of anti-MHC class II specific effector cells is that the maturation of T lymphocytes in a thymic environment lacking class II determinants results in a failure to recognize these antigens as self. On the other hand, we cannot exclude that these antigens provide a differentiation signal so that during CsA treatment, these cells are immaturely released into the peripheral circulation without appropriate selection or differentiation. Experimental evidence suggests that CsA therapy does result in the early release of immature (CD4+ CD8+ Thy 1.1+) T cells (15). It is possible that these immature T cells differentiate extrathymically without the exquisite thymic control in the elimination of autoreactive cells. Such an organ to allow extra thymic differentiation may be the skin associated lymphoid tissue as proposed by Streilein (17). The data presented in the current studies implicate a differentiation process which is characterized by predominantly acute GVHD early, followed by the development of a more chronic type GVHD. This is also reflected by a change in the predominant phenotype of the cells infiltrating the tissue site (CD8+, CD4+ to CD4+). It is unknown if the cells underwent maturation at the tissue site or if the change in the phenotypic pattern is due to purely a different cell population infiltrating the tissue. If differentiation does occur at the tissue site, it will be of interest to assess the role of class II MHC antigens in this setting.

At present many problems remain unresolved regarding syngeneic GVHD. In any case, this model at least, will allow us to probe into the mechanisms accounting for self:non-self discrimination. It may also change our concepts of the immunobiology of GVHD occurring after allogeneic BMT.

ACKNOWLEDGEMENTS

The authors acknowledge the excellent secretarial assistance of Ms. Pauline Divel. The work was supported by grants CA 15396 and AI 24319 from that National Institutes of Health. Dr. Allan D. Hess is a scholar of the Leukemia Society of American, Inc.

REFERENCES

1. Santos GW, Hess AD, Vogelsang GB. (1985) Graft-versus-Host Reactions and Disease. Immunol Rev 88:169-191
2. Tutschka PJ, Hess AD, Beschorner W, Santos GW (1981) Suppressor cells in tranplantation tolerance. I. Suppressor cells in the mechanism of tolerance in radiation chimeras. Transplantation 32:203
3. Tutschka PJ, Ki P, Beschorner W, Hess AD, Santos GW (1981) Suppressor cells in transplantation tolerance. II. Maturation of suppressor cells in the bone marrow chimera. Transplantation 32:321
4. Billingham RE (1966-67) The biology of graft-versus-host reactions. Harvey Lectures 62:21
5. Glazier A, Tutschka PJ, Farmer ER, Santos GW (1983) Graft-versus-host disease in cyclosporin A treated rats after syngeneic and autologous bone marrow reconstitution. J Exp Med 158:1
6. Glazier A, Tutschka PJ, Farmer ER (1983) Studies on the immunobiology of syngeneic and autologous graft-versus-host disease in cyclosporine treated rats. Transplant. Proc. 15:3035
7. Hess AD, Horwitz L, Beschorner WE Santos GW (1985) Development of graft-versus-host disease-like syndrome in cyclosporine treated rats after syngeneic bone marrow transplantation I. Development of cytotoxic T lymphocytes with apparent polyclonal anti-Ia specific including autoreactivity. J Exp Med 161:718
8. Sorokin R, Kimura H, Schroder K, Wilson DH, Wilson DB (1986) Cyclosporine-induced autoimmunity. Conditions for expressing disease, requirement for intact thymus, and potency estimates of autoimmune lymphocytes in drug-treated rats. J Exp Med 164:1615

9. Tutschka PJ, Hutchins GM Santos GW (1979) Suppressor cells as possible mediators of immune function after marrow transplantation in Experimental Hematology Today 1978 (ed. S.J. Baum and G.D. Ledney) Springer-Verlag, New York pp. 113-121
10. Beschorner WE, Tutschka PJ, Santos GW (1982) Sequential morphology of graft-versus-host disease in the rat radiation chimera. Clin Immunol Immunopathol 22:203
11. Parfrey NA, Mann RB, Selonick SE, Beschorner WE (1985) Malignant large cell lymphoma of B cell type with multilobated nuclei: Report of a case and review of the literature. Cancer 55:1913-1917
12. Burnet F (1959) The clonal selection theory of acquired immunity (Cambridge University Press, Cambridge)
13. Dorsh S, Roser B (1975) T cells mediate transplantation tolerance. Nature, Lond 258:233
14. Holan V, Chutna J, Hasek M (1978) Specific suppression of antigen reactive cells in neonatal transplantation tolerance. Nature, Lond 274:895
15. Cheney RT, Sprent J (1985) Capacity of cyclosporine to induce autograft-versus-host disease and impair intrathymic T cell differentiation. Transplant Proc 17:528
16. Hess AD, Vogelsang GB, Heyd J, Beschorner WE (1987) Cyclosporine induced syngeneic graft-versus-host disease: Assessment of T-cell differentiation. Trans Proc 19:2683
17. Streilein JW (1983) Skin-associated lymphoid tissue (SALT): Orgins and functions. J Invest Dermatol 80:125

Table 1: Histological Characterization of Syngeneic GVHD Following Syngeneic Marrow Transplantation and CsA Therapy[a]

Days Post Onset of Syngeneic GVHD	Incidence Acute GVHD	Chronic GVHD
1 (n=6)	4	2
3-4 (n=4)	1	3
6-8 (n=2)	0	2

Animals were sacrificed at various intervals after the onset of clinical symptoms of syngeneic GVHD and evaluated histologically for acute and/or chronic GVHD.

Table 2: Phenotypic Characterization of Mononuclear Cell Infiltrates In Epidermis and Submucosa of Tongue (Syngeneic GVHD)[a]

Days Post Onset of Syngeneic GVHD	Epidermis Phenotype W3/25 (CD4)	Epidermis OX8 (CD8)	Submucosa Phenotype W3/25 (CD4)	Submucosa OX8 (CD8)
1	62 ± 5 (n=5)	65 ± 4 (n=5)	50 ± 5 (n=5)	48 ± 3 (n=5)
3-4	54 ± 17 (n=4)	30 ± 20 (n=4)	50 ± 4 (n=4)	28 ± 5 (n=4)
6-8	70 (n=1)	20 (n=1)	75 ± 15 (n=2)	17 ± 20 (n=2)

[a] Animals were sacrificed at various intervals after the onset of clinical syngeneic GVHD. Frozen sections of tongue were analyzed for phenotypic characterization of the mononuclear cell infiltrates by immunoperoxidase. Assessment of T cells by expression of Ox19 revealed that >90-95% of the infiltrating cells expressed this T cell marker.

Table 3: Drug and Radiosensitivity of Autoregulatory Suppressor Cells in Normal Lewis Rats[a]

Treatment of Secondary Recipients	Incidence of Syngeneic GVHD In Secondary Recipients
Untreated	0/8
Irradiation	
Total Body	
500R	0/4
1000R	8/8
Upper Body (1000R)	6/8
Lower Body (1000R)	0/8
Busulfan (30 mg/kg)	1/7[b]
Cyclophosphamide (100 mg/kg)	4/4

[a] Secondary Lewis rats were either untreated, irradiated, or treated with busulfan or cyclophosphamide prior to infusion of $3x10^7$ spleen cells from animals with active syngeneic GVHD together with $6x10^7$ marrow cells from normal Lewis rats.

[b] Syngeneic GVHD developed late - 4 weeks post therapy in one animal

Table 4: Adoptive Transfer of Autoregulatory Suppressor Cells [a]

Normal Spleen Cells Adoptively Transferred with Syngeneic GVHD Effector Cells	Incidence of Syngeneic GVHD in Secondary Recipients
No Normal Spleen Cells	8/8
Unfractionated Normal Spleen Cells ($6x10^7$)	0/8

[a] Spleen cells ($3x10^7$) from animals with active syngeneic GVHD and/or normal spleen cells were adoptively transferred along with fresh normal Lewis marrow into irradiated (1000R) Lewis rats.

3: Transfusion-Induced Allosensitization in Marrow Transplant Recipients: Mechanisms and Preventive Measures

H. Joachim Deeg, Sherrill J. Slichter, and Rainer Storb

Many patients treated by bone marrow transplantation have received blood transfusions (Tx) pretransplant, and virtually all require Tx for several weeks post transplant (1,2). The aim of Tx is to provide blood components that are lacking or deficient in the recipient. However, there are undesired Tx effects that are dependent upon factors such as composition of the Tx product, histocompatibility differences between donor and recipient, the immune status of the recipient, the functional capacities of the transfused cells, and the frequency of Tx (3,4,5). In an immunocompetent Tx recipient, transfused cells are generally recognized and destroyed by the recipient's immune system, leading to allosensitization. This may result in Tx refractoriness and an increased risk of rejecting a subsequent marrow graft. In an immunosuppressed recipient, in addition, transfused cells may become engrafted, replicate and initiate a graft-vs-host reaction (6). Consequently, in the setting of marrow transplantation, the activation of both donor and host immunocompetent cells in response to Tx is undesirable.

We will first discuss attempts at the prevention of pretransplant Tx induced sensitization, and then consider post transplantation Tx 'support.

TRANSFUSION SUPPORT BEFORE MARROW TRANSPLANTATION

Blood Tx given before marrow transplantation increase the risk for graft rejection even when donor and recipient are genotypically identical for the major histocompatibility complex (HLA, DLA, etc.) antigens (7-10). In previously transfused patients with severe aplastic anemia conditioned with cyclophosphamide in preparation for HLA identical marrow transplantation, the probability of rejection in early reports was 25-60% (11). Subsequently, with the use of more immunosuppressive regimens or the infusion of marrow donor buffy coat cells, engraftment was achieved more consistently (11). In recent years, for reasons not completely understood, the risk of graft rejection has decreased further (12). At the same time rejection has occurred in §1% of patients with leukemia given HLA identical marrow grafts. These patients are usually given Tx at a time when they also receive antileukemic chemotherapy. Since chemotherapy is immunosuppressive it may modify an active host response to Tx (3). Furthermore, patients with leukemia are generally conditioned for transplantation with more aggressive combination chemotherapy or with regimens including the use of total body irradiation (TBI), which may be more effective in abrogating sensitization (13). Finally, the nature of the underlying disease by itself may have an effect on the patient's immune response to Tx.

PREVENTION OF TRANSFUSION-INDUCED SENSITIZATION

The simplest way of preventing Tx induced sensitization is that of avoiding Tx (14). Therefore, patients with severe aplastic anemia who are likely to be candidates for marrow transplantation, whenever possible, should not receive pretransplant Tx. However, since Tx can not always be avoided, it may be important to determine which cells in the Tx product are responsible for sensitization. This in turn might allow the development of techniques to eliminate or inactivate such cells, and thus prevent sensitization.

Experimental Studies

Whole blood. Untransfused dogs given 9.2 Gy of TBI followed by the infusion of marrow and buffy coat cells from a DLA non-identical unrelated donor generally achieve sustained engraftment (91%) while a single pretransplant Tx of 50 ml of whole blood from the intended marrow donor (given 1 to 90 days pretransplant) is associated with a significantly increased risk (86-50%) of marrow graft rejection (15).

Untransfused dogs given 9.2 to 12 Gy of TBI followed by hemopoietic grafts from DLA identical littermate donors almost uniformly (98%) achieve sustained engraftment (7). With a single Tx of 50 ml of whole blood from the intended marrow donor given 10 days pretransplant approximately 75% of dogs reject their graft (16). With three Tx of whole blood given 24, 17 and 10 days pretransplant dogs uniformly reject their graft (7,18). Even with three Tx from unrelated DLA nonidentical donors, three of 11 dogs (27%) rejected their graft (17). Sensitization and subsequent graft rejection was then by definition, due to "minor" (non-DLA) antigens, presumably, two polymorphic systems expressed on cells contained in the Tx product and on donor marrow cells (7).

Platelets. Subsequent studies were aimed at preparing highly purified red blood cells (RBC) and platelets, the two most widely used Tx products, and testing their immunogenicity in vivo (7). Dogs were given three Tx of "leukocyte and RBC poor" platelets from the prospective marrow donor 24, 17, and 10 days pretransplant (7). Platelets were depleted of 99.9% of leukocytes. Among fifteen dogs transplanted, seven rejected their graft and eight (53%) achieved sustained engraftment (18).

Red blood cells. Fourteen dogs were given three Tx of "leukocyte and platelet poor" RBC from the intended marrow donor (7,18), depleted of 99.8% of leukocytes. Only five dogs rejected their graft and nine (64%) had sustained engraftment strongly suggesting that leukocyte depletion had rendered the Tx less immunogenic, thus implying a role for leukocytes in the sensitizing process.

Leukocytes. RBC or platelet Tx described above contained on the average 12.5 x 10^3 leukocytes/kg recipient body weight. In subsequent experiments (unless indicated otherwise) this was the total number of leukocytes given in 3 Tx to the recipient dog, i.e. 4,166 cells/kg/Tx (18). Results are summarized in Table 1.

Only dogs given peripheral blood mononuclear cells obtained from Ficoll-Hypaque gradients and transfused without further fractionation became sensitized and rejected their marrow graft. The possibility of a dose/response relationship rather than an all or none phenomenon cannot be excluded. Passage over cotton-wool columns, removing monocytes and other Ia positive cells (18,19) yielded a cell population that no longer was able to induce sensitization. It was surprising, therefore, that Tx of neither peripheral blood monocytes nor alveolar macrophages induced sensitization. However, as described previously (19,20) in vitro studies revealed that methods used for monocyte enrichment, although significantly increasing the purity of monocytes, resulted in a loss of accessory function of these cells as determined in mitogen stimulated T cell proliferation. Instead, accessory function was contained among light buoyant density cells eliminated in the process of monocyte enrichment. These cells had the characteristics of dendritic cells (21). Since dendritic cells function as potent stimulator cells in mixed leukocyte culture, accessory cells in T cell activation and passenger leukocytes in organ transplantation (21-26), we hypothesized that dendritic cells might also be responsible for transfusion-related sensitization. It was disappointing, therefore, that two dogs given dendritic cells failed to become sensitized (Table 1).

UV-irradiation of whole blood. However, enrichment and purification of dendritic cells is difficult. We, therefore, chose an indirect approach. Dendritic cells are highly sensitive to ultraviolet (UV) light (27,28), which abrogates accessory function and stimulating ability in mixed leukocyte culture. We postulated that, similar to the abrogation of in vitro stimulating ability of leukocytes, exposure of blood to UV light could also prevent its in vivo stimulating (i.e. sensitizing) function (27). This was indeed the case (Table 2). Dogs transfused with UV-exposed blood consistently achieved sustained engraftment while dogs given sham-exposed or unmanipulated blood consistently rejected their grafts. Survival of 51Cr labelled UV-exposed RBC was only insignificantly shortened as compared to unmanipulated RBC (Deeg et al. unpublished observations).

In a follow-up experiment dogs were transfused with UV-exposed blood to which normal dendritic cells or monocytes (from the same donor) were added. While dogs given dendritic cells rejected their grafts, dogs given monocytes generally did not (Deeg et al. unpublished observations). These results indicate that antigen presenting cells, specifically dendritic cells, play a central role in the sensitization process.

Clinical Studies

No clinical studies on the effect of purified cell populations on engraftment have been carried out. Nevertheless, the probability of marrow graft rejection in patients with aplastic anemia who have not been transfused prior to transplantation is lower than in patients who have been transfused (14). A recent analysis, however, suggests that Tx per se is not the most important risk factor (12). Rather, the number of units of platelets transfused before transplantation showed a positive correlation with probability of graft rejection. The reason for this is not clear. Conceivably, leukocytes contaminating platelet preparations were involved, and consequently an increased number of Tx would imply exposure to increased numbers of foreign antigens, and an increased probability of these being shared with antigens expressed on donor marrow. A concurrent analysis of refractoriness to platelet Tx in patients with aplastic anemia indicated that the most strongly correlated factor was the development of lymphocytotoxic antibodies in the recipient, followed by the number of platelet units given in excess of 40 (29). It is of interest in this context that in the canine model the Tx of UV exposed histoincompatible blood prevented the development of lymphocytotoxic antibodies in the recipient (30).

ABROGATION OF TRANSFUSION-INDUCED SENSITIZATION

Experimental Studies

The recipient's immune response to Tx is thought to be mediated by T lymphocytes (17,30,31). At the time of marrow infusion, memory T cells are likely to recognize antigens to which they were previously exposed. Consequently, efforts at abrogating sensitization have been directed at T lymphocytes (Table 3). Methotrexate, used widely as an anti T cell reagent for the prevention of GVHD, had no beneficial effect in a model of DLA nonidentical unrelated dogs
(17). However, the use of antithymocyte serum (ATS) or procarbazine given pretransplant (but after Tx) reduced the probability of graft rejection to 50%. When procarbazine and ATS were combined, only one of 10 dogs given three Tx from non-identical unrelated donors 20 and 13 days before transplantation, rejected a graft, and 2 of 15 dogs given 6 Tx 15-50 days before transplantation, failed to engraft (17). We then tested cyclosporine, another T cell directed agent for its usefulness in abrogating Tx induced sensitization (32). Dogs were given Tx of whole blood 24, 17 and 10 days before transplantation from a DLA identical littermate. Cyclosporine was given i.m. in doses of 20 mg/kg/d on days -5 to 0. Among 9 evaluable dogs, two failed to engraft and seven had sustained engraftment. These data clearly support the hypothesis that rejection was T cell mediated.

Tx of histoincompatible cells results in phenotypic and functional changes of circulating recipient lymphocytes (30), including an increase in cells expressing class II (Ia-like) histocompatibility antigens. We postulated that these cells were involved in marrow graft rejection. Consequently, dogs were given three Tx of whole blood from the marrow donor 24, 17 and 10 days pretransplant, and on days -6 through -1 they were injected with anti-class II monoclonal antibody 7.2, at 0.5 mg/kg/d (33). However, none of the five dogs so treated showed engraftment, and all died with marrow aplasia. Apparently anti-Ia antibody alone was insufficient to eliminate or inactivate cells responsible for graft rejection.

Clinical Studies

Results with cyclosporine in the canine model (32) were in agreement with a clinical study which had shown that the use of cyclosporine given with the intent of preventing graft-vs-host disease also significantly reduced the incidence of graft rejection in previously transfused patients with severe aplastic anemia. A pilot study in our own institution, however, did not confirm that impression (34), and a retrospective analysis failed to identify cyclosporine as a prognostic factor for engraftment (27).

TRANSFUSION AFTER MARROW TRANSPLANTATION

As discussed above, patients undergoing marrow transplantation require intensive cytoreductive/immunosuppressive treatment pretransplant. Until the transplanted marrow begins to function, patients are RBC and platelet Tx dependent, usually for a period of 4-6 weeks (1). During that interval patients remain immunosuppressed and Tx of allogeneic cells, similar to transplanted marrow cells, can result in engraftment and Tx-induced graft-vs-host disease. Consequently, all blood products should be irradiated with approximately 1500-2000 rad to prevent engraftment and proliferation of transfused leukocytes (6). However, gamma-irradiation does not prevent sensitization of the recipient.

Experimental Studies

Only limited data on experimental post transplant Tx support are available. However, interesting studies have been carried out in a canine platelet Tx model (35). Dogs were given weekly Tx of platelets from DLA different unrelated donors. The median time to sensitization was 3.1 weeks, and approximately 85% of dogs became refractory after eight Tx. We studied three protocols aimed at reducing the rate of sensitization. Dogs were given either daily oral cyclosporine, or they received platelets that had been irradiated with UV C light in vitro, or incubated with cyclosporine in vitro (35). Nine dogs were given oral cyclosporine and all remained responsive to platelet Tx during the entire eight week study. Twelve dogs were given UV-irradiated platelets, and eleven remained Tx responsive. Nine were given cyclosporine loaded donor platelets, and five remained Tx responsive. These results clearly showed a beneficial effect for both cyclosporine and UV-irradiation on Tx-related sensitization. It was, furthermore, of interest that 44-67% of the non-immunized recipients remained responsive to continued platelet Tx from the original donor even after discontinuing experimental treatment, i.e. with the Tx of normal unmanipulated platelets.

Clinical Studies

Many patients transfused with platelets obtained from random donors become refractory, i.e. no longer show a Tx increment (3,36). At that point an attempt is made to obtain platelets via apheresis from family members, ideally the bone marrow donor. In some instances HLA matched unrelated donors can be used (37,38).

The extent of Tx support required varies widely. In a recent analysis in 82 patients with severe aplastic anemia, the Tx requirement during the first 100 days after transplantation was 1-82 (mean 9) units of RBC, and 6-468 (mean 44) units of platelets (39). Most of those Tx were required during the first month after transplantation.

The clinical usefulness of UV or cyclosporine treated platelets remains to be determined. However, as described above, dogs transfused with UV irradiated blood products failed to develop cytotoxic antibodies (30). If this can be extrapolated to the clinical situation, one might well expect a decrease in the rate of refractoriness with UV exposed platelets. It is not clear whether UV light results in a modification of platelet associated antigens or exerts its' beneficial effect via inactivation of leukocytes, for example, dendritic cells contaminating the platelet preparations.

TABLE 1: **Results in Dogs Given 9.2 Gy of TBI and Hemopoietic Grafts From DLA Identical Littermates Following Three Tx with Marrow Donor Leukocytes**

Pretransplant Tx Type of Tx[2]	Number of Cells[3]	Number of Dogs Studied	% of Dogs With Sustained Graft
PBMC (FH)	- 12.5×10^3	7	43
	- 75×10^6	2	0
PBMC (FH-CWNA)	- 12.5×10^3	7	100
Alveolar	12.5×10^3	7	100
PBMC-MO	- 12.5×10^3	3	
	- 12.5×10^4	3	100
	- 12.5×10^5	2	
PBMC-DC	- 12.5×10^3	2	100

[1]Transfusions were given 24, 17 and 10 days pretransplant
[2]Tx = transfusion; PBMC = peripheral blood mononuclear cells; FH = Ficoll-hypaque interphase cells (88±5% lymphocytes; 3±3% monocytes); FH-CWNA = FH cells that were also cotton wool adherent (97±3% lymphocytes; 0.5±0.8% monocytes); Alveolar MO = bronchoalveolar lavage cells (10±9% lymphocytes; 88±7% macrophages); PBMC-MO = peripheral blood monocytes (3±4% lymphocytes; 89±6% monocytes); DC = dendritic cells (70±12% lymphocytes; 2±3% monocytes; 25±13% dendritic cells).
[3]Cells/kg/3Tx given 24, 17 and 10 days pretransplant

TABLE 2: **Results in Dogs Given 9.2 Gy TBI and Hemopoietic Grafts From DLA Identical Littermates With or Without Preceding Tx From The Marrow Donor**

Pretransplant Tx[1]	Number of Dogs Studied	% of Dogs With Sustained Graft
None	60	98
Whole Blood	21	0
UV-irradiated blood[2]	10	100
Sham-irradiated blood[3]	4	0

[1]Transfusions were given 24, 17 and 10 days pretransplant
[2]Whole blood exposed to 1.35 J/cm^2 of UV light (27).
[3]Whole blood exposed to visible light

TABLE 3: Abrogation of Tx Induced Sensitization in Dogs Given 9.2 GY TBI and Hemopoietic Grafts

Donor/Recipient Combination	Preceding Whole Blood Tx from Marrow Donor	Additional Treatment	Number of Dogs Studied	% of Dogs With Engraftment
DLA Nonidentical Unrelated	None	None	7	100
		MTX[1]	11	91
	1 Tx day -10	None	5	0
		MTX[1]	5	0
	2 Tx days -20, -13	None	10	30
		ATS[2]	10	50
		Procarbazine[3]	8	50
		ATS[2] + Procarbazine[3]	10	90
DLA Identical	3 Tx days -24,-17,-10	None	21	0
		Cyclosporine[4]	9	78
		mAb 7.2[5]	5	0

[1]Methotrexate 0.4 mg/kg i.v. on days 1, 3, 6 and 11 post transplant.
[2]Rabbit antithymocyte serum 0.6 ml/kg s.c. on days -7, -5, -3.
[3]Procarbazine 12.5 mg/kg i.v. on days -8, -6 and -4.
[4]Cyclosporine 20 mg/kg/day i.m. on days -5 to 0.
[5]Monoclonal antibody 7.2 (anti-Ia), 0.5 mg/kg/d i.v. on days -6 to -1.

CONCLUSIONS

Tx recipients can become sensitized to minor and major histocompatibility antigens. Available evidence suggests that sensitization is mediated by leukocytes, specifically class II antigen positive antigen presenting cells, most importantly dendritic cells. UV treatment of Tx products in vitro reduces or eliminates Tx induced sensitization presumably by abrogating antigenicity of the Tx product. Conceivably, similar results can be obtained by selectively eliminating the responsible cell population from the Tx product. If UV exposure can also prevent the graft-vs-host effect, as is likely based on in vitro studies, UV exposure could replace gamma irradiation of Tx products post transplantation, i.e. UV treatment would prevent both the risk of Tx-induced graft-vs-host disease as well as refractoriness.

ACKNOWLEDGEMENTS

This study was supported in part by grants HL33859, CA31787, CA18221, CA15704, HL36444, and HL33775, awarded by the National Institutes of Health, DHHS.

REFERENCES

1. Storb R and Weiden PL (1981) Transfusion problems associated with transplantation. Seminars in Hematology 18:163.
2. Brand A, Claas FHJ, Falkenburg JHF et al. (1984) Blood component therapy in bone marrow transplantation. Seminars in Hematology 21:141.
3. Slichter SJ (1986) Prevention of platelet alloimmunization. In Transfusion Medicine Recent Technological Advances, K. Murawski; F. Peetoom (eds.) A.R. Liss, New York, pp 83.
4. Eernisse JG, Brand A (1981) Prevention of platelet refractoriness due to HLA antibodies by administration of leukocyte-poor blood components. Exp Hematol 9:77.
5. Herzig RH, Herzig GP, Bull MI et al. (1975) Correction of poor platelet transfusion responses with leukocyte-poor HL-A-matched platelet concentrates. Blood 46:743.
6. Pflieger H (1983) Graft-versus-host disease following blood transfusions. Blut 46:61.
7. Storb R, Weiden PL, Deeg HJ et al. (1979) Rejection of marrow from DLA-identical canine littermates given transfusions before grafting: Antigens involved are expressed on leukocytes and skin epithelial cells but not on platelets and red blood cells. Blood 54:477.
8. Storb R, Prentice RL, Thomas ED et al. (1983) Factors associated with graft rejection after HLA-identical marrow transplantation for aplastic anaemia. Br J Haematol 55:573.
9. da Costa H, Amiel JL, Mathe G et al (1964) Immunisation contre des greffes de cellules hematopoietiques allogeniques par des transfusions de sang anterieures. Vox San 9:420.
10. van Putten LM, van Bekkum DW, de Vries MJ et al. (1967) The effect of preceding blood transfusions on the fate of homologous bone marrow grafts in lethally irradiated monkeys. Blood 30:749.
11. Storb R, Thomas ED, Buckner CD et al. (1984) Marrow transplantation for aplastic anemia. Seminars in Hematology 21:27.
12. Deeg HJ, Self S, Storb R et al. (1986) Decreased incidence of marrow graft rejection in patients with severe aplastic anemia: changing impact of risk factors. Blood 68:1363.
13. Feig SA, Champlin R, Arenson E et al (1983) Improved survival following bone marrow transplantation for aplastic anaemia. British J Haematol 54:509.
14. Anasetti C, Doney KC, Storb R et al. (1986) Marrow transplantation for severe aplastic anemia. Annals of Internal Med 104:461.
15. Weiden PL, Storb R, Kolb HJ et al. (1975) Effect of time on sensitization to hemopoietic grafts by preceding blood transfusion. Transplantation 19:240.
16. Storb R, Epstein RB, Rudolph RH et al. (1970) The effect of prior transfusion on marrow grafts between histocompatible canine siblings. J Immunol 105:627.
17. Storb R, Deeg HJ (1986) Failure of allogeneic canine marrow grafts after total-body irradiation. Allogeneic resistance versus transfusion-induced sensitization. Transplantation 42:571.
18. Deeg HJ, Torok-Storb B, Storb R et al. (1981) Rejection of DLA-identical canine littermate marrow after transfusion-induced sensitization: Antigens involved are expressed on cotton-wool adherent but not on nonadherent mononuclear cells, granulocytes, or thoracic duct lymphocytes. In Baum SJ, Ledney GD, Khan A (eds): "Experimental Hematology Today 1981" Basel: S. Karger, pp 31-37.
19. Aprile JA, Deeg HJ, Wulff JC et al. (1984) Purified canine monocytes fail to confer concanavalin-A responsiveness to accessory-cell-depleted lymphocytes. Exp Hematol 12:45.
20. Aprile J, Deeg HJ (1986) UV irradiation of canine dendritic cells prevents mitogen induced cluster formation and lymphocyte proliferation. Transplantation 42:653.
21. Nussenzweig MC, Steinman RM (1980) Contribution of dendritic cells to stimulation of the murine syngeneic mixed leukocyte reaction. J Exp Med 151:1196.
22. Tew JG, Thorbecke GH, Steinman RM (1982) Dendritic cells in the immune-response: Characteristics and recommended nomenclature. J Reticuloendothel Soc 31:371.

23. Van Voorhis W, Valensky J, Hoffman E et al. (1983) Relative efficiency of human monocytes and dendritic cells as accessory cells for T cell replication. J Exp Med 158:174.
24. Steinman RM, Gutchinov B, Witmer MD et al. (1983) Dendritic cells are the principal stimulators of the primary mixed leukocyte reaction in mice. J Exp Med 157:613.
25. Lechler RI, Batchelor JR (1982) Restoration of immunogenicity to passenger cell-depleted kidney allografts by the addition of donor strain dendritic cells. J Exp Med 155:31.
26. Crow NK, Kunkel HG (1982) Human dendritic cells: Major stimulators of the autologous and allogeneic mixed leukocyte reactions. Clin Exp Immunol 49:338.
27. Deeg HJ, Aprile J, Graham TC et al. (1986) Ultraviolet irradiation of blood prevents transfusion-induced sensitization and marrow graft rejection in dogs. Blood 67:537.
28. Lau H, Reemtsma K, Hardy MA (1984) Prolongation of rat islet allograft survival by direct ultraviolet irradiation of the graft. Science 223:607.
29. Klingemann HG, Self S, Banaji M et al. (1986) Refractoriness to random donor platelet transfusions in patients with aplastic anaemia: a multivariate analysis of data from 264 cases. Br J Haematol 66:115.
30. Deeg HJ, Aprile J, Severns E et al. (1987) Phenotypic and functional alterations of recipient lymphocytes after transfusion of UV-irradiated and normal blood - Implications for marrow transplantation. Transplant Proc 19:2709.
31. Torok-Storb B, Deeg HJ, Storb R (1980) Functional subsets of peripheral blood mononuclear cells in transfused dogs separated by size with the fluorescence activated cell sorter. Exp Hematol 8:906.
32. Storb R, Deeg HJ, Atkinson K et al. (1982) Cyclosporin-A abrogates transfusion-induced sensitization and prevents marrow graft rejection in DLA-identical canine littermates. Blood 60:524.
33. Storb R, Deeg HJ, Appelbaum FR et al. Anti-Ia monoclonal antibody fails to abrogate transfusion-induced sensitization and prevent marrow graft rejection in DLA-identical canine littermates. Transplantation, in press.
34. Deeg HJ, Shulman HM, Schmidt E et al. (1986) Marrow graft rejection and veno-occlusive disease of the liver in patients with aplastic anemia conditioned with cyclophosphamide and cyclosporine. Transplantation 42:497.
35. Slichter SJ, Deeg HJ, Kennedy MS (1987) Prevention of platelet alloimmunization in dogs with systemic cyclosporine and by UV-irradiation or cyclosporine-loading of donor platelets. Blood 69:414.
36. Schiffer CA, Dutcher JP, Aisner J et al. (1983) A randomized trial of leukocyte-depleted platelet transfusion to modify alloimmunization in patients with leukemia. Blood 62:815.
37. Yankee RA, Grumet FC, Rogentine GN (1969) Platelet transfusion therapy. The selection of compatible platelet donors for refractory patients by lymphocyte HLA typing. N Eng J Med 281:1208.
38. Tosato G, Appelbaum FR, Deisseroth AB (1978) HLA-matched platelet transfusion therapy of severe aplastic anemia. Blood 52:846.
39. Wulff JC, Santner TJ, Storb R et al. (1983) Tranfusion requirements after HLA-identical marrow transplantation in 82 patients with aplastic anemia. Vox Sang 44:366.

II. Experimental Bone Marrow Transplantation: J.P. OKunewick and Y. Kodera, Chairpersons

4: Utilization of Monoclonal Antibodies for Autologous Bone Marrow Transplantation

Y. Kodera, Y. Morishima, Y. Moriyama, T. Mori, A. Kanamaru, K. Shinohara, T. Ito, H. Mugishima, and T. Masaoka

ABSTRACT

At nine institutes in Japan, from 1983 to 1986, autologous bone marrow transplantation (BMT) was carried out in 21 patients with null-cell type acute lymphocytic leukemia (Null-ALL) and in 2 Burkitt's lymphoma patients after depletion of leukemia or lymphoma cells from transplanted bone marrow with monoclonal antibodies.

Patients' autologous bone marrow cells were harvested and treated in vitro with either the combination of BA-1, BA-2 and BA-3 or the combination of NL-1, NL-22 and HL-47 and complement, then cryopreserved.

In Null-ALL patients, 9 received the treated marrow during the first remission period, 6 received it during the second remission period and 6 were transplanted at a more advanced stage of the disease.

Engraftment was confirmed in all the cases. Six out of 9 (67%) patients transplanted during the first remission, 2 out of 8 (25%) patients grafted at the 2nd or 3rd remission and 2 Burkitt's lymphoma patients continued in remission for more than 5-31 months after the BMT, suggesting autologous BMT with these monoclonal antibodies may be an effective mode of therapy for Null-ALL and Burkitt's lymphoma especially when applied at an early stage of the disease.

INTRODUCTION

Recent advances of allogeneic BMT in leukemia treatment have resulted in a high rate of patients' disease free survivals (1,2,3,4), suggesting that high dose chemo-radiotherapy followed by marrow rescue procedure is potentially a curative treatment for leukemia. Allogeneic BMT is, however, generally indicated only for patients who have HLA identical donors and also some of the patients may suffer from variable complications based on complications based on graft vs. host disease (GvH-D) after BMT (5). The development of mouse monoclonal antibodies which are predominantly reactive to leukemia cells (6-10) offered a possibility of autologous BMT in leukemia by depleting the contaminated leukemia cells in patients' autologous marrow with these monoclonal antibodies. Ritz et al (6) have used J-5 monoclonal antibodies plus rabbit complement to deplete the contaminating leukemia cells in marrow of patients with Null-ALL. Ramsey et al (7) also applied three monoclonal antibodies, BA-1, BA-2 and BA-3 (anti-CALLA) for autologous BMT in the same type of disease. Since 1983, such autologous BMT utilizing mouse monoclonal antibodies has been also carried out in Japan and so far, 23 cases have been registered by the BMT Study Group. In this symposium, the summary of these 23 cases experienced in 9 institutes will be presented.

Send reprint requests to Yoshihisa Kodera, M.D., The 4th Dept. of Int. Med., Japanese Red Cross Nagoya First Hospital, 3-35 Mitchishita-cho, Nakamura-ku, Nagoya, Japan

MATERIALS AND METHODS

Patients (Table #1.)

Twenty one Null-ALL patients and 2 Burkitts's lymphoma patients were subjected to autologous BMT. None of them had HLA identical donors. In 11 of 21 Null-ALL patients, the bone marrow cells were harvested during the first remission stage of the disease and in 7 patients during the second remission (from 1 of the 6, the marrow cells were also harvested during the third remission.) In the other 3 patients harvest was performed during the fourth remission (8,9). In 2 Burkitt's lymphoma patients (10), there was no evidence of lymphoma cell invasion to their bone marrow when the cells were harvested.

MONOCLONAL ANTIBODIES (MoAbs)

For 13 Null-ALL patients and 2 Burkitt's lymphoma patients in 7 institutes, BA-1, BA-2 and BA-3 MoAbs were used for in vitro treatment of autologous bone marrow.

Table #1. Patients' Profiles, MoAbs and Preconditioning Regimens.

CASE NO.	DIAGNOSIS	AGE (SEX)	MARROW HARV-ESTED DURING	CELL NUMBERS HARVESTED d).	MoAbs	PRECONDITIONING REGIMENS
1.	Null-ALL	28 (M)	4th CR[a]	22	BA-1,2,3	CY[b] TBI(10Gy)[c]
2.	Null-ALL	33 (M)	2nd CR	33	BA-1,2,3	CY,TBI(10Gy)
3.	Null-ALL	12 (F)	1st CR	9.3	BA-1,2,3	CY,TBI(10Gy)
4.	Null-ALL	42 (M)	2nd CR	17	BA-1,2,3	CY,TBI(10Gy)
5.	Null-ALL	32 (F)	1st CR	7.7	BA-1,2,3	CY,TBI(12Gy)
6.	Null-ALL	36 (F)	1st CR	18	BA-1,2,3	CY,TBI(12Gy)
7.	Null-ALL	5 (M)	4th CR	4.5	BA-1,2,3	VP-16,BCNU,CY,TBI(10Gy)
8.	Null-ALL	6 (M)	2nd CR	12	BA-1,2,3	VP-16,CY,TBI(10Gy)
9.	Null-ALL	32 (M)	2nd CR	21	BA-1,2,3	ADR[e],CY,TBI(12Gy)
10.	Null-ALL	25 (F)	2nd&3rd CR	15(TOTAL)	BA-1,2,3	CY,TBI
11.	Null-ALL	11 (F)	1st CR	21	BA-1,2,3	CA[f],CY,TBI(10Gy)
12.	Null-ALL	10 (F)	2nd CR	6	BA-1,2,3	CY,TBI(10Gy)
13.	Null-ALL	8 (F)	1st CR	7.7	BA-1.2.3	CA,CY,TBI(12Gy)
14.	Null-ALL	30 (M)	1st CR	20	NL-1,HL-47	CA,CY,TBI(12Gy)
15.	Null-ALL	20 (M)	1st CR	13	NL-1,22,HL-47	CA,CY,TBI(12Gy)
16.	Null-ALL	17 (M)	1st CR	26	NL-1,HL-47	CA,CY,TBI(12Gy)
17.	Null-ALL	6 (M)	2nd CR	14	NL-1,22,HL-47	CA,CY,TBI(12Gy)
18.	Null-ALL	11 (F)	1st CR	35	NL-1,22,HL-47	CA,CY,TBI(12Gy)
19.	Null-ALL	40 (M)	1st CR	12	NL,1,22,HL-47	CA,CY,TBI(12Gy)
20.	Null-ALL	9 (M)	4th CR	23	NL-1,HL-47	CA,CY,TBI(12Gy)
21.	Null-ALL	20 (M)	1st CR	18	NL-1,22,HL-47	CA,CY,TBI(12Gy)
22.	BURKITT'S[h]	13 (M)	1st CR	16	BA-1,3	CA,TBI(12Gy),TI[g]
23.	BURKITT'S	5 (M)	1st CR	72	BA-1,3	CA,TBI(10Gy)

a). complete remission b). cyclophosphamide c). total body irradiation d). $x10^9$ per patient
e). adriamycine f). cytosine arabinoside g). tumor irradiation h). Burkitt's lymphoma

For the other 8 Null-ALL patients in 2 institutes, NL-1,NL-22 and HL-47 MoAbs (12,13) were used. The serological specificities and the safety for clinical use of the latter 3 MoAbs were described in the previous reports (8,14).

COMPLEMENT (C)

Baby rabbit serum (Pel-Freeze, Roger, Ariz., USA) was used as a source of C. in all the 9 institutes. The higher C activity for cytotoxicity by MoAbs and the lower non-specific cytotoxicity to hematopoietic stem cells were screened before clinical use (14).

C-DEPENDENT CYTOTOXIC TEST

In 13 out of 23 cases, the activity of MoAbs and C to the corresponding autologous leukemia cells was tested in vitro according to the procedure described previously. (14).

HEMATOPOIETIC STEM CELL ASSAY

In 17 out of 23 cases, granulocyte-macrophage colony forming units (CFU-GM) and erythroid burst forming units (BFU-E) were assayed before and after the in vitro treatment of bone marrow cells. The standard procedure of the assay were described in the preceding study (14).

BONE MARROW HARVEST AND IN VITRO TREATMENT WITH MOABS AND C

Between 4.5 and 72 x 10^9 nucleated cells were harvested from patients' bone marrow. When the number of cells was not enough for MoAb treatment and back-up, a second harvest of bone marrow was carried out.

In the senior author's institute, mononuclear cells were, then, purified by Ficoll-Hypaque density centrifugation, washed and adjusted for MoAb treatment and back-up storage. The cells to be treated were incubated at 4°C with an appropriate combination of MoAbs at a cell density of 1-2 $x10^6$ per ml in 50ml tubes, then, the same volume of rabbit C was added. The mixture was incubated for 60 minutes at 37°C. After the incubation, the cells were washed, suspended in RPMI 1640 medium with 10% dimethyl-sulfoxide and 10% autologous serum, then transferred into freezer bags (Delmed, Canton, Mass., USA).

They were frozen down to -80°c at a freezing rate of -1°C per minute using an automated program freezer and stored in liquid nitrogen (8).

PRECONDITIONING REGIMENS AND SUPPORTIVE FOR BMT

The combination of high dose chemotherapy and radiotherapy was employed to eradicate the residual leukemia or lymphoma cells in a patient's body (Table 1.). Patients received intensive care including gut decontamination and platelet transfusion and were isolated in clean rooms until hematological recovery was obtained.

TRANSPLANTATION OF BONE MAROW

The frozen-bags stored in liquid nitrogen were quickly thawed in a 37°C waterbath and the bone marrow cells were immediately transfused intravenously without washing.

MAINTENANCE THERAPY

When patients achieved hematological recovery after the BMT, some of them received relatively weak chemotherapy to prevent leukemic relapse.

RESULTS

CYTOTOXIC EFFECT OF MoAbs ON PATIENTS' AUTOLOGOUS LEUKEMIA CELLS (Table 2.)

In twelve of 21 Null-ALL cases and 1 of 2 Burkitt's lymphoma cases, the tumoricidal effect of MoAbs plus C was examined in vitro against the corresponding autologous tumor cells which had been, in most cases, cryopreserved at the time of first diagnosis. (In one Burkitt's lymphoma case, the tumor cells to be target cells derived from the specimen obtained from the patient's lymph node on the neck.) As shown in Table 2., the combination of BA-1, BA-2 and BA-3 or that of NL-1, NL-22 and HL-47 revealed more than 90% killing except case No. 20), which indicated that most of tumor cells should be depleted if one considers the possible contamination of up to 10% of normal cells in the samples tested.

Table #2.
IN VITRO CYTOTOXICITY OF MoAbs

CASE #	MOABS	% CTX[a] ON AUTOLOGOUS TUMOR CELLS
5.	BA-1,2,3	99%
8.	BA-1,2,3	95%
9.	BA-1,2,3	98%
11.	BA-1,2,3	90%
14.	NL-1,HL-47	97%
15.	NL-1,22,HL-47	98%
16.	NL-1,HL-47	98%
17.	NL-1,22,HL-47	98%
18.	NL-1,22,HL-47	97%
19.	NL-1,22,HL-47	95%
20.	NL-1,HL-47	71%
21.	NL-1,22,HL-47	98%
23.	BA-1,3	(++)[b]

a). cytotoxicity b). strong CTX was observed but %CTX was not calculated.

RECOVERY OF VIABLE BONE MARROW CELLS AND HEMATOPOIETIC STEM CELLS AFTER TREATMENT WITH MOABS AND CRYOPRESERVATION.

The numbers of bone marrow nucleated cells harvested from 23 patients ranged from 4.5 to 72 x 10^9 (Median: 17 x 10^9) and the numbers of viable nucleated cells transfused at BMT time ranged from 0.16 to 8.1 x 10^9 (Median: 1.2 x 10^9) per patient. The recovery rate of viable nucleated cells after the entire procedure (Ficoll-Hypaque separation, MoAbs plus C treatment, cryopreservation and thawing) were, thus, approximately 7% in 23 cases. In 23 cases, the influence of MoAb treatment and cryopreservation on hematopoietic stem cells was investigated.

As appears in table #3., CFU-GM and BFU-E per viable bone marrow nucleated cells did not significantly decrease during the in vitro procedure.

Table #3.
PRESERVATION OF CFU-GM AND BFU-E AFTER IN VITRO TREATMENT WITH MOABS AND CRYOPRESERVATION.

Case #	RECOVERY RATE[a] OF CFU-GM	BFU-E
2.	199%	231%
3.	168%	N.T.[b]
4.	811%	430%
10.	89%	200%
11.	170%	N.T.
12.	84%	N.T.
13.	86%	N.T.
14.	126%	61%
15.	113%	200%
16.	169%	90%
17.	130%	82%
18.	97%	104%
19.	180%	166%
20.	77%	N.T.
21.	87%	N.T.
22.	111%	121%
23.	127%	109%

a). calculated by the following formula:

$$\frac{\text{CFU per a unit of nucleated cells before in vitro procedure.}}{\text{CFU per the same unit of nucleated cells after the procedure.}} \times 100$$

b). not tested.

BMT: ENGRAFTMENT AND FUNCTIONING OF GRAFT

Among 21 patients with Null-ALL, 9 were transplanted at the first complete remission (CR) period, 6 were transplanted at the second CR period, 2 were done at the third CR, 3 were done at fourth CR and the other one was transplanted at the time of the disease relapse. In 2 Burkitt's lymphoma patients, there was suggestive evidence of tumor residue (such as swelling of the lymph node or high lactic dehydrogenase level in serum) when they were transplanted. General clinical conditions of 23 patients at the time of BMT were relatively good (Clinical score: 1-2 by Thomas's criteria (1).

Engraftment was confirmed in all the cases (Table 4.), nevertheless, insufficient granulocyte recovery (staying below 500/cmm) and poor platelelet recovery (staying below 50,000/cmm) were observed at 2 out of 23 and 6 out of 23 cases respectively. Among the recovery cases, the required time period for granulocyte recovery ranged from 15 to 60 (Median: 23) days and that for platelet recovery ranged from 22 to 84 (Median: 35) days.

Table #4. BMT: Engraftment and Functioning of Graft

CASE #	TIME OF BMT	(CLINICAL SCORE)	CELL #'S TRANSPLANTED[a].	ENGRAFTMENT	HEMATOLOGICAL RECOVERY Gl>500[b].	Pl>50,000[c]	MAINTENANCE THERAPY
1.	4th CR	(1)	0.16	YES	43	39	+
2.	3rd CR	(1)	0.37	YES	35	35	−
3.	1st CR	(1)	0.74	YES	49	47	+
4.	2nd CR	(1)	1.51	YES	18	44	−
5.	1st CR	(0)	0.8	YES	N.E.[f].	N.E.	−
6.	1st CR	(0)	2.0	YES	23	22	+
7.	4th CR	(1)	4.3	YES	60	70	+
8.	2nd CR	(1)	2.0	YES	54	N.E.	+
9.	2nd CR	(1)	2.2	YES	24	25	+
10.	3rd CR	(1)	0.46	YES	15	N.E.	−
11.	2nd CR	(1)	1.5	YES	N.E.	N.E.	−
12.	2nd CR	(1)	0.72	YES	21	25	−
13.	1st CR	(0)	0.6	YES	43	43	+
14.	1st CR	(1)	0.8	YES	13	26	+
15.	1st CR	(1)	1.2	YES	20	25	+
16.	1st CR	(1)	1.2	YES	22	31	+
17.	2nd CR	(1)	0.65	YES	27	84	+
18.	1st CR	(1)	0.36	YES	22	75	+
19.	1st CR	(1)	0.7	YES	15	25	−
20.	4th CR	(1)	1.6	YES	19	N.E.	−
21.	RELAPSE	(2)	0.5	YES	15	N.E.	−
22.	TUMOR(+)[d].	−	3.4	YES	55	61	−
23.	HIGH LDH[e].	−	8.1	YES	25	35	−

a). transplanted cell number x 10^{-9} per patient. b). days required for granulocyte count exceeding 500/cmm. c). days required for platelet count exceeding 50,000/cmm. d). presence of lymph node swelling. e). lactic dehydrogenase in serum. f). not evaluable.

Table #5. Patient's Outcome After BMT.

CASE #	DURATION[a] OF CR	DURATION[a] OF SURVIVAL	RELAPSE	P.S.[b]	LEADING CAUSE OF DEATH
1.	5	12	+	0	Pulmonary embolism
2.	10	17+	+	100	
3.	25+	25+	−	100	
4.	5	5	+	0	Relapse
5.	N.E.[c]	0.5	−	0	Sepsis
6.	25+	25+	−	100	
7.	3	6	+	0	Relapse
8.	2	4	+	0	Relapse
9.	5+	5+	−	100	
10.	0.7	4	+	0	Relapse
11.	N.E.	0.9	−	0	Intraabdominal bleeding
12.	6	11	+	0	Relapse
13.	1.7	1.7	−	0	Interstitial pneumonia
14.	7	10	+	0	Relapse
15.	31+	31+	−	100	
16.	18+	18+	−	100	
17.	6	7	+	0	Relapse
18.	10+	10+	−	100	
19.	13+	13+	−	100	
20.	N.E.	2	−	0	Cerebral bleeding
21.	N.E.	1	−	0	Hepatic failure
22.	15+	15+	−	100	
23.	6+	6+	−	100	

a). months after the BMT. b). performance status by Karnofsky scale. c). not evaluable.

Table #6. Analysis of Factors in Association with the Patients' Prognosis in Null-ALL

FACTORS	DISEASE-FREE SURVIVAL CASE (N=7)	RELAPSED CASE (N=9)	EARLY DEATH CASE (N=5)	EVALUATION
AGE (Median)	20	25	11	N.S.[a]
SEX (M/F)	4/3	7/2	2/3	N.S.
BM HARVEST at 1st CR	6/7 (86%)	1/9 (11%)	4/5 (80%)	Sig.[b]
BMT at 1st CR	6/7 (86%)	1/9 (11%)	2/5 (40%)	Sig.
LAST CR-BMT	8 months	4 months	6 months	N.S.
MARROW DOSE (Median X 10^{-9}/body)	1.2	0.8	0.8	N.S.
WBC RECOVERY	22 days	27 days	18.5 days	N.S.
Pl RECOVERY	25 days	39 days	43.5 days	N.S.
MAINTENANCE CHEMOTHERAPY (yes)	100%	67%	0%	N.S.
OBSERVATION PERIOD (Median)	5-31 (25)mos.	4-17 (7)mos.	0.5-2 (1)mo.	

a). not significant b). significant between disease-free survival case and relapsed-case.

PATIENTS' OUTCOME AFTER THE BMT. (Table #5.)
Among 21 Null-ALL patients, 8 (38%) are surviving for more than 5-31 months in good clinical condition. Among 8 survivors, one relapsed at 10 months after the BMT but he achieved remission again by systemic chemotherapy. The other 7 have survived without the recurrence of disease so far (as of Oct. 1986). Two Burkitt's lymphoma patients also continue in disease-free survival for 6 and 15 months. Nine out of 21 (43%) Null-ALL patients relapsed at 0.7-10 months after the BMT and all except one (Case #2.) died within five months after the relapse. The other 5 of 21 (24%) Null-ALL cases were the cases of early death and they died from sepsis, intraabdominal hemorrhage, interstitial pneumonitis, brain hemorrhage or hepatic failure within 2 months after the BMT.

FACTORS CONTRIBUTING TO DISEASE-FREE SURVIVAL AFTER BMT. (Table #6.)
Several variables such as the timing of marrow harvest and transplantation, the duration from the last remission to the BMT time or the period of time required for hematological recovery were compared among the patient groups to disease-free survivals, relapsed cases and early death cases. So far as analyzed, the timing of transplantation (to be transplanted during the first remission period, which means the marrow harvest during the first remission) appeared to be a significantly contributing factor for disease-free survivals after BMT, in Null-ALL patients.

DISCUSSION
Autologous BMT with the depletion of contaminated tumor cells from transplanted bone marrow by using mouse MoAbs, BA-1, BA-2, BA-3 or NL-1, NL-22, HL-47 combinations was carried out in 21 Null-ALL patients. These patients were subjected to autologous BMT treatment because adult Null-ALL (12 out of 21) and Burkitt's lymphoma in stage-3 belong to a high-risk group of hematologic malignancies. Nine out of 21 Null-ALL patients were under age 15, nevertheless, 5 of them were the cases with the history of leukemia relapse and the other 4 had relatively refractory disease when they achieved the first remission with conventional chemotherapy, thus BMT was chosen to maintain the remission.

As previously reported (6,7,8,14), the results of C-dependent cytotoxic test and hematopoietic stem cell assay in these cases revealed that the MoAbs used were highly active to Null-ALL and Burkitt's lymphoma cells but did not significantly affect hematopoietic stem cells.
Infused nucleated cell numbers at BMT time ranged from 0.16 to 8.1 x 10^9 (Median: 1.2 x 10^9), which were approximately 1/10 of the usual marrow dose for allogeneic BMT (3). Nevertheless, engraftment was confirmed in all the cases and there were no correlations between the infused cell numbers and the period required for hematological recovery. From this observation, we feel it can be stated that the procedures of in vitro marrow treatment by our hand were clinically acceptable in terms of engraftment, even though initially harvested cell numbers (Median: 17x10^9) decreased to less than 1/10 during the procedures.

As it was reported that the relapse rate of leukemia after BMT was higher in syngeneic BMT, which is considered to be equivalent to autologous BMT (15), most of the participant institutes applied more stronger preconditioning regimens than those of allogeneic BMT, such as cytosine arabiniside or etoposide in addition to cyclophosphamide plus total body irradiation. So far as we experienced, these strengthened regimens were tolerable ones for patients without inducing critical complications.

Among 21 Null-ALL patients, 7 were the disease-free survivors with good performance status. We thus compared these disease-free survivors with the patients who had leukemia relapse and also with the patients of early death at several variables to see any contributing factors for disease-free survival. As appears in Table #6., the timing of BMT (which was the same for the timing of marrow harvest in the disease-free survivors group but different from it in the early-death patient group) was a significant factor which affected the patients' prognosis. When analyzed in more detail, 6 out of 9 patients (67%) who were transplanted during the 1st CR and 1 out of 6 patients (17%) who were transplanted during the 2nd CR have survived for more than 5-31 months without the recurrence of disease. On the other hand, the relapse rate in these patients were 1 out of 9 (11%) and 4 out of 6 (67%) respectively. It might be concluded that autologous BMT in Null-ALL should be applied during the first remission period to be a radical cure-oriented treatment.

Another factor that contributes to disease-free survival seems to be the maintenance chemotherapy after BMT. All of 7 disease-free survivors received some maintenance chemotherapy. On the other hand, 3 out of 9 patients who had leukemia relapse did not receive chemotherapy after the BMT. These 3 patients (case #2,4,and 12) had continued remission for 5-10 months before the relapse, thus it can be speculated that certain maintenance chemotherapy might have changed their clinical course if it had been applied during those remission periods.

Two Burkitt's lymphoma patients have continued remission with good performance status (10). The results of allogeneic BMT in Burkitt's lymphoma in the senior author's hospital was also excellent (16). This information suggests that Burkitt's lymphoma is supersensitive to chemo-radiotherapy, thus a good indication for autologous as well as allogeneic BMT.

Several groups have reported the results of autologous BMT in leukemia with monoclonal antibody treatment. In 1984, Ramsay et al (7) reported that 13 child Null-ALL cases in 2nd to 4th remission period were treated by autologous BMT with BA-1, BA-2 and BA-3 MoAbs plus rabbit C and that 4 of 13 (31%) were disease-free survivors and 8 of 13 (62%) relapsed. Ritz et al (6) treated 16 children Null-ALL by autologous BMT after the depletion of leukemia cells with J-5 MoAbs plus rabbit C. There, six of 16 (38%) were in clinical remission at 4-30 months and another 6 of 16 (38%) relapsed at 2-8 months after BMT. The relatively high relapse rate in these studies and ours seems to be a major problem in autologous BMT for leukemia treatment. Weiden et al (17) reported that the presence of GvH-D, which is hazardous immunological complication in allogeneic BMT, might be beneficial to patients in terms of leukemia relapse after BMT (graft vs.leukemia phenomenon). Certain immunotherapeutic maneuvers, such as adjuvant immunotherapy (18,19) or adoptive transfer of in vitro activated lymphoid cells to patients (20), as well as maintenance chemotherapy might reveal prophylactic effects on leukemia relapse after autologous BMT.

REFERENCES

1. Thomas ED, Buckner CD, Banaji M, Clift RA, Fefer A, Flournoy N, Sale GE, Sanders JE, Singer J, Stevens M, Storb R, Weden PL (1977) One hundred patients with acute leukemia treated by chemotherapy, total body irradiation and allogeneic marrow transplantation. Blood 49:511
2. Gale RP, UCLA Bone Marrow Transplantation Unit (1979) Current status of bone marrow transplantation in acute leukemia. Transplant Proc 11:1920
3. Kodera Y, Morishima Y, Morishita Y, Murase T, Okumura M, Yamada H, Minami S, Kato Y, Ogura M, Nagura E, Kawashima K, Ohno R, Mizuno S, Yokomaku S, Iwamura H, Kato K, Yoshida M, Yamada K (1984). Sixteen adult patients with leukemia treated by chemotherapy, total body irradiation and allogeneic marrow transplantation. Japan J. Clin. Oncol. 14 (Suppl. 1):479
4. Yoshikawa S, Kodera Y (1985) Bone marrow transplantation Jpn. J. Clin. Hematol. 26:841. (in Japanese)
5. Yoshikawa S, Adao Y, Hiraiwa A, Sao H, Yamauchi T, Tahara T, Yoshikawa H, Matsuyama K, Kimura S, Kitayama S, Tanabe S, Uno H (1984) Graft-vs-host disease following allogeneic bone marrow transplantation. 14 (Suppl. 1):509
6. Ritz J, Sallan SE, Bast RC, Lipton JM, Clavell LA, Feeney M, Hercent YN, Nathan DG, Schlossman SF (1982) Autologous bone marrow transplantation in CALLA positive acute lymphoblastic leukemia after in vitro treatment with J5 monoclonal antibody and complement. Lancet ii:60
7. Ramsay N, LeBien T, Nesbit M, McGlave P, Goldman A, Kim T, Kercy S (1984) Autologous bone marrow transplantation (BMT) for acute lymphoblastic leukemia (ALL) following marrow treatment with BA-1, BA-2, Ba-3 and rabbit complement (C'). Exp. Hematol. 12:461
8. Morishima Y, Sao H, Ueda R, Morishita Y, Murase T, Kodera Y, Ohno R, Tahara T, Yoshikawa S, Kato Y, Yokomaku S, Takahashi T, Saito H (1985) Preliminary clinical trial of autologous bone marrow transplantation after in vitro monoclonal antibody and complement treatment in null cell-type acute lymphocytic leukemia. Jpn. J. Cancer Res. 76:1222
9. Ito T, Ishikawa Y, Noda M, Fujii R (1987) Autologous bone marrow transplantation in acute lymphoblastic leukemia following in vitro treatment with monoclonal antibodies and with complement: Analysis for two cases of failure. Jpn. J. Clin. Oncol. 17:63
10. Mugishima H, Fujisawa T, Sato E, Kohira R,

Kawada K, Okuni M, Baba K, Momoki T (1986) Monoclonal antibody and complement treatment in autologous bone marrow transplantation for a Burkitt's lymphoma. Acta Haematologica Japonica 49 (2):444 (The 48th Annual Meeting of Japan Haematological Society in Japanese)
11. Ramsey N, LeBien T, Nesbit M, McGlave P, Weisdorf D, Kenyon P, Hurd D, Goldman A, Kim T, Kersey J (1985) Autologous bone marrow transplantation for patients with acute lymphoblastic leukemia in second or subsequent remission: results of bone marow treated with monoclonal antibodies BA-1, BA-2, BA-3 plus complement. Blood 66:508
12. Ueda R, Tanimoto M, Takahashi T, Ogata S, Nishida K, Namikawa R, Nishizuka Y, Ota K (1982) Serological analysis of cell surface antigens of null cell acute lymphocytic leukemia by mouse monoclonal antibodies. Proc. Natl. Acad. Sci. USA, 79:4386
13. Namikawa R, Ogata S, Ueda R, Tsuge I, Nishida K, Minami S, Koike K, Suchi T, Ota K, Iijima S, Takahashi T (1983) Serological analysis of cell surface antigens of HL-60 cells before and after treatment with a phorbol ester tumor promotor. Leuk.Res. 7:375
14. Sao H, Morishima Y, Veda R, Yoshikawa S, Kodera Y, Ohno R, Takahashi T (1985) Serological study for in vitro use of monoclonal antibody for autologous bone marrow transplantation in null cell-type acute lymphocytic leukemia. Jpn. J. Cancer Res. 76:1212
15. Buckner CD, Steward PB, Bensinger W, Clift R, Appelbaum F, Martin P, Sanders J, Fefer A, Lum L, Storb R, Hill R, Thomas ED (1983) Clinical issues in autologous marrow transplantation for hematopoietic malignancies. In: Gale RP (ed) Recent advances in bone marrow transplantation. New York, Alan R. Liss, Inc.
16. Hiraiwa A, Yoshikawa S, Sao H, Yamauchi T, Minami S, Yoshikawa H, Kodera Y, Akao H, Naito K, Yamada K (1986) A successful case of Burkitt's lymphoma treated with allogeneic bone marrow transplantation. Jpn. J. Clin. Hematol. 27:600 (in Japanese)
17. Weiden PL, Sullivan MK, Fluornoy N (1981) Antileukemic effect of chronic graft-vs-host disease. Contribution to improved survival after allogeneic marrow transplantation. N. Engl. J. Med. 304:1529.
18. Ota K, Kurita S, Yamada K, Masaoka T, Uzuka Y, Ogawa N (1986) Results of investigation into prognosis after immunotherapy with bestatin for acute lymphocytic leukemia in adults. Jpn. J. Cancer Chemother. 13 (4): Part 1:1017
19. Ohno R, Kodera Y, Ogura M, Yamada H (1984) Induction of transplantation resistance to murine L-1210 leukemia cells in BCG-primed mice by immunization with tuberculin protein-coupled L-1210 cells. Jpn.J. Cancer Res. 75:187.
20. Rosenberg SA (1984) Adoptive immunotherapy of cancer: Accomplishments and prospects. Cancer Treatment Report 68:233.

5: Characterization of Malignant Lymphoma in Dogs and Use as a Model for the Development of Treatment Strategies

Frederick R. Appelbaum, Paul A. Brown, Theodore C. Graham, Brenda M. Sandmaier, Friedrich W. Schuening, and Rainer Storb

INTRODUCTION

Malignant lymphoma develops spontaneously in dogs with an annual incidence of 24 per 100,000 [1]. Since these dogs are frequently seen by veterinarians they can, with the cooperation of the veterinarian and owner, be referred for study providing a unique model of a spontaneously occurring lymphoma in an out-bred species. We and others have carried out a series of studies in which the disease has been characterized pathologically and immunologically and has been shown to resemble human lymphoma in many ways. We have used this model to develop methods designed to improve and broaden the application of marrow transplantation to the treatment of malignant lymphoma. These strategies have included the use of alternative sources of stem cells including peripheral blood and the development of better methods of eradicating disease from the patient with the use of antibody-isotope conjugates.

CLINICAL PRESENTATION

The disease usually presents in middle-aged dogs (mean = 6.5 years) with equal frequency in both sexes [2]. There is no clear preference for breed, and there is no know association with a viral etiology [3]. By far the most common clinical presentation is diffuse adenopathy which is the presenting feature in 85% of cases [4]. Frequently in these cases bone marrow or peripheral blood may also be involved. In our series, 43 of 95 animals with malignant lymphoma presenting in lymph nodes had evidence of hematologic dissemination at the time of diagnosis [5]. Other less common presenting syndromes include primary gastrointestinal lymphoma (7%), primary cutaneous lymphoma (6%), and primary mediastinal lymphoma (2%). The common presenting syndrome of diffuse, apparently painless, lymphadenopathy with frequent marrow and peripheral blood involvement mimics the human situation.

HISTOLOGY AND IMMUNOLOGIC DESCRIPTION

Until recently there has been a lack of agreement among investigators as to the histopathologic categorization of canine lymphoma and a complete lack of knowledge as to the immunologic background of the tumor. These deficiencies existed, in part, because there have been few histologic reviews carried out by pathologists familiar with human lymphomas and because the reagents necessary to define the antigens expressed on normal canine lymphocytes and their malignant counterparts simply did not exist. Recently a series of monoclonal antibodies have been shown to react with particular subsets of canine cells, and these can be used along with other conventional reagents to categorize lymphoma cell type. Thus, with the use of goat-anti-dog surface immunoglobulin, monoclonal antibody 7.2 (an anti-Ia antibody), and monoclonal antibody DT-2 (an anti-T cell reagent), it is possible to describe the immunological background of the tumors. We previously reported on 40 consecutive cases of canine malignant lymphoma categorized by pathologists experienced in human lymphomas and immunophenotyped using these reagents [6]. Interestingly, we found no cases of Hodgkin's disease and no cases of nodular lymphoma. Rather, all cases were within the broad category of diffuse non-Hodgkin's lymphoma. Within this category the disease histology very much resembled that in man with diffuse large cell, diffuse mixed and immunoblastic lymphomas being the most common categories (see Table 1). Also, the distribution of immunophenotypes was similar to that seen in man in that 78% of tumors were of B-cell origin (SIg+ and Ia+), 10% were of

Table 1. Histologic and Immunologic Classification of Canine Lymphoma

B-cell (SIg+, Ia+) tumors (N=31)

11 - Diffuse mixed small & large cell
5 - Diffuse large noncleaved
15 - Lymphoblastic

T-cell (SIg-, DT2+) tumors (N=4)

1 - Diffuse mixed small & large cell
3 - Lymphoblastic

Non-B,non-T-cell (SIg-, DT2-) tumors (N=5)

3 - Diffuse mixed small & large cell
1 - Diffuse large noncleaved
1 - Lymphoblastic

apparent T-cell origin (SIg- and DT2+), and 12% were of non B-cell, non T-cell origin. Ia-like antigens were restricted to B-cell neoplasms. Surface markers correlated well with histologic type with 85% of the diffuse large cell and diffuse mixed cell lymphomas appearing to be of B-cell origin, while the lymphoblastic tumors reacted only with the anti-T-cell reagent DT2. A large number of apparent B-cell tumors (Ia+ and SIg+) also reacted with the T-cell marker DT2. We have been unable to detect a population of lymphocytes in normal dogs which are both SIg+ and DT2+. The expression on malignant B-cells of antigens normally restricted to T-cells has precedence in the human situation where T-cell markers have been found on immunoglobulin bearing cells in most patients with chronic lymphocytic leukemia. These studies thus provide a histologic and immunologic classification of the canine lymphomas and suggest an analogy between canine lymphomas and human disease.

CHEMOTHERAPY AND MARROW TRANSPLANTATON FOR CANINE LYMPHOMA

Treatment of dogs suffering from malignant lymphoma with combination chemotherapy results in complete responses in approximately 60% of cases [7,8]. Using induction chemotherapy alone we showed that all dogs relapsed within 250 days (median remission duration = 85 days) [8]. We then demonstrated that if dogs which have achieved a complete remission have autologous marrow stored and are then treated with 8.4 Gy of total body irradiation (TBI) delivered at 4 cGy/minute followed by infusion of their autologous marrow, 24% of animals can be cured, results very similar to that seen in autologous transplantation for human lymphomas [5,9-11]. The reasons for failure in this model are death prior to engraftment (5%), death due to late transplant complications (21%), or relapse (50%). Higher doses of TBI did not improve results because of a higher incidence of both early and late complications.

REQUIREMENTS FOR SUCCESSFUL ENGRAFTMENT AND ALTERNATIVE SOURCES OF HEMATOPOIETIC STEM CELLS

Without hematopoietic stem cell support, doses of TBI of 5 Gy or higher are invariably fatal to dogs and probably to man as well [12]. We have previously studied the effects of marrow cell dose on engraftment. If either fresh or short-term (less than 5 months) frozen marrow is used, a marrow cell dose of 0.5×10^8 mononuclear cells/kg ensures engraftment and long-term survival [13]. At lower doses some animals do not engraft and those that do engraft at a slower pace. If peripheral blood mononuclear cells are used instead of marrow, approximately 1 log more cells ($\geq 6 \times 10^8$ peripheral blood mononuclear cells/kg) are required to ensure engraftment [14]. Others have shown that the blood content of committed hematopoietic precursors (CFU-C, CFU-E, and BFU-E) can be increased by pretreatment with dextran sulfate, endotoxin or carefully timed chemotherapy [15,16]. We tested whether these manipulations could lower the number of cells necessary for engraftment. Pretreatment with dextran sulfate doubled the number of circulating peripheral blood mononuclear cells and led to a five-fold increase in circulating CFU-C but did not lower the number of cells necessary for engraftment [14]. Treatment with cyclophosphamide 14 days prior to collection led to a 16-fold increase in circulating CFU-C and allowed for engraftment with as few as 0.5×10^8 peripheral blood mononuclear cells/kg [17]. With this background we then studied the outcome of treatment of lymphoma dogs with 8.4 Gy TBI at 4 cGy/minute and peripheral blood stem cells collected following cyclophosphamide pretreatment [18]. Twelve lymphoma dogs in remission had an average of $10.43 \pm 9.75 \times 10^8$ peripheral blood mononuclear cells/kg collected and stored. All animals were then treated with TBI and reinfusion of their stored cells. There was one early death, three deaths due to late transplant complications and five relapses. Three dogs remain alive in remission at 2-1/2, 3, and 4 years posttransplant. These results are virtually identical to those obtained using autologous marrow and suggest that peripheral blood stem cells collected following chemotherapy pretreatment can be used as a substitute for autologous marrow.

USE OF ANTIBODY ISOTOPE CONJUGATES AS TREATMENT FOR MALIGNANT LYMPHOMA

No matter the source of hematopoietic stem cells (marrow or peripheral blood; autologous, allogeneic or syngeneic), the major problem following the clinical use of marrow transplantation in man for malignant lymphoma is recurrence of malignancy. If transplantation is carried out at first relapse or second remission, approximately 40% of patients relapse. If transplantation is delayed until patients are in end-stage relapse, recurrence rates of 70% or more are seen. The high recurrence rates are despite the use of very intensive treatment regimens such as cyclophosphamide and TBI which result in approximately 10% mortality due to treatment-associated toxicities. One possible way to deliver more radiotherapy to the tumor and thereby decrease relapse rates, and at the same time spare important normal organs and thus decrease toxicity, is to use monoclonal antibodies as carriers for radioisotopes which deliver their energy locally.

Biodistribution

In order to use antibody-conjugates safely and effectively, the amount of radiation delivered to different parts of the body and the tumor (i.e. the internal radiation dosimetry) must be determined. Biodistribution studies in dogs were performed by labeling selected antibodies with trace amounts of I-131 and I-125 and injecting them intravenously into anesthetized animals [19]. Following injection, blood clearance curves were measured and individual organ distributions over time were determined by external gamma camera scanning followed by sacrifice of animals and measurement of actual tissue isotope concentrations. Initial studies demonstrated rapid decline over three hours of both antibody 7.2 (anti-Ia) and antibody S5 (anti-myeloid) to approximately 20% of initial levels while an irrelevant control antibody remained at $\geq$90% blood levels over the same time period. This rapid decline presumably reflects antigen-specific binding of the relevant antibodies. Localization of antibody 7.2 and antibody S5 in normal dogs is shown in Table 2. In vivo distribution correlated well with in vitro immunoperoxidase staining. Based on a dose of 10 Gy delivered to blood, I-131-labeled 7.2 would deliver 32.7 Gy to spleen, 16.3 Gy to marrow, and 9.8 Gy to liver, while I-131-labeled S5 would deliver 38.6 Gy to spleen, 52.5 Gy to marrow, and 16 Gy to liver. These experiments, therefore, support the hypothesis that radiotherapy delivered via isotope conjugates can be directed to organs of interest. We next determined the distribution of antibody S5 in dogs with lymphoma either in remission or relapse. These results are shown in Table 3 and demonstrate that dogs with lymphoma in remission behave almost identically to normal dogs but that it is difficult to deliver isotope to large tumor masses in dogs who are in relapse. An important qualification, however, is that these studies were performed using a relatively low dose of antibody, 1 mg/kg, and that we have shown in other models that higher doses of antibody may allow better tumor penetration and thereby improve dosimetry [20].

Table 2. Localization of Antibodies 7.2 and S5 24 Hours After Injection

Tissue	Tissue/Blood		
	7.2	S5	Irrelevant
Blood	1.00	1.00	1.00
Muscle	0.06	0.03	0.04
Lung	0.46	1.31	0.23
Liver	0.93	1.87	0.24
Lymph Node	1.87	1.17	0.20
Spleen	4.08	5.88	0.19
Marrow	1.96	7.48	0.22

Table 3. Localization of Antibody S5 in Normal Dogs and in Dogs with Lymphoma both in Remission and in Relapse

Tissue	Tissue/Blood		
	Normal	Remission	Relapse
Blood	1.00	1.00	1.00
Muscle	0.03	0.01	0.04
Lymph Node	1.17	1.25	0.39
Spleen	5.88	2.71	1.50
Marrow	7.48	9.80	3.96

Treatment

Following these initial biodistribution studies, we carried out preliminary experiments measuring the toxicity of increasing doses of I-131 linked to 1 mg/kg of S5 antibody. Based on the biodistribution studies, we estimated that a dose of 2 mCi/kg of I-131 linked to S5 should deliver a dose of approximately 2 Gy to marrow. When this dose was given, the white count and platelet count nadirs (600/mm^3 and 5000/mm^3) and time to recovery were similar to that seen with 2 Gy external beam total body irradiation, demonstrating that our dose estimates were reasonably correct. We have since shown that 6 mCi/kg I-131 (a dose estimated to deliver 6 Gy to marrow) is lethal without marrow support but that with autologous marrow support, complete and sustained hematologic recovery results.

SUMMARY

The series of studies briefly reviewed above demonstrate that canine lymphoma represents a unique model of a spontaneously occurring hematologic neoplasm in an outbred species which can be used to develop and test new treatment strategies. The disease is predominantly a B-cell neoplasm which closely resembles the diffuse non-Hodgkin's lymphomas of man. Using this model, we have demonstrated the following: 1) The use of high-dose total body irradiation (8.4 Gy) followed by autologous marrow transplantation can cure roughly 25% of cases not cured by conventional dose chemotherapy. 2) Autologous peripheral blood stem cells collected after chemotherapy-induced expansion of the peripheral blood stem cell pool can be substituted for marrow with roughly equivalent results. 3) Biodistribution studies suggest that monoclonal antibodies can be used to direct radiotherapy to sites of disease and away from potential sites of dose-limiting toxicity. 4) Marrow is particularly accessible to antibody while large bulky lymph nodes are more difficult to penetrate. 5) Dosimetry estimates of antibody-isotope directed radiotherapy can be made with accuracy. 6) Marrow engraftment after antibody-isotope-induced marrow ablation is possible.

ACKNOWLEDGEMENTS

This work was supported in part by grants CA 18105 and CA 31787 from the National Cancer Institute of the National Institutes of Health, DHHS.

REFERENCES

1. Squire RA (1969) Spontaneous hematopoietic tumors of dogs. Natl Cancer Inst Monogr 32:97-116

2. Squire RA, Bush M, Melby EC, Neeley LM, Yarbrough B (1973) Clinical and pathologic study of canine lymphoma: clinical staging, cell classification, and therapy. J Natl Cancer Inst 51:565-572

3. Dorn CR, Tayler DO, Hibbard HH (1967) Epizootiologic characteristics of canine and feline leukemia and lymphoma. Am J Vet Res 28:993-1001

4. Weller RE, Holmberg CA, Theilen GH, Madewell BR (1980) Histologic classification as a prognostic criterion for canine lymphosarcoma. Am J Vet Res 41:1310-1314

5. Appelbaum FR, Deeg HJ, Storb, R, Self S, Graham TC, Sale GE, Weiden PL (1985) Marrow transplant studies in dogs with malignant lymphoma. Transplantation 39:499-504

6. Appelbaum FR, Sale GE, Storb R, Charrier K, Deeg HJ, Graham T, Wulff JC (1984) Phenotyping of canine lymphoma with monoclonal antibodies directed at cell surface antigens: classification, morphology, clinical presentation and response to chemotherapy. Hematol Oncol 2:151-168

7. Bowles CA, Bull M, McCormick K, Kadin M, Lucas D (1980) Autologous bone marrow transplantation following chemotherapy and irradiation in dogs with spontaneous lymphomas. J Natl Cancer Inst 65:615-620

8. Weiden PL, Storb R, Deeg HJ, Graham TC, Thomas ED (1979) Prolonged survival in dogs with lymphoma after total body irradiation and autologous marrow transplantation consolidation of combination-chemotherapy-induced remissions. Blood 54:1039-1049

9. Appelbaum FR, Herzig GP, Ziegler JL, Graw RG, Levine AS, Deisseroth AB (1978) Successful engraftment of cryopreserved autologous bone marrow in patients with malignant lymphoma. Blood 52:85-95

10. Appelbaum FR, Thomas ED (1983) Review of the use of marrow transplantation in the treatment of non-Hodgkin's lymphoma. J Clin Oncol 7:440-447

11. Appelbaum FR, Sullivan KM, Buckner CD, Clift RA, Deeg HJ, Fefer A, Hill R, Mortimer J, Neiman PE, Sanders JE, Singer J, Stewart P, Storb R, Thomas ED (1987) Treatment of malignant lymphoma in one hundred patients with chemotherapy, total body irradiation and marrow transplantation. J Clin Oncol, in press

12. Thomas ED, LeBlond R, Graham T, Storb R (1970) Marrow infusions in dogs given midlethal or lethal irradiation. Radiat Res 41:113-124

13. Appelbaum FR, Herzig GP, Graw RG, Bull MI, Bowles C, Gorin NC, Deisseroth AB (1978) Study of cell dose and storage time on engraftment of cryopreserved autologous bone marrow in a canine model. Transplantation 26:245-248

14. Appelbaum FR (1979) Hemopoietic reconstitution following autologous bone marrow and peripheral blood mononuclear cell infusions. Exp Hematol 7:7-11

15. Ross WM, Koerbling M, Nothdurft W, Fliedner TM (1978) The role of dextran sulfate in increasing the CFUc concentration in dog blood. Proc Soc Exp Bio Med 157:301-305

16. Richman CM, Weiner RS, Yankee RA (1976) Increase in circulating stem cells following chemotherapy in man. Blood 47:1031-1039

17. Abrams RA, McCormack K, Bowles C, Deisseroth AB (1981) Cyclophosphamide treatment expands the circulating hematopoietic stem cell pool in dogs. J Clin Invest 67:1392-1399

18. Appelbaum FR, Deeg HJ, Storb R, Graham TC, Charrier K, Bensinger W (1986) Cure of malignant lymphoma in dogs with peripheral blood stem cell transplantation. Transplantation 42:19-22

19. Appelbaum FR, Badger CC, Deeg HJ, Nelp WB, Storb R (1987) Use of Iodine-131-labeled anti-immune response-associated monoclonal antibody as preparative regimen prior to bone marrow transplantation: initial dosimetry. NCI Monogr 3:67-71

20. Press OW, Appelbaum F, Ledbetter JA, Martin PJ, Zarling J, Kidd P, Thomas ED (1987) Monoclonal antibody 1F5 (anti-CD20) serotherapy of human B cell lymphomas. Blood 69:584-591

6: Hematopoietic Cell Transplantation in Murine Globoid Cell Leukodystrophy (The Twitcher Mouse)—A Model of a Human Sphingolipidosis (Krabbe Disease)

Andrew M. Yeager, Takao Ichioka, Eitoku Toyoshima, Yasuo Kishimoto, Susan Brennan, Hugo W. Moser, Richard F. Mayer, and George W. Santos

Human lysosomal storage diseases are associated with significant morbidity and mortality, and the management of these conditions has been limited to symptomatic supportive care. Allogeneic bone marrow transplantation (BMT) may be therapeutic in these disorders by repopulating the lymphohematopoietic and reticuloendothelial systems with enzymatically normal donor-derived cells, thus providing a stable, self-renewing source of enzyme(s) in which the recipient is deficient [1,2]. Despite several favorable preliminary clinical reports [3-10], the long-term therapeutic effects of BMT in patients with genetic storage diseases are not well known. In particular, the ability of enzyme replacement by BMT to stabilize or reverse the central nervous system (CNS) manifestations of storage diseases has not been conclusively demonstrated. The lack of appropriate animal models of genetic storage diseases has hitherto limited the preclinical studies of enzyme replacement by BMT.

The "twitcher" mouse (murine globoid cell leukodystrophy; GCL) exhibits an autosomal recessive neurodegenerative syndrome with demyelination in both the peripheral nerves and the CNS [11]. Characteristic globoid cells accumulate in the central nervous system; these monocyte-derived cells [12] contain myelin breakdown products and stain positive with the periodic acid-Schiff (PAS) technique [11]. Affected twitcher mice appear normal at birth but develop progressive neurological dysfunction by approximately 3 weeks of age, fail to thrive, and die by 6 to 7 weeks of age, even with intensive supportive care [11]. Twitcher mice lack the lysosomal hydrolase galactosylceramidase (galactosylcerebrosidase). In contrast to other lysosomal storage diseases, the substrate (galactosylceramide) does not accumulate in neural tissues of mice with GCL; instead, psychosine (galactosylsphingosine), its deacylated derivative, is present in extremely high levels [13]. Psychosine is highly toxic to cells, especially oligodendroglia and Schwann cells, which are responsible for the formation and maintenance of the myelin sheath [13,14]. The twitcher is the first murine model of a neurodegenerative disease with which the deficiency of a specific lysosomal enzyme is associated. From clinical, neuropathological, and biochemical standpoints, the twitcher is an authentic model of human galactosylceramidase deficiency (Krabbe disease) [15].

Because of its homology with the human sphingolipidosis, murine GCL is an appropriate model in which to study the effects of enzyme replacement by BMT. In this report, we describe the clinical, histopathological, neurophysiological, and biochemical alterations following transplantation of enzymatically normal congenic marrow and spleen cells (hematopoietic cell transplantation; HCT) in the twitcher mouse.

MATERIALS AND METHODS

Mice. Breeding pairs of C57BL/6 mice that were heterozygous carriers for the twitcher mutation (+/twi) were obtained from the Jackson Laboratory, Bar Harbor, Maine. Inbred congenic C57BL/6 mice that were homozygous for the A isoenzyme of glucose phosphate isomerase-1 (GPI-1A) had normal levels of galactosylceramidase and were used as HCT donors. Normally, mice of the C57BL/6 strain, including those that carry the twitcher mutation, are homozygous for the codominant B isoenzyme of GPI-1 (GPI-1B); hematopoietic engraftment was thus assessed in the post-transplant period by electrophoretic analysis of small (5-10 ul) samples of blood from recipient mice to detect the presence of donor GPI isoenzyme [16]. Animals were housed in sterilized microisolator shoebox-type plastic cages and were given tap water and sterilized standard laboratory chow ad libitum. Identification of the genetic status (affected twitcher, heterozygous carrier, or enzymatically normal homozygote) of 7-day-old offspring was made by determination of galactosylceramidase activity in homogenates of clipped tail tips [17]. Behavioral observations provided clinical identification of affected (twi/twi) offspring, in which the onset of neurological symptoms and signs occur at approximately 3 weeks of age.

Hematopoietic cell transplantation (HCT) procedure. Twenty-four hours before HCT, cohorts of twitcher and control littermates received total body irradiation (TBI) in a ^{137}cesium irradiator at a dose rate of 120 rad/min and a total dose of 900 rad. Each recipient mouse was given an intraperitoneal injection of 10-15 x 10^6 bone marrow and 35-50 x 10^6 spleen cells freshly obtained from donor GPI-1A congenic C57BL/6 mice. For 14 days after HCT, animals received acidified drinking water (pH 2.5) to which was added neomycin (500 ug/ml), polymyxin B (13 ug/ml), and trimethoprim-sulfa (100 ug/ml as trimethoprim). At selected ages and/or times after HCT, untreated and transplanted twitcher mice and control normal littermates were killed, and tissues were obtained for biochemical and histological studies.

Neuropathological studies. Sciatic nerves from untreated and HCT-treated twitcher mice and normal control animals were fixed in 4% paraformaldehyde and then 5% glutaraldehyde, dehydrated in graded alcohols, embedded in Epon, cut in 1 um longitudinal sections, and stained with the Luxol fast blue technique to assess myelination [18]. Thin transverse sections of sciatic nerves were stained with lead citrate and uranyl acetate for electron microscopic studies.

Neurometric studies. Nerve-conduction studies were carried out on untreated and HCT-treated twitcher mice and enzymatically normal or heterozygous littermates at various ages and/or at selected times after HCT. Under light methoxyflurane anaesthesia and at a body surface temperature maintained at 36°C with a temperature-controlled heating pad, animals received percutaneous stimulation of the sciatic-tibial nerves at the sciatic notch or sacral region and at the ankle. A pulse generator provided a supramaximal strength square-wave pulse of 50-100 us duration, and recordings were obtained from the plantar foot muscles [19]. The evoked compound muscle action potentials (CMAPs) were amplified with an AC amplifier, displayed on a storage oscilloscope and photographically recorded with a Polaroid instant camera. The motor conduction velocity (MCV), distal latency (DL), amplitudes and durations of proximal and distal CMAPs, and number of phases of CMAPs were determined.

Biochemical assays. Galactosylceramidase activity was assayed in aqueous homogenates of tail tips from 7-day-old mice and samples of spleen, brain, and kidney from untreated and HCT-treated twitcher and control mice, using ^{3}H-galactosylceramide as the substrate [20]. Psychosine levels were determined in total lipid extracts of aqueous homogenates of brain and sciatic nerve of untreated and transplanted twitcher and control mice by acetylation with ^{3}H-acetic anhydride, benzoylation, isolation by thin-layer chromatography densitometric scanning on silica-gel plates, and quantitation of ^{3}H radioactivity in the N-acetyl-psychosine spot [21]. This method allowed detection of as little as 5 pmol of psychosine.

RESULTS

Effect of HCT on survival of twitcher mice. The median survival of untreated twitcher mice was 40 days (range, 28-47). Affected twitchers appeared normal for the first 2 to 3 weeks of life, then failed to thrive and developed progressive neurological deterioration with head drop, truncal tremor, and limb paralysis (most apparent in the hindlimbs). When HCT was carried out in twitcher mice with apparent neurological manifestations (19 days and older) or immediately before onset of these signs (age 14 days), no significant prolongation of survival was noted (Table 1), suggesting that HCT did not appreciably alter the neurodegeneration in these animals. In addition, many of these mice were too clinically impaired to tolerate the immunosuppression and aplasia associated with the HCT procedure.

Subsequent studies examined the role of HCT in presymptomatic 10-day-old twitcher mice that received 900 rad TBI 24 hours before transplantation. Electrophoretic analysis of glucose phosphate isomerase-1 (GPI-1) isoenzymes in peripheral blood samples obtained from HCT-treated twitcher mice indicated that hematopoietic engraftment, as assessed by the presence of donor erythrocyte GPI-1A, was

TABLE 1: HEMATOPOIETIC CELL TRANSPLANTATION (HCT) IN TWITCHER MICE

Age at HCT (Days)	Number of Animals	Median Age (Days) at Death (Range)
10	19	91 (56-155)*
14	6	29 (27-30)
19	4	24 (23-38)
24	2	28, 29
35	2	39, 40
Untreated Twitchers	51	40 (28-47)

Animals were given total body irradiation (900 rad) 24 hours before HCT. Each animal received 10-15 x 10^6 bone marrow and 35-50 x 10^6 spleen cells i.p. from enzymatically normal congenic donors.

* $p<0.001$ by Wilcoxon rank-sum test.

detected by 2 to 3 weeks after HCT; complete conversion to donor erythropoiesis occurred by 6 to 7 weeks after transplantation. In contrast to the observations in untreated or transplanted symptomatic twitchers, the lifespan of 19 twitcher mice that received HCT at age 10 days was significantly prolonged: the median survival was 91 days (range, 56-155; p< 0.001 by Wilcoxon rank-sum test) (Table 1). To our knowledge, this is the first report of significant prolongation of survival after HCT in an animal model of a human genetic storage disease [22].

Gait, foraging, and grooming behaviors were qualitatively less impaired in transplanted twitcher mice, which did not develop the characteristic hindlimb paralysis observed in untreated animals. However, the magnitude of truncal tremor was similar in HCT-treated and untreated twitchers. Despite a 2- to 3-fold prolongation of lifespan, the weights of HCT-treated twitcher mice were similar to those of untreated affected animals (Figure 1). The HCT procedure did not appreciably affect the growth and development of enzymatically normal or heterozygous littermates, which gained weight normally after transplantation (Figure 1). To exclude the possibility that TBI and attendant immunosuppression (and not transplantation of enzymatically normal donor cells) might be responsible for the prolonged survival in HCT-treated twitcher mice, 2 experiments were carried out in which affected 35- to 40-day old twitcher mice served as donors for HCT into 10-day-old twitchers. The median lifespan of the 6 recipients of twitcher-into-twitcher HCT was 34 days (range, 22-52), not significantly different from that of untreated twitcher mice.

Effects of HCT on histopathology of twitcher peripheral nerves. Light-microscopic studies of sciatic nerves from untreated or HCT-treated normal C57BL/6 mice demonstrated positive staining of myelin sheaths by the Luxol fast blue (LFB) technique. In

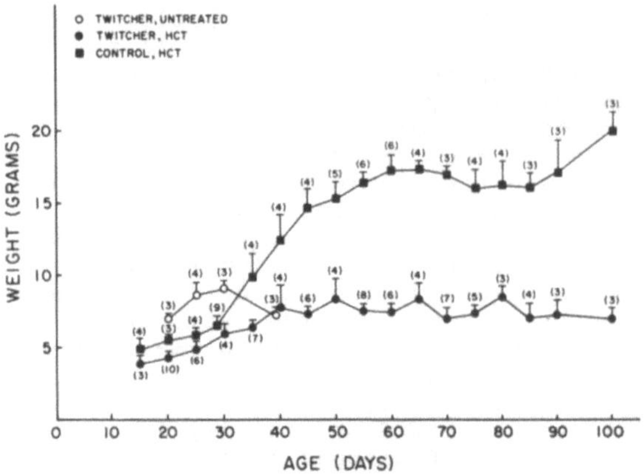

Figure 1. Weights of untreated twitcher mice and HCT-treated twitchers and control littermates. Numbers in parentheses indicate the number of animals studied; the mean # standard error is shown. From [22], © AAAS.

untreated clinically affected twitcher mice, the peripheral nerves showed perineurial edema, interstitial inflammatory reaction with mononuclear cells, and no staining with LFB, consistent with total loss of myelin sheaths (Figure 2A). Sciatic nerves from 90-day-old HCT-treated twitcher mice (80 days after HCT) had substantial but incomplete remyelination; although some inflammatory changes persisted, perineurial edema was decreased (Figure 2B) [22]. Electron-microscopic studies confirmed the loss of normal myelin lamellae and deterioration of Schwann cells in the sciatic nerves of untreated twitchers (Figure 2C). By 80 days after HCT, twitcher sciatic nerves had areas of well-myelinated axons and normal-appearing Schwann cells (Figure 2D).

Effect of HCT on neurophysiologic status of twitcher mice. The motor conduction velocities (MCVs) in sciatic nerves of untreated twitcher and normal control mice were similar until age 15-19 days, when significant reduction in MCV was detected in twitcher mice, even in the absence of clinical manifestations. The MCV in 15- to 19-day-old twitchers was 12.8 + 2.8 m/s, compared with 18.1 + 2.6 m/s in age-matched control mice. As untreated twitcher mice developed neurodegenerative signs, MCV decreased substantially; in preterminal 35- to 39-day-old twitchers, MCV fell to 5.8 + 1.0 m/s whereas it had increased to 29.3 + 2.6 m/s in enzymatically normal littermates (Figure 3A) [19]. Additional neurometric abnormalities in untreated twitchers included prolonged distal latency (DL), decreased distal

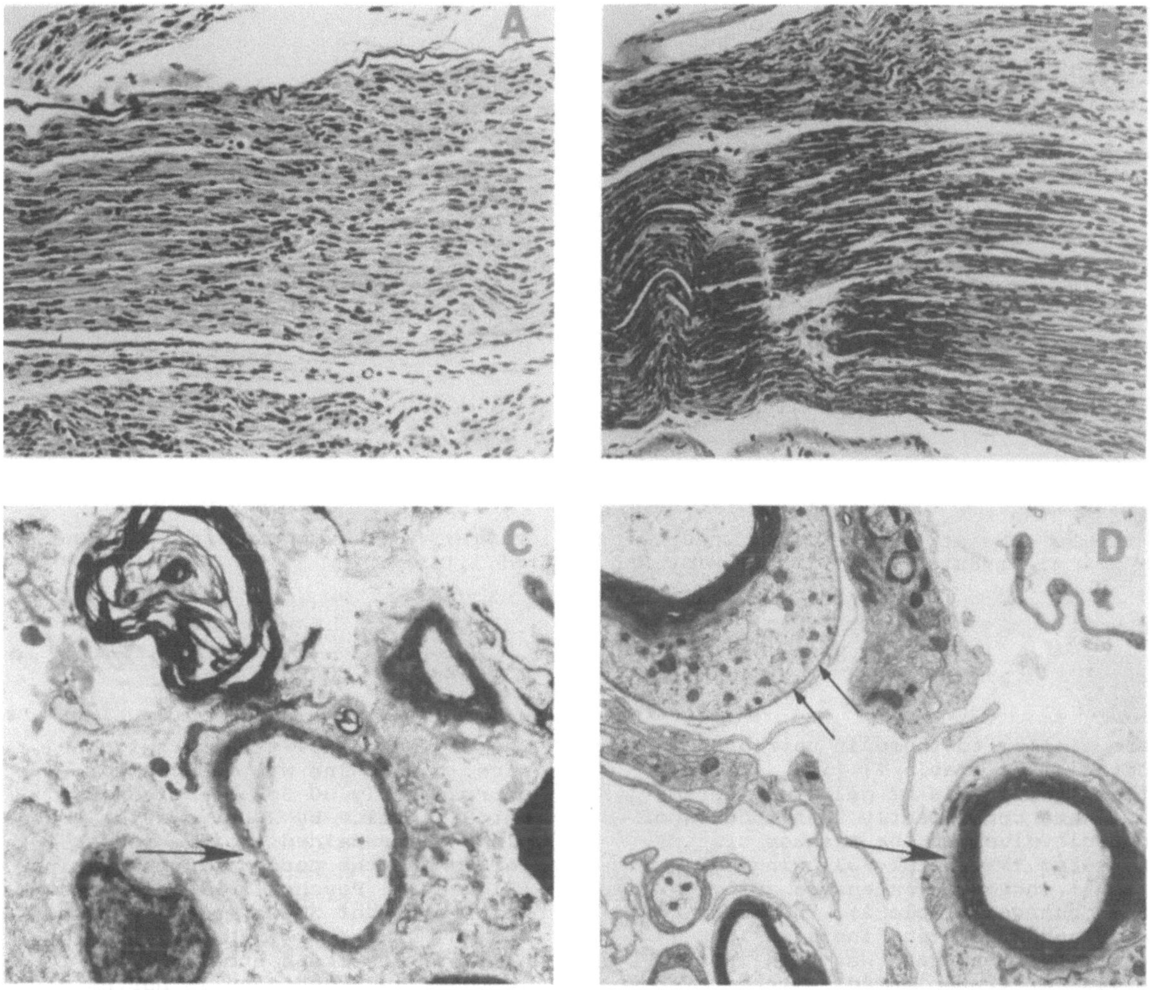

Figure 2. A. Sciatic nerve from untreated 40-day-old twitcher mouse; myelin sheaths are absent. B. Sciatic nerve from HCT-treated 90-day-old twitcher; dark LFB-positive areas indicate remyelination. C. Electron micrograph of sciatic nerve from untreated twitcher; myelin lamellae are decreased (arrow). D. Electron micrograph of sciatic nerve from HCT-treated twitcher; myelin lamellae (arrow) and Schwann cell (double arrow) appear normal. (Figures 2A and 2B reprinted by permission of [22], © AAAS.)

compound muscle action potential (dCMAP), and increased number of phases of the dCMAP, consistent with partial conduction block in proximal nerve fibers and slowed conduction in both distal and proximal nerve segments [19].

In HCT-treated twitcher mice, serial evaluations indicated a stabilization of MCV at subnormal levels (6.7 + 1.2 m/s vs. 34.5 + 3.9 m/s) throughout the period of observation after transplantation (Figure 3B). The DL was also prolonged in HCT-treated twitchers, but to a lesser degree than in untreated twitcher mice [19]. Since HCT-treated twitchers did not develop the characteristic hindlimb paralysis seen in affected untreated mice, the subnormal but stable MCVs in transplanted animals were sufficient to allow neuromuscular transmission and prevent paralysis.

Effects of HCT on galactosylceramidase and psychosine in twitcher tissues. After HCT at age 10 days from enzymatically normal congenic donors, the levels of galactosylceramidase in the kidneys of 50-day-old normal littermates were reduced to approximately 35% of values in untransplanted control mice, although enzyme activity in brains and spleens was relatively unchanged. By 60 days after HCT, tissue galactosylceramidase levels in transplanted normal animals

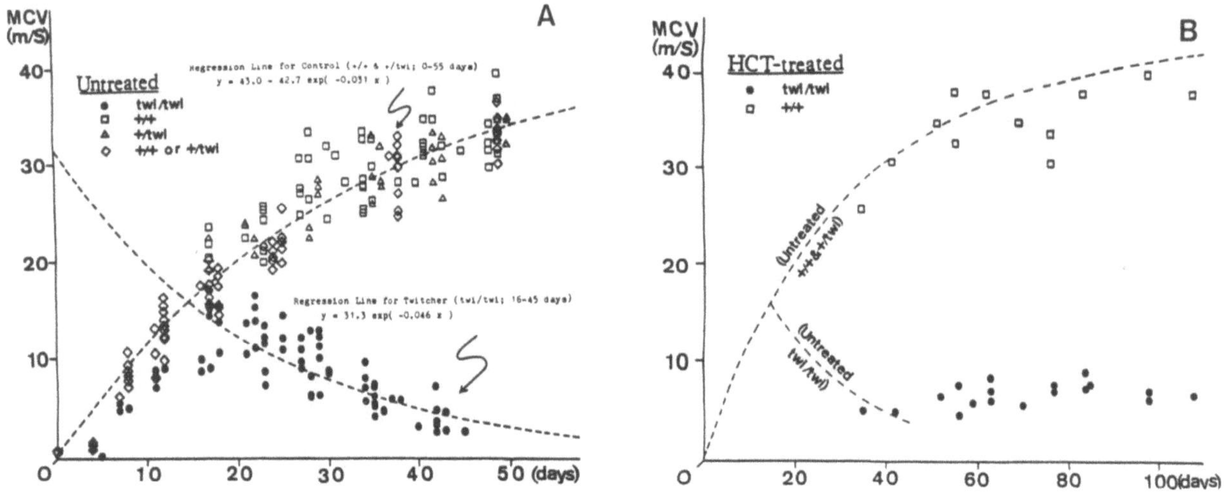

Figure 3. Sciatic nerve motor conduction velocities (MCVs) in untreated (A) and HCT-treated (B) twitcher mice and control littermates.

were similar to those in untreated control mice (Table 2) [21]. In contrast, the levels of galactosylceramidase were consistently less than 8% of control values in the tissues of untreated twitchers. Following HCT, gradual increases in enzyme activity were observed (Table 2). The most rapid and consistent increase in galactosylceramidase was seen in the spleens of transplanted twitcher mice: enzyme activity was 30-40% of control values in 50- and 70-day-old mice and exceeded normal levels in 100-day-old animals. In twitcher mouse kidneys, the levels of galactosylceramidase gradually increased to 15-25% of normal in 50- to 70-day-old mice and reached only 20-30% of control in 100-day-old twitchers. Most striking was the observation that galactosylceramidase activity in the brains of HCT-treated twitcher mice was practically absent before HCT, rose to 15-25% of control in 50- to 70-day-old mice, and reached normal values in 100-day-old transplanted twitchers [21]. It is of interest that normal enzyme activity was attained in the twitcher CNS even though no specific techniques were used to induce or maintain permeability of the blood-brain barrier after irradiation and HCT.

Psychosine was barely detectable in the tissues of untreated or transplanted enzymatically normal mice. In untreated twitchers, the levels of psychosine were elevated by approximately 70-fold in the brains and 80-fold in the sciatic nerves [21]. In the brains of HCT-treated twitcher mice, psychosine was reduced to approximately 30-35% of values in untreated mice by 20 days after transplant and remained in this range throughout the period of observation (Figure 4). Psychosine levels in sciatic nerves of 30-day-old untreated and HCT-treated twitcher mice were similar; despite a much slower increase in psychosine in nerves of transplanted twitchers, the levels of the compound in sciatic nerves of 100-day-old HCT-treated twitchers were similar to those in preterminal 40- to 45-day-old untreated animals (Figure 4) [21].

TABLE 2: GALACTOSYLCERAMIDASE ACTIVITY AFTER HEMATOPOIETIC CELL TRANSPLANTATION (HCT)

Status	Age.days	Enzyme Activity (nmol/hr/mg protein)* Kidney	Spleen	Brain
Twitcher				
Non-HCT	40 (n=10)	0.0176±0.005	0.002±0.0001	0.0186±0.007
HCT	50 (n=4)	0.023±0.012	0.21±0.07	0.075±0.018
	70 (n=4)	0.146±0.083	0.31±0.01	0.090±0.061
	100 (n=4)	0.30±0.10	1.90±1.25	0.341±0.173
Control				
Non-HCT	40 (n=10)	1.005±0.117	0.70±0.02	0.223±0.04
HCT	50 (n=3)	0.34±0.06	0.69±0.15	0.28±0.10
	70 (n=3)	1.20±0.12	0.74±0.07	0.59±0.48
	100 (n=5)	1.62±0.65	1.17±0.02	0.39±0.18

* Mean values ± 1 standard error are shown. Animals received HCT at age 10 days.

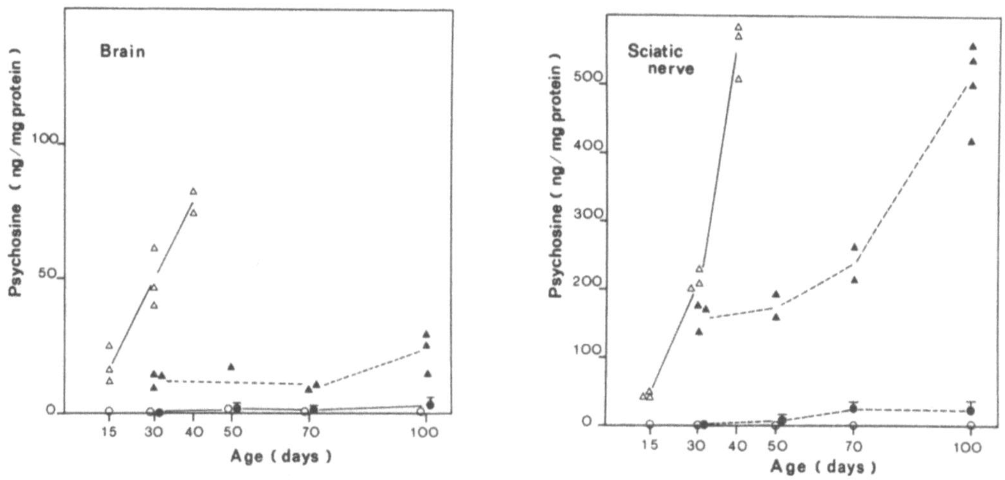

Figure 4. Levels of psychosine in brains (left panel) and sciatic nerves (right panel) of twitcher mice (triangles) and normal littermates (circles). Untreated and HCT-treated mice are indicated by open and solid symbols, respectively.

DISCUSSION

Our studies in this murine model of a human sphingolipid storage disease have shown that transplantation of enzymatically normal hematopoietic cells is associated with prolonged lifespan [22], objective stabilization to improvement in the peripheral demyelinating neuropathy [19,22], and favorable biochemical alterations (including appearance of hydrolase and decreases in the levels of the major toxic metabolite) in the CNS [21]. Although enzyme replacement by BMT has been demonstrated in other murine models of lysosomal storage disease such as β-glucuronidase deficiency, these animals have no neurological symptoms and have a normal lifespan [23,24]. When BMT from enzymatically normal donors is performed in 4-week-old mice with sphingomyelinase deficiency (a model of human Niemann-Pick disease), reduction of sphingomyelin in liver and spleen occurs, but the neurodegenerative process is not altered and survival is not prolonged [25]. These findings and our experience with HCT in clinically affected twitcher mice suggest that HCT or BMT must be undertaken in young presymptomatic animals to favorably affect survival and symptomatology in murine sphingolipidoses. One study of BMT in twitcher mice failed to demonstrate either increased tissue galactosylceramidase activity or prolonged survival [26]. Since the recipient animals in this report did not receive irradiation or immunosuppressive/myeloablative chemotherapy before BMT, it is unlikely that any mice had sustained engraftment of enzymatically normal donor cells. In contrast, we have been able to demonstrate sustained engraftment after preparation with 900 rad TBI and an intraperitoneal injection of congenic hematopoietic cells.

The observation that HCT was associated with remyelination and stabilization of motor nerve conduction velocities in peripheral nerves is of interest. Orthotopic transplantation of demyelinated sciatic nerves from twitchers into normal congenic recipient mice leads to repair of myelin sheaths and appearance of galactosylceramidase in the nerves [27]. These studies and our findings indicate that these transplantation methods provide effective enzyme replacement, in a manner sufficient to repair demyelinated peripheral nerves and maintain neurological function. The exact mechanism by which HCT leads to repair of peripheral nerves is not clear. After transplantation of twitcher sciatic nerves into normal mice, there is no evidence for migration of donor Schwann cells into the demyelinated twitcher grafts [27]. Conceivably, the remyelination observed after HCT in twitcher mice may be effected by replacement of the inflammatory cells in the demyelinated nerves by enzymatically normal donor macrophages, and galactosylceramidase produced by these donor cells may then be taken up by twitcher Schwann cells. Despite these favorable clinical, histological, and neurometric observations, however, the levels of psychosine in twitcher sciatic nerves continued to increase after HCT, albeit at a slower rate than that seen in untreated animals [21]. Furthermore, levels of this toxic metabolite increased in peripheral neural tissues while remaining stable in the central nervous system after HCT. The reasons for this discrepancy have not been elucidated.

A major question in the treatment of human lysosomal storage diseases by BMT is whether adequate enzyme replacement can occur in the CNS because of the relative impermeability of the blood-brain barrier to hydrolase in the circulation. In bovine mannosidosis, hematopoietic chimerism with enzymatically normal donor cells and favorable effects on the visceral manifestations of this glycoprotein storage disease are contrasted with lack of improvement in the CNS, suggesting that circulating donor mannosidase does not cross the blood-brain barrier [28]. Similarly, BMT into irradiated β-glucuronidase-deficient mice leads to normalization of enzyme activity in both non-neural and peripheral nervous tissues, but not in the CNS [24]. The gradual attainment of normal levels of galactosylceramidase and the associated decrease in psychosine in the brains of HCT-treated twitcher mice are encouraging observations; although no specific techniques were used to induce permeability of the blood-brain barrier in twitcher mice undergoing HCT, donor enzyme was nevertheless effectively transferred into the CNS. In support of these findings in twitcher mice, recent studies in canine fucosidosis (a glycoprotein storage disease characterized by neurological abnormalities and a deficiency of the lysosomal hydrolase α-L-fucosidase) also indicate that enzyme activity may be detected in the CNS following allogeneic BMT after total lymphoid irradiation and without any strategy to disrupt the blood-brain barrier [29]. Taken together, these preclinical findings suggest heterogeneity among the various lysosomal storage diseases with regard to the degree of enzyme replacement in the CNS after BMT.

It is not known whether the appearance of galactosylceramidase in the brains of transplanted twitchers is due to the entry of enzyme or of donor mononuclear cells into the CNS. Studies in murine radiation-induced chimeras indicate that a substantial population of Ia-antigen-bearing cells derived from donor bone marrow can be identified in the brains of recipient mice [30] after BMT. The appearance of donor mononuclear cells in the cerebrospinal fluid of a child who underwent BMT for metachromatic leukodystrophy supports these observations [6]. The characteristic PAS-positive globoid cells in the CNS of twitcher mice have immunohistochemical characteristics of macrophages and probably arise (at least in part) from the monocytes in the peripheral blood [13]. It is therefore possible that infiltration of the CNS with exogenous circulating mononuclear cells occurs primarily as a consequence of the neurodegenerative processes in the brains of twitcher mice. This phenomenon may be due to the elaboration from the CNS of monocyte chemotactic factors and/or alterations in the permeability of the blood-brain barrier of affected animals. At this time, no studies of the integrity of the blood-brain barrier in murine or human GCL have been conducted.

Allogeneic marrow transplantation has been carried out in several human lysosomal storage diseases [3-10]. Although the biochemical and clinical improvement observed in some of these patients has been encouraging, the period of follow-up is short. Multisystem long-term evaluation of the clinical outcome in patients undergoing BMT for genetic storage diseases and comprehensive studies of transplantation in animal models such as the twitcher mouse will be necessary to provide information about efficacy of and problems associated with enzyme replacement by BMT in these conditions. Ultimately, the treatment of lysosomal hydrolase deficiency states will probably entail the transplantation of autologous bone marrow cells into which the specific cloned hydrolase gene has been inserted [31]. Therefore, the need for myeloablative and/or immunosuppressive regimens in preparation for engraftment of genetically modified autologous hematopoietic stem cells must also be addressed in preclinical model systems.

ACKNOWLEDGMENTS

This work was supported in part by grant nos. K08 HD00535 and R01 NS24097 (A.M.Y.), NS13559 and NS13569 (Y.K.), and P01 CA15396 (G.W.S.), and P30 CA06973 from the National Institutes of Health, grant no. BNS 8314777 from the National Science Foundation (Y.K.), and Basil O'Connor Starter Research Grant no. 5-485 from the March of Dimes Birth Defects Foundation (A.M.Y.).

REFERENCES

1. Hobbs JR (1981) Bone marrow transplantation for inborn errors. Lancet 2:735-739
2. Barranger JA (1984) Marrow transplantation in genetic disease. N Engl J Med 311:1629-1631
3. Hugh-Jones K, Hobbs J, Chambers D, White S, Byron N, Williamson S, Barrett J, Henry K, Patrick D

(1984) Bone marrow transplantation in mucopolysaccharidoses. In: Barranger JA, Brady RO (eds) Molecular Basis of Lysosomal Storage Disorders. Orlando, FL: Academic Press, pp. 411-428
4. Hobbs JR (1985) Correction of 34 genetic diseases by displacement bone marrow transplantation. Plasma Ther Transfus Technol 6:221-246
5. Krivit W, Pierpont ME, Ayaz K, Tsai M, Ramsay NKC, Kersey JH, Weisdorf S,Sibley R, Snover D, McGovern MM, Schwartz MF, Desnick RJ (1984) Bone marrow transplantation in the Maroteaux-Lamy syndrome (mucopolysaccharidosis type VI). N Engl J Med 311:1606-1611
6. Bayever E, Ladisch S, Philippart M, Brill N, Nuwer M, Sparkes RS, Feig S (1985) Bone-marrow transplantation for metachromatic leukodystrophy. Lancet 2:471-473
7. Rappeport JM, Ginns E (1984) Bone-marrow transplantation in severe Gaucher's disease. N Engl J Med 311:84-88
8. Svennerholm L, Mansson JE, Nilsson O, Tibblin E, Eriksson A, Groth C-G, Lundgren G, Ringden O (1984) Bone marrow transplantation in the Norrbottnian form of Gaucher disease. In: Barranger JA, Brady RO (eds) Molecular Basis of Lysosomal Storage Disorders. Orlando, FL: Academic Press, pp. 441-459
9. Lundgren G, Eriksson A, Groth C-G, Gahrton G, Lonnqvist B, Myrenfors P, Nilsson O, Ringden O, Sundelin P, Svennerholm L (1984) Bone marrow transplantation in juvenile Gaucher's disease. Exp Hematol 12(Suppl 15):99-100
10. Lipton M, Lockman LA, Ramsay NKC, Kersey JH, Jacobson RI, Krivit W (1986) Bone marrow transplantation in metachromatic leukodystrophy. Birth Defects 22:57-67
11. Suzuki K, Suzuki Y (1983) The twitcher mouse: A model of human globoid cell leukodystrophy (Krabbe's disease). Am J Pathol 111:394-397
12. Kobayashi S, Katayama M, Bourque E, Suzuki K, Suzuki K (1985) The twitcher mouse: Positive immunohistochemical staining of globoid cells with monoclonal antibody against Mac-1 antigen. Develop Brain Res 20:49-54
13. Igisu H, Suzuki K (1984) Progressive accumulation of a toxic metabolite in a genetic leukodystrophy. Science 244:753-755
14. Taketomi T, Nishimura K (1964) Physiological activities of psychosine. Japan J Exp Med 34: 255-265
15. Suzuki K, Suzuki K (1982) Galactosylceramide lipidosis: Globoid cell leukodystrophy (Krabbe's disease). In: Stanbury JB, Wyngaarden JB, Frederickson DS, Goldstein JL, Brown MS (eds) The Metabolic Basis of Inherited Disease, 5th edn. New York: McGraw-Hill, pp. 857-880
16. Eicher EM, Washburn LL (1978) Assignment of genes to regions of mouse chromosomes. Proc Natl Acad Sci USA 75: 946-950
17. Kobayashi T, Nagara H, Suzuki K, Suzuki K (1982) The twitcher mouse: Determinations of genetic status by galactosylceramidase assays on clipped tail. Biochem Med 27:8-14
18. Kluver H, Barrera E (1953) A method for the combined staining of cells and fibers in the nervous system. J Neuropath Exp Neurol 12: 400-403
19. Toyoshima E, Yeager AM, Brennan S, Santos GW, Moser HW, Mayer RF (1986) Nerve conduction studies in the twitcher mouse (murine globoid cell leukodystrophy). J Neurol Sci 74: 307-318
20. Suzuki K (1978) Enzymic diagnosis of sphingolipidoses. Methods Enzymol 50: 456-488
21. Ichioka T, Kishimoto Y, Brennan S, Santos GW, Yeager AM (1987) Hematopoietic cell transplantation in murine globoid cell leukodystrophy (the twitcher mouse): Effects on levels of galactosylceramidase, psychosine, and galactocerebrosides. Proc Natl Acad Sci USA 84:4259-4263
22. Yeager AM, Brennan S, Tiffany C, Moser HW, Santos GW (1984) Prolonged survival and remyelination after hematopoietic cell transplantation in the twitcher mouse. Science 225: 1052-1054
23. Yatziv S, Weiss L, Morecki S, Fuks Z, Slavin S (1982) Long-term enzyme replacement therapy in β-glucuronidase deficient mice by allogeneic bone marrow transplantation. J Lab Clin Med 99: 792-797
24. Hoogerbrugge PM, Poorthuis BJHM, Mulder AH, Wagemaker G, Dooren IJ, Vossen JMJJ, van Bekkum DW (1987) Correction of lysosomal enzyme deficiency in various organs of β-glucuronidase deficient mice by allogeneic bone marrow transplantation. Transplantation 43: 609-614
25. Sakiyama T, Tsuda M, Owada M, Joh K, Miyawaki S, Kitagawa T (1983) Bone marrow transplantation for Niemann-Pick mice. Biochem Biophys Res Comm 113: 605-610
26. Seller MJ, Perkins KJ, Fensom AH (1986) Galactosylcerebrosidase

activity in tissues of twitcher mice with and without bone marrow transplantation. J Inher Metab Dis 9: 234-238

27. Scaravilli FM, Jacobs JM (1981) Peripheral nerve grafts in hereditary leukdystrophic mutant mice (twitcher). Nature 290: 56-58
28. Jolly RD, Thompson CE, Murphy CE, Manktelow BW, Bruere AN, Winchester BG (1976) Enzyme replacement therapy - experiment of nature in a chimeric mannosidosis calf. Pediatr Res 10: 219-224
29. Taylor RM, Farrow BRH, Stewart GJ, Healy PJ (1986) Enzyme replacement in nervous tissue after allogeneic bone-marrow transplantation for fucosidosis in dogs. Lancet 2: 772-774
30. Ting JP-Y, Nixon DF, Weiner LP, Frelinger JA (1983) Brain Ia antigens have a bone marrow origin. Immunogenetics 17: 295-301
31. Anderson WF (1984) Prospects for human gene therapy. Science 226:401-409

7: Experimental Basis of Bone Marrow Purging with Chemical and Photodynamic Agents

A. Porcellini, A. Manna, M.T. Marchetti-Rossi, F. Centis, N. Talevi, G. Sparaventi, C. Pazzaglia, A. Bocconcelli, and M. Palazzi

The major stumbling-block in ABMT is the high relapse rate compared to that observed in both allogeneic and syngeneic marrow transplant (1). This is possibly due to occult leukemic cells contaminating the remission marrow. Although the efficacy of the ex-vivo purging procedure has yet to be definitely established in clinical practice, there are indications that cleansing the marrow is associated with improved survival in some cases (1,2). To meet the obvious need for methods capable of eliminating these cells from autologous marrow, several techniques have been investigated (3-7).

Studies on in vitro active derivatives of cyclophosphamide (CY) have shown that these drugs, 4-HC and mafosfamide (AZ), may purge marrow of clonogenic cells while sparing the pluripotential stem cells (8-10).

The exhaustive work of Sieber and coll. has shown that photolysis mediated by the lipophilic fluorescent dye merocyanine 540 (MC-540) causes death of leukemia cells more rapidly than pluripotential hemopoietic stem cells (day 11/12 CFU-S) and human committed progenitors (CFU-GEMM, CFU-GM) (11-13).

A major problem in ex-vivo cleansing strategies is the evaluation of their efficacy in terms of residual clonogenic cell removal.

We have recently developed a highly sensitive in vitro clonogenic assay which involves mixing 5% of established leukemia cell lines with an excess of normal human bone marrow. This assay permitted detection of as much as 6 log reduction in simulated remission marrows purged with either mafosfamide (AZ) or MC-540.

In the present paper we report the results of preclinical studies which examine the efficacy of several distinct purging protocols in which AZ, MC-540 or hyperthermia (43°C) are used either singly or in combination and the frequency of leukemia cells persisting after purging is estimated by limiting dilution analysis.

MATERIALS AND METHODS

Details of preparation of bone marrow cell suspensions, leukemic cell lines, purging agents (MC-540 and AZ), decontamination procedures have been described previously (14).

CLEANSING PROCEDURE

Three different purging protocols were investigated in these experiments.

In Protocol I, cleansing agents were used singly; a remission leukemia bone marrow was simulated by mixing 2×10^5 (MC-540 studies) or 10^6 (AZ studies) leukemia cells of the CCRF-SB or K-562 lines with a 19-fold excess of normal human bone marrow mononuclear cells (HBMMC), and incubated with the aforesaid agents as previously described.

In Protocol II a combination of AZ + MC-540 was investigated by contaminating a HBMMC suspension with 10 or 15% (2 or 3×10^6) clonogenic cells.

In Protocol III, a combination of AZ and hyperthermia was tested on HBMMC suspensions contaminated with 10% clonogenic cells.

LIMITING DILUTION ASSAY (LDA)

The ability of the purging protocols used to eliminate clonogenic cells from the marrow suspensions was tested by means of a clonogenic assay which utilizes continuous human leukemia cell lines and involves mixing these cells with an excess of HBMMC and treating the cell mixtures with either one of the aforesaid cleansing protocols.

TABLE 1. Enumeration of residual leukemic cells after in vitro purging

Leukemia cell line	In vitro treatment	Residual blasts/well	C.E. %
CCRF-SB 5%	AZ	0	22
	MC-540	0	13.4
K-562 5%	AZ	0.08	44
	MC-540	0.11	40.3

The number of calculated residual blasts/well is represented by the X-intercept of the regression line of best fit, as determined by the maximum likelihood regression analysis. Data were originated by Minuit computer program (C.E.R.N. Geneva) in a Vax-750 computer (see Results).

TABLE 2. Survival of day 11 CFU-S after in vitro treatment

Treatment	Day 11 CFU-S % of controls
AZ	44.3
MC-540	69.7
43°C	49.3
AZ (at 43°C)	34.5
AZ + MC-540	47.9
MC-540 + AZ	52.1
43°C + AZ	45.9

Effect of different treatment protocols on murine day 11 CFU-S. Values are ± 1 SE from 3-6 experiments. CFU-S are derived from spleen colony assays in 22-31 surviving recipient mice. Results are expressed as percentage of values from control suspension. $P < 0.05$

In our microtray assay system, after AZ or MC-540 treatment no acute leukemia CCRF-SB lymphoblasts were detectable in the cell mixtures, while the figure for K-562 cells corresponded to 99.97% decontamination, in all the experiments in which the clonogenic cell contamination was 5% of the total cell number.

The clonogenic cell frequency was increased to 15% and 10% to define the decontaminating efficiency of AZ alone or in combination with the photosensitizer MC-540 or hyperthermia.

All the combinations tested were equally ineffective. Although treatment with AZ followed by MC-540 photosensitization seemed to give better results than either AZ or MC-540 used alone on the CCRF-SB line, this improvement is most probably only apparent: it must be noted, in fact, that limiting dilution analysis of the frequency of leukemic cell lines has a technical limit. When an excessive amount of residual leukemic cells remains in the wells after cleansing, medium supply may become a limiting factor, owing to the excessive proliferation rate, and hence an unexpectedly high proportion of negative wells results. This technical limit was more evident in the hyperthermia alone experiments, in which the number of residual blasts was so high that it was not possible to enumerate them reliably. Likewise, preliminary results using AZ at 43°C indicated that decontamination was not attained (data not shown).

In conclusion, our data show that LD analysis for determination of established leukemic cell frequency is a reliable method with a sensitivity threshold of 1 leukemic blast x 10^4 HBMMC, i.e. 0.001%, provided that the clonogenic cell contamination does not exceed 5% of HBMMC.

With higher blast contamination levels (15% or 10%), residual clonogenic cells remaining in the cell mixture after treatment cause an excessive cell proliferation which undermines the reliability of this method. At these contamination levels, combined treatments (AZ with MC-540 or hyperthermia) are not able to decrease the cell frequencies detectable with our LD analysis. This finding suggests that there might be a critical leukemic cell frequency limit, beyond which any cleansing procedure whatsoever is completely ineffective.

TABLE 3. Enumeration of residual leukemic cells after in vitro purging

Leukemia cell line	Leukemia cell contamination %	In vitro treatment	Residual blasts/well
CCRF-SB	15	AZ	0.6
	15	AZ+MC-540	0.25
	10	AZ	0.8
	10	43°C	–
	10	AZ+43°C	–
K-562	15	AZ	1.75
	15	AZ+MC	1.83
	10	AZ	0.5
	10	43°C	no purging
	10	AZ+43°C	1.35

Results obtained from limiting dilution analysis of HBMMC contaminated with 15% or 10% CCRF-lymphoblasts or myelogenous K-562 cells and subsequently treated with AZ alone or in combination with MC-540 or hyperthermia. Details as in Table 1.

After treatment, aliquots of 10^4 cells were dispensed in microwell plates to which graded cell numbers of the same cell line were added by the limiting dilution assay (LDA) and incubated for 13 days. Cells previously pulse-labelled with ^{3}H-Tdr were harvested and incorporated thymidine was determined by scintillation counting.

PLURIPOTENTIAL STEM CELL STUDIES

The effects of the purging combinations on normal pluripotential stem cells were defined on murine CFU-S. After incubation with either one of the cleansing protocols, 10^5 normal marrow cells were injected into lethally-irradiated mice that had received 850 rads from a Ce gamma-ray apparatus. Spleen colonies were evaluated on day 11 (15).

RESULTS

The strategy of LDA to evaluate the frequency of leukemic cells surviving after treatment with either one of the purging protocols, involves defining a threshold 3 SD above the mean of the 24 microwells in which no leukemic cells were added. Wells with ^{3}H-Tdr uptake greater than this threshold were scored as responders. It is assumed that the clonogenic cells are distributed randomly amongst the culture wells, according to the Poisson probability distribution; hence for the 0 term of the Poisson distribution equation, the proportion of nonresponders is a logarithmic function of the number of leukemic cells added to each well. Accordingly, the x-intercept calculated from the maximum likelihood regression line will represent an estimate of the number of leukemic cells which would have to be removed from the feeders to obtain 100% nonresponders (i.e. complete purging). The cloning efficiency (CE) of leukemic cells was obtained from the slope of the regression line when the ordinate is the natural log of the percent nonresponders. Table 1 shows the data obtained from LDAs of cleansed mixtures of HBMMC and 5% leukemic cells. As shown in our model system, decontamination with a single agent completely eliminated CCRF-SB lymphoblasts, while 0.08 and 0.11 K-562 cells survived the exposure to AZ and to MC-540 respectively. The CEs in these experiments were 22% and 13.4% (CCRF-SB), and 44% and 40.3% (K-562).

To test whether is was possible to improve the cleansing efficiency we used Protocols II and III, which adopt different combinations or schedules of cleansing agents.

In order to assess how far these drug combinations could be harmful to normal hematopoietic stem cells, murine bone marrow cells were incubated in the same way as the contaminated cell mixture, and survival of pluripotential stem cells was tested in the day 11 CFU-S assay. As shown in Table 2 incubation of murine marrow cells with a single agent (AZ, MC-540 or 43°C) decreased day 11 CFU-S of about 50% of controls. Surprisingly, the results were not significantly different when these agents were used in combination.

In Protocol II the leukemic cell frequency was increased to 15% and cell mixtures were exposed to AZ, MC-540 or both. The results are shown in Table 3. The number of calculated residual clonogenic lymphoblasts CCRF-SB in each well containing 10^4 cell mixtures was 0.6 after incubation with AZ and decreased to 0.25 after exposure to both agents (AZ followed by MC-540). K-562 cells proved more resistant, in that 1.75 cells survived the treatment with a single agent and 1.83 with both agents.

As it proved impossible to attain total purging when the contaminating leukemic cell frequency was increased to 15%, we had to back down to 10% contamination. The purging protocol in this case involved using AZ in combination with hyperthermia (43°C). Hyperthermia per se has been shown to have a selective killing effect on clonogenic cells (16). Table 3 presents the results obtained by exposing HBMMC suspensions containing 10% of CCRF-SB lymphoblasts or K-562 cells to AZ, hyperthermia (43°), or both. After incubation with AZ at 37°, 0.8 CCRF-SB cells and 0.5 K-562 cells survived. Hyperthermia alone did not prove able to produce an adequate cleansing effect detectable by our LDA. As the table shows, no purging of K-562 cells was attained; after exposure to AZ following 60 min. incubation at 43° C, the number of residual K-562 cells in the wells was 1.35, and the C.E. was very low at 10.7%. When incubation with AZ was preceded or followed by hyperthermia, the results did not improve, nor did they by incubating the test cells with AZ at 43°C (data not shown).

DISCUSSION

To improve the efficacy of autologous BMT in acute leukemia, it may be important to remove malignant cells from the inoculum. However, as a test for pluripotential stem cells in man is not currently available, a major complication in this procedure is the impossibility of evaluating the effects of in vitro treatment both on cells responsible for engraftment and on clonogenic cell removal. To partially overcome this problem we have tested the effect of our cleansing protocols on murine day 11 CFU-S. Our results show that incubation with AZ alone spared about 50% of pluripotential stem cells. Combined treatment with AZ followed by MC-540 or hyperthermia yielded surprisingly comparable results.

REFERENCES

1. Gorin NC, Aegerter P (1987) Autologous bone marrow transplantation for acute leukemia in remission: 4th EBMT survey. Bone Marrow Transplantation 2 (suppl. 1):320-21

2. Yeager AM, Kaizer H, Santos GW, Saral R, Colvin OM, Stuart RK, Braine HG, Burke PJ, Ambinder RF, Burns WH, Fuller DJ, Davis JM, Karp JE, Stradford May W, Rowley SD, Sensenbrenner LL, Vogelsang GB, Wingard JR (1986) Autologous bone marrow transplantation in patients with acute nonlymphocytic leukemia, using ex vivo marrow treatment with 4-hydroperoxycyclophosphamide. N Eng J Med 315:141-47

3. Bast RC, De Fabritiis P, Lipton J, Gelber R, Maver C, Nadler L, Sallan S, Ritz J (1985) Elimination of malignant clonogenic cells from human bone marrow using multiple monoclonal antibodies and complement. Cancer Res 45: 499-506

4. Leonard JE, Taetle R, To D, Rhyner K(1985) Preclinical studies on the use of selective antibody-ricin conjugates in autologous bone marrow transplantation. Blood 65:1149-53

5. Uckun FM, Ramakrishnan S, Houston LL (1985) Increased efficiency in selective elimination of leukemia cells by a combination of a stable derivative of cyclophosphamide and a human B-cell- specific immunotoxin containing pokeweed antiviral protein. Canc Res 45:69-75

6. Berenson RJ, Bensinger WI, Kalamasz D, Martin P (1986) Elimination of Daudi lymphoblasts from human bone marrow using avidin-biotin immune adsorption. Blood 67:509-15

7. Uckun FM, Gajl-Peczalska K, Meyers DE, Ramsay NC, Kersey JH, Colvin M, Vallera DA (1987) Marrow purging in autologous bone marrow transplantation for T-lineage acute lymphoblastic leukemia: Efficacy of ex-vivo treatment with immunotoxins and 4- hydroperoxycyclophosphamide against fresh leukemic marrow progenitor cells. Blood 69:361-65

8. Sharkis SJ, Santos GW, Colvin M (1980) Elimination of acute myelogenous leukemic cells from marrow and tumor suspensions in the rat with 4-hydroperoxycyclophosphamide. Blood 55:521-23

9. Sarpel SC, Epstein RB (1979) Chemoseparation of cell populations in dogs by activated cyclophosphamide. Blood 54:230a (abstr.)

10. Porcellini A, Manna A, Talevi N, Sparaventi G, Marchetti-Rossi MT, Baronciani D, De Biagi M (1984) Effect of two cyclophos - phamide derivatives on hemopoietic progenitor cells and pluripotential stem cells. Exp Hematol 12:863-66

11. Sieber F, Meagher RC, Spivak JL (1981) Differential sensitivity of mouse hematopoietic stem cells to merocyanine-540. Differentiation 19:65-69

12. Meagher RC, Sieber F, Spivak JL (1983) Susceptibility to merocyanine-540-mediated photosensitization: a differentiation marker on murine hematopoietic progenitor cells. J Cell Physiol 116:118-24

13. Sieber F, Spivak JL, Sutcliffe AM (1984) Selective killing of leukemic cells by merocyanine-540 - mediated photosensitization. Proc Natl Acad Sci USA 81:7584-87

14. Porcellini A, Talevi N, Marchetti-Rossi MT, Manna A, Sparaventi G, Palazzi M (1985) Selective elimination of leukemic cells from marrow cell suspensions by mafosfamide (AZ) or merocyanine-540 (MC). Blood 66(suppl.1): 270 (abstr.)

15. Magli MC, Iscove NN, Odartchenko N (1982) Transient nature of early haematopoietic spleen colonies. Nature 295:527-29

16. Moriyama Y, Narita M, Sato K, Urushiyama M, Koyama S, Hirosawa H, Kishi K, Takai K, Takahashi M, Shibata A (1986) Application of hyperthermia to the treatment of human acute leukemia: purging human leukemic progenitor cells by heat. Blood 67 :802-04

III. Leukemia: R.P. Gale and T. Masaoka, Chairpersons

8: Oncogenes in Acute Myelogenous Leukemia

Robert Peter Gale and Anna Butturini

Normal eukaryotic DNA contain a family of genes termed proto-oncogenes thought to regulate normal cell growth and development (1). Expression of viral analogues of cellular proto-oncogenes in the context of acutely transforming retroviruses, is responsible for neoplastic transformation. Possible mechanisms by which viral or cellular oncogenes can cause neoplastic transformation have been recently reviewed (2,3). Since qualitative and quantitative alterations of oncogene expression can result in neoplastic transformation in experimental models, expression of cellular oncogenes in human leukemias is the subject of intense investigation. Recently we reviewed the role of oncogenes in human leukemias (4). In this review we focus on oncogene abnormalities in acute myeloid leukemia (AML).

Many acutely transforming retroviruses increase leukemia in animals (reviewed in 5). However, there is little evidence that AML is caused by viruses. Thus, if cellular oncogenes are involved in the development of AML, they are likely activated by mechanisms other than viral transduction or insertion.

Activation of cellular oncogenes at the level of DNA has been described by three basic mechanisms: changes in primary structure such as point mutation, deletion or insertion; gene amplification; and gene rearrangement. In AML, the most common alterations at the DNA level are point mutations involving predominately genes of the ras family. ras oncogene abnormalities have been detected using the NIH/3T3 transfection assay and subsequent restriction enzyme mapping or DNA sequencing (6). ras mutations have been detected in three AML derived cell lines, HL-60, KG-1 and Rc2a (7,8). Recently with more sensitive assays, such as hybridization to synthetic oligonucleotide probes, leukemia cells from one third of patients with AML are reported to have point mutation in N-ras or Ki-ras oncogenes (9-13). About one half of N-ras gene mutations in AML occur in codon 13; the others occur in Codon 12 and 61; this is in contrast with N-ras mutations in other cancers, where codon 13 is rarely involved. Ki-ras is usually mutated in codons 12 and 61. ras oncogene mutations were not detected in normal bone marrow cells from one AML patient in remission, nor in other non-hematological tissues. These data imply that these are acquired mutations, limited to the neoplastic cells.

Oncogene amplification has been reported in some myeloid leukemia cell lines, but is rarely detected in fresh AML cells (14). c-myc was reported to be amplified in the HL-60 promyelocytic cell line and in fresh leukemia cells from the patient from whom this cell line was derived (15,16). c-myc was also amplified in one patient with the M2 form of AML characterized by presence of double minute chromosomes (17). c-myb is amplified in three myeloid cell lines, ML1, ML2 and ML3, derived from a patient with the M2 form of AML with multiple chromosome abnormalities including 6q-, which developed after a T cell malignant lymphoma (18). This c-myb amplification was present in early and late passages in culture; fresh leukemia cells from the patient were not tested (19). Hu-ets 1 was reportedly amplified in a case of M4 form of AML (20).

In most cases of chronic myelogenous leukemia (CML) and in some cases of acute lymphoblastic leukemia (ALL) chromosome translocations are consistently associated with oncogene rearrangement and related alterations of oncogene transcription and/or expression (for review see 5). In contrast, although chromosome translocations are common in AML, few involve known oncogenes or other identified genes. In 5 patients with the M4 and M5 subtypes of AML and the t(9;11) (p22;q23) translocation, Hu-ets 1 was reported to be translocated from chromosome 11 to chromosome 9 near the alpha interferon locus (21). In two patients with M2 subtype of AML and the t(8;21) (q22;a22) translocation, Hu-ets 2 was reported to be translocated from chromosome 21 to chromosome 8 (22). A small number of cases of AML with the t(9;22) (q34;q11) and translocation of c-abl oncogene from chromosome 9 to 22 have been reported. In these cases the rearrangement involves the bcr gene and the product of the chimeric bcr/abl gene is similar to that in CML.

As indicated, most chromosome translocations in AML do not involve known oncogenes. The t(8;21) translocation typical of the M2 form of AML does not involve the c-mos and c-myc oncogenes (23); c-abl is not rearranged in the t(6;9) (p22;q23) typical of AML with basophilia (24); erb-A, c-fes and the p53 gene are not rearranged in the M3 form of AML associated with the t(15;17) translocation (25,26). There have been relatively few studies that correlate the above reported alteration at DNA levels with changes in RNA transcription. Increased levels of ras related RNA are reported in some cases of AML with point mutation of ras genes (9). Levels of c-myb and c-myc related RNA are increased in the ML1-3 and HL-60 cell lines respectively. This increase is likely related to the oncogene amplification (19,27). Several surveys of oncogene related mRNA by northern analyses, dot-blots or in situ hybridization have been reported. c-myc, c-myb, c-abl, and c-fos transcripts are usually present and commonly increased in AML cells. In one study, c-fos RNA were reported mostly in the M4 and M5 subtypes of AML. In almost all the cases studied, increased levels of oncogene related transcripts were observed without a corresponding detectable DNA rearrangement or amplification (27-35).

Few studies of oncogene related protein expression have been reported. A c-fes related protein has been studied in normal and leukemic cells (36). A 92 kd c-fes protein (P92) has been identified in normal bone marrow cells particularly monocyte/macrophages and granulocytes. P92 has also been detected in the HL-60 and KG1 myeloid cell lines and in fresh leukemia cells from 3 patients with AML. There are no qualitative or quantitative difference in P92 in leukemia and normal cells at the same stage of differentiation. The KG1a cell line, which differs from KG1 in relative independence from granulocyte-macrophage colony stimulating factor (GM-CSF), lacks P92 protein. These and other data have led to the hypthesis that this protein may be involved in the response to myeloid growth factors, probably as a component of receptor for one or more colony stimulating factors (CSF).

Discussion

The precise role of oncogene abnormalities in the etiology of AML is unknown. In contrast to CML, where virtually all patients exhibit a consistent alteration in expression of c-abl, AML is heterogeneous, and most cases show no detectable oncogene abnormailties. Although initial data suggested a relatively specific mutational locus in N-ras codon 13, it is no longer certain that this change is AML specific or etiologic.

In some instances, specific translocation are associated with specific AML subtypes; examples are discussed in the section on cytogenetics and include t(8;21) in M2, t(15;17) in M3, t(6;9) in M2 with basofilia. Other structural abnormalities, such as -5/-5q or -7/-7q, 11q-, and inv or del (16) are correlated with therapy linked AML, M5 and M2 with eosinophilia respectively. Although one might expect specific oncogene abnormalities in these instances, these were found in few cases. The table reviews involvement of oncogenes and growth factor related genes in chromosome abnormalities typical of AML (21-26, 37-40). Although it is possible that not all oncogenes have been identified, it is likely that genes other than conventional oncogenes, as defined by transduction by acutely transforming retroviruses, are involved. Thus, it may be necessary to broaden the operational definition of oncogene, to include any gene or regulatory sequence whose abnormal expression can cause or maintain the transformed state. These include genes for ligands and receptors that regulate hematopoietic cell growth. In this context it is noteworthy that cytogenetic abnormalities in AML include long arm of chromosome 5, site of GM-CSF gene and c-fms oncogene, whose gene product is part of CSF-1 receptor (41) and short arm of chromosome 3, putative site of one or more thrombopoietin growth factor or receptors (37). Precisely how deletion or rearrangement of such genes might eventuate in AML is uncertain. However, abnormal G-CSF expression in transgenic mice results in a malignant proliferation of myeloid cells (Metcalf D, presented at Australian Haematological Society Meeting, Hamilton Island, July 6, 1987).

Some data indicate that transcription of some oncogenes is increased in AML. These observations should be tempered by several considerations. First the oncogenes studied are different than those implicated by cytogenetic abnormalities. Second, Transcription of the c-myb, c-myc, c-abl and c-fos oncogenes have also been reported in other types of leukemias and in other types of leukemias and in normal myeloid cells during proliferation or differentiation (42-46). Thus oncogene transcription may result from, rather than cause AML. Finally, appropriate cell type and cell cycle specific controls are mostly lacking.

In summary, oncogenes, as broadly defined, must be involved in the pathogenesis of AML. Whether the genetic abnormalities of AML correspond to regulatory regions of conventionally defined oncogenes or to other genes is unknown; there are no convincing data of a role of known oncogenes in AML, except for th relatively high proportion of of AML with ras gene mutations. Clearly additional data are needed to critically evaluate the role of oncogenes in AML and to establish their value in diagnosis, prognosis or therapy.

REFERENCES

1. DeFeo-Jones D, Tatchell K, Robinson LC, Sigal IS, VAss WC, Lowy DR, Scolnick EM (1985) Mammalian and Yeast ras gene products: biological function in their heterologous systems. Science 228:179-184
2. Bishop MJ, VArmus H (1985) Function and origins of retroviral transforming genes. In: Weiss R, Teich N, Varmus H, Coffin J (eds) RNA Tumor Viruses. Cold Spring Harbor Laboratory Publications p 249-256

3. Wyke J (1986) Principles of viral leukemogenesis. Sem Hematol 23:189-200
4. Butturini A, Gale RP (1987) Oncogenes in human leukemias. Blood (In Press)
5. Pierce JH, Eva A, Aaronson SA (1986) Interactions of oncogenes with hematopoietic cells. Clin Haematol 15:573-596
6. Copeland NG, Cooper GM (1979) Transfection by exogenous and endogenous murine retrovirus DNAs. Cell 16:347-351
7. Murray MJ, Cunningham JM, Parad LF, Dantry F, Leibowitz P, Weinberg RA (1983) A ras oncogene coexisting with alterated myc genes in hematopoietic tumors. Cell 33:749-752
8. Janssen WG, Steenvoorden ACM, Collard JG, Nusse R (1985) ONcogene activation in human myeloid leukemia. Cancer Res 45:3262-3267
9. Bos JL, Toksoz D, Marshall CJ, Verland-de Vries M, van der Erb A, Van Boom JH, Jannsen JWG, Tenvaaden ACM (1985) Aminoacid sustituttion at codon 13 of the N-ras oncogene in human acute myelogenous leukemia. Nature 315: 726-730
10. Bos JL, Verland de Vries M, van der Erb A, Janssen JWG, Delwel R, Lowenberg B, Colly LP, (1987) Mutation in N-ras predominate in cute myeloid leukemia. Blood 69: 1237-1241
11. Gambke C, Signer E, Moroni C (1984) Activation of N-ras gene in bone marrow cells from a patient with acute myeloblastic leukemia. Nature 307:476-478
12. Hirai H, Tanaka S, Azuma M, Kubayshi Y, Fujisawa M, Okaba T, Urabe A, Tataku F (1985) Transforming genes in human leukemia cells. Blood 66(6): 1371-1378
13. Needleman SW, Kraus MH, Srivastava SK, Levine PH, Aaronson SA (1986) High frequency of N-ras activation in acute myelogenous leukemia. 67:753-757
14. Yokota J, Tsumestugo-Yokota Y, Battiflora H, Slamon D, Cline M (1986) Alteration of myc, myb and rasHa proto-oncogenes in cancer are frequent and show clinical correlation. Science 231:2615
15. Collins S, Groudine M (1982) Amplification of endogenous myc related DNA sequences in a human myeloid leukemia cell line. Nature 298:679-681
16. Dalla Favera R, Wong-Staal F, Gallo RC (1982) Oncogene amplification in promyelocytic leukemia cell line HL-60 and primary leukemia cells of the same patient. Nature 299:61-63
17. Alitalo K, Saksela K, Winqvist R, Alitalo R Keski-Oja J, Laiho M, Ilvonen M, Knuutila S, de la Chapelle A (1985) Acute meyelogenous leukemia with c-myc amplification and double minute chromosome. Lancet ii:1035-1038
18. Ohyashiki K, Ohyashiki JH, Snadberg AA (1986) Cytogenetic characterization of putative human origin of the cells. Cancer Res 46: 3642-3647
19. Pelicci PG, Lanfrancone L, Brathwarte MD, Wolman SR, Dalla Favera R (1984) Amplification of the c-myb oncogene in a case of acute myelogenous leukemia. Science 224: 1117-1121
20. Rovigatti U, Watson D, Yunis JJ (1986) Amplification and rearrangement of Hu-ets-1 in leukemia and lymphoma with involvement of 11q23. Science 232:398-400
21. Diaz MO, Le Beau MM, Pitha P, Rowley JD (1985) Interferon and c-ets-1 genes in the translocation (9;11) (p22;q23) in human acute monocytic leukemia. Science 231: 265-267
22. Sacchi N, Watson DK, van Kessel HMG, Hagenmeijer A, Kersey J, Drabkin HD, Patterson D, Papas TS (1986) Hu-ets-1 and Hu-ets-2 genes are transposed in acute leukemia with (4;11) and (8;21) translocation. Science 231:379-382
23. Diaz MO, Le Beau MM, Rowley JD, Drabkin HD, Patterson D. (1985) The role of the c-mos gene in the 8;21 translocation in human acute myeloblastic leukemia. Science 229:767-769
24. Westbrook CA, Le Beau MM, Diaz MO, Graffin J, Rowley JD (1985) Chromosomal localization and characterization of c-abl in the t(6;9) of acute nonlymphocytic leukemia. Proc Natl Acad Sci USA 82:8742-8746
25. Dayton AI, Seldon J, Laws G, Dernay DJ, Finan J, Tripputi D, Enamel BS, Rovera G, Nowell PC, Croche CM (1984) A human erb-A oncogene homologue is closely proximal to the chromosome 17 breakpoint in acute promyelocytic leukemia. Proc Natl Acad Sci USA 81: 4495-4499
26. Isobe M, Enamel BS, Givoli D, Oren M, Croce CM (1986) Localization of gene for human p53 tumor antigen to ban 17p 13. Nature 320: 93-85
27. Westin EH, Gallo RC, Arya SK, Eva A, Souza LM Baluda MA, Aaronson SA, Wong-Staal F (1982) Differential expression of the amv gene in human hematopoietic cells. Proc Natal Acad Sci USA 79:2194-2198
28. Blick M, Westin E, Gutterman J, Wong-Staal F, Gallo R, McCredie K, Keating M, Murphy E (1984) Oncogene expression in human leukemia. Blood 64:1234-1239
29. Slamon DJ, De Kernon JB, Verna IM, Cline M (1984) Expression of cellular oncogenes in human malignancies. Science 224:256-262
30. Ferrari S, Torelli U, Selleri L, Donelli A, Venturelli D, Narni F, Moretti L, Torelli G (1985) Study of the levels of expression of two oncogenes, c-myc, ans c-myb in acute and chronic leukemias of both lymphoid and myeloid lineage. Leukemia Res 9:833-842
31. Slamon D, Boone TC, Murdock DC, Keith DE, Press MF, Larson RA, Souza LM (1986) Studies of the human c-myb gene and its predict in human acute leukemias. Science 223:347-351
32. Romero P, Blick M, Talpaz M, Murphy E, Hester J, Gutterman J (1986) c-sis and c-abl expression in chronic myelogenous leukemia and other hematologic malignancies. Blood 67:839-841
33. Preisler HD, Kinniburgh AJ, Wei-Dong G, Khan S (1987) Expression of the proto-oncogenes c-myc, c-fos, and c-fms in acute myelocytic leukemia at diagnosis and in remission. Cancer Res 47:874-880
34. Birnie GD, Warnock AM, Burns JH, Clark P (1986) Expression of the myc gene locus in population of leukocytes from leukemia patients and normal individuals. Leuk Res 10:515-526

35. Mavilio F, Testa U, Sposi MN, Petrini M, Pelosi E, Bordignon C, Amadori S, Mandelli F, Peschle C (1987) Selective expression of fos proto-oncogene in human acute myelomonocytic and monocytic leukemias: a molecular marker of terminal differentiation. Blood 69:160-164
36. Feldman RA, Gabrilove JL, Tam JP, Moore MAS, Hanafusa H (1985) Specific expression of the human cellular fps/fes encoded protein NCP92 in normal and leukemic cells. Proc Natl Acad Sci USA 82:2379-2383
37. Pinto MR, King MA, Goss GD, Bezwoda WR, Fernandes-Costa F, Mendelow B, McDonald TP, Dowdle E, Bernstein R (1985) Acute megacaryoblastic leukemia with 3q inversion and elevated thrombopoietin (TSF): an autocrin role for TSF? Br J Haematol 61:687-693
38. Nienhuis AW, Bunn HF, Turner P, Gopal TV, Nash WG, O'Brien SJ, Sherr CJ (1986) Expression of the human c-fms proto-oncogene in hematopoietic cells and its deletion in the 5q- syndrome. Cell 42:421-428
39. Le Beau MM, Westbrook CA, Diaz MO, Larsen RA Rowley J, Gasson JC, Golde DW, Sherr CJ (1987) Evidence for the involvement of GM-CSF and c-fms in the deletion (5q-) in myeloid disorders. Science 231:984-987
40. Diaz MO, Le Beau MM, Harden H, Rowley JD (1985) Trisomy 8 in human hematologic neoplasia and the c-myc and c-mos oncogenes. Leukemia Res 9:1437-1442
41. Sherr JC, Rottemier CW, Sacca R, Roussel MF, Look AT, Stanley ER. The c-fms proto-oncogene product is related to the receptor for the mononuclear phagocyte growth factor, CSF1. Cell 41:665-676
42. Gowda SD, Koler RD, Bagby GC (1986) Regulation of c-myc expression during growth and differeentation of normal and leukemic human myeloid progenitor cells. J Clin Invest 77: 271-178
43. Duprey SP, Boettinger D (1985) Developmental regulation of c-myb in normal myeloid progenitor cells. Proc Natl Acad Sci USA 82: 6937-6941
44. Lee J, Metha K, Blick MB, Gutterman JU, Lopez Berestein G (1987) Expression of c-fos, c-myb and c-myc in human monocytes: correlation with monocytic differentation. Blood 69:1542-1545
45. Muller R, Curran T, Muller D, Guilbert D (1986) Induction of c-fos during myelomonocytic differentiation and macrophage proliferation. Nature 314:546-548
46. Mitchell RL, Zokas L, Schreiver RD, Verma IM (1985) Induction of the expression of proto-oncogene fos during human monocytic differentiation. Cell 40:209-217

CHROMOSOMAL ABNORMALITIES AND ONCOGENE INVOLVEMENT IN AML

Type of AML	Chromosome Abnormality	Oncogene[1]	Growth Factor[2] Gene	Abnormality[3]	References
M1 M2	inv(3)(q21; q25-27)	NR	Thrombopoietin[2]		37
M2	t(3;5)(q26;q22)	NR	Thrombopoietin		37
M2 M4	+4	c-raf2 (4q27)	NR		
M1 M2 M4 M5 M6	-5, -5q (q13q35)	c-fms (5q34)	GM-CSF (5q23q31)	deletion	38,39
M1 M2	t(6;9) (q22.2;q34)	c-myb (6q23) c-abl (9q34)		NR No rearrangement	24
M1 M2 M4 M5 M6	+8	c-myc (8q24) c-mos (8q11-22)		Extracopy Rare rearrangement Extracopy No rearrangement	40 40
M2	t(8;21) (q22.1;q22.3)	Hu-ets-2 (21q22) c-mos (8q11-22) c-myc (8q24)		Translocation No rearrangement No rearrangement	22 23 23
M2 M4 M5a	t(9;11)	Hue-ets 1 (11q23)		Translocation[4]	21
M1 M2	t(9;22) (q34;q11)	c-abl (9q34)		Fusion gene (bcr-abl)	
M3	t(15;17) (q22;q11)	erb A (17q21) p53 gene (17q13) c-fes (15q24-26)		No rearrangement No rearrangement No rearrangement	25 26 25
M2 M4 M5b	inv(16) (q13;q22) 16q-	- -	Methallothionine (16q22)	NR	
M1 M2 M4	-7/-7q	erb b (7p14) met (7q22) kit (7q31)		NR NR NR	

Note
1 Oncogenes or growth factor genes located near the chromosome rearrangement
2 Proposed location of thrombopoietin gene; GM-CSF, granulocyte-macrophage colony stimulating factor
3 NR = Not Reported
4 Near alpha-interferon locus

9: Optimal Timing of Marrow Transplantation for Patients with Acute Nonlymphoblastic and Acute Lymphoblastic Leukemia

C. Dean Buckner, Reginald A. Clift, Frederick R. Appelbaum, Jean E. Sanders, Kristine Doney, and E. Donnall Thomas

INTRODUCTION

Marrow transplantation has become an important therapeutic modality in the management of patients with acute non-lymphoblastic (ANL) and acute lymphoblastic leukemia (ALL). However, the optimal time for intervention in a patient's disease course with marrow transplantation is yet to be determined. The following will briefly review the current situation.

ACUTE NON-LYMPHOBLASTIC LEUKEMIA

Chemotherapy for patients with ANL produces long-term disease-free survival in a proportion of patients (20% or greater) who achieve a complete remission. Once a patient has relapsed there is little prospect of cure without marrow transplantation. Transplantation for patients with resistant disease results in the cure of 20% of such patients with currently used regimens. Transplantation has been employed earlier in the course of the disease and the outcome for patients transplanted in first remission is considerably better with 40-70% of patients surviving disease free for 3 or more years [1]. Table 1 shows the probabilities of relapse and survival at 3 years following allogeneic marrow transplantation from HLA matched siblings. Similar data have been reported from the International Bone Marrow Transplant Registry (IBMTR) [2].

The largest body of experience is for patients transplanted in first remission because of the superior results of transplantation at this stage of the disease. Attempts have been made to identify pretransplant factors predictive for success or failure of outcome of transplantation during first remission which might assist in decision making concerning management of an individual patient. Obviously, the risk factors for survival from transplantation have to be weighed against those associated with chemotherapy. Unfortunately risk factors for surviving a transplant may be similar to those for survival from chemotherapy. Table 2 shows the effects of age on survival from transplantation.

The probability of relapse post-transplant is independent of age. An analysis of the IBMTR data involving 447 patients identified FAB subtype M 5 vs M 1-4 as an adverse risk factor for survival.[2] However, this could not be confirmed in the Seattle experience for patients transplanted in 1st remission. In addition to age the only pretransplant prognostic factors found in the Seattle analysis was donor sex and number of circulating blasts [1]. Posttransplant risk factors obviously do not assist in decision making.

TABLE 1

ALLOGENEIC MARROW TRANSPLANTATION FOR PATIENTS WITH ANL - Seattle Experience

	Number	Relapse	Survival
First remission	227	23%	51%
Untreated			
1st relapse	52	27%	32%
2nd remission	49	35%	30%
Resistant			
1st relapse	25	60%	19%

TABLE 2

EFFECTS OF AGE ON SURVIVAL FOR PATIENTS WITH ANL TRANSPLANTED IN 1ST CR - Seattle Experience

AGE	NUMBER	SURVIVAL
<10	20	80%
11-20	52	65%
21-30	89	42%
31-40	44	40%
>40	22	40%

The results of allogeneic marrow transplants for patients with ANL shown in Table 1 are informative and assist in designing a study of transplant intervention. These data suggest that for patients with a suitable marrow donor who are not transplanted in first remission the optimal time is as soon as possible after relapse. There is no advantage to being transplanted in second remission as compared to untreated relapse and many patients will become treatment resistant or die during remission induction attempts.

Several studies have prospectively compared the outcome of marrow transplantation to that of continued chemotherapy for patients with ANL in first remission. These studies have shown either a marginal or clear advantage for marrow transplantation [3-5]. These studies have not, however, compared the outcome of transplantation in first remission to that of chemotherapy with those failing chemotherapy being offered subsequent transplantation at first relapse. For patients with ANL in first remission who have a marrow donor this is the more relevant question. Only by the use of a controlled randomized trial can the impact of marrow transplantation in first remission be determined. If the sum of chemotherapy cures plus cures from transplantion in untreated first relapse is no worse than the survival expectation for patients transplanted in first remission, then first relapse would be the best time for intervention by marrow transplantation. This is because such timing would avoid transplanting patients already cured or who could be cured by conventional chemotherapy, and because subsequent improvements in conventional therapy could be easily accommodated within such a treatment strategy. Such a study would necessarily involve a multi-center trial in order to accrue adequate numbers of patients. All patients with suitable marrow donors should be randomized when they enter complete remission. One group would receive immediate transplant while the other group would receive continued chemotherapy and be transplanted at the first sign of relapse. This study design would permit comparison of allografts in first remission versus first relapse plus chemotherapy cures.

The previous discussion relates to transplantation from HLA identical donors. The results of transplantation from donors mismatched for one HLA antigen have been very similar, but transplantation from other categories of donor has been less successful. The optimal timing for intervention by marrow transplantation in the treatment of patients with ANL will vary according to the origin and HLA compatibility of the marrow.

Several recent studies have documented long-term disease-free survival following autologous marrow transplantation for patients with ANL in first remission. These studies are difficult to evaluate without a contemporaneous control group since some of these patients may have been cured prior to transplant. Further, it is uncertain how many patients can be salvaged with autologous marrow transplantation at first relapse. The combination of initial chemotherapy plus autologous transplantation at first relapse, as outlined above for allogeneic transplantation, could be equal to or better than transplantation in first remission. As for allogeneic marrow transplantation this can only be answered in a prospective randomized trial. Until the answers from these studies are forthcoming all patients without marrow donors should have marrow stored while in first remission for use in first relapse since salvage chemotherapy produces no long-term survivors.

ACUTE LYMPHOBLASTIC LEUKEMIA

Marrow transplantation of children with ALL in first remission is controversial due to the increasing survival rate of poor risk patients, as defined by age and WBC, receiving intensive chemotherapeutic regimens. With the exception of infants, children with high risk ALL have a survival of 46 - 67% following intensive treatment regimens [6-8]. In addition to age and WBC, patients with translocation type of chromosome abnormalities have a poor prognosis as do patients with extramedullary relapse [9-11]. Comparable patients transplanted in first remission from HLA matched siblings in Seattle have a 60% disease-free survival [Sanders, unpublished observations]. At the present time it is reasonable to consider marrow transplantation in first marrow remission for children with ALL who are less than 12 months of age, who have translocation type of chromosome abnormalities at diagnosis, who have more than one extramedullary relapse and perhaps for those who have an overt testicular relapse on therapy or a CNS relapse after previous cranial irradiation. For adults with ALL the probability of remaining in first C.R. with continued chemotherapy is as high as 60% [12], which is similar to that reported for patients transplanted in 1st C.R. Transplantation of adults with ALL in 1st remission is probably not warranted at the present time except as incorporated into a prospective study.

The most important determinant of survival following 1st relapse is whether the relapse occurred on or off therapy. Of 80 children who had relapses after therapy had been discontinued, life-table estimated survival was 75%, in contrast to a projection of less than 20% survival for 231 patients whose relapse occurred while on chemotherapy [11]. The next most important determinant was the site of relapse. The ultimate survival following chemotherapy for those with an isolated marrow relapse was projected to be less than 5%, whereas a survival for an isolated testicular relapse was 25%, and for those with an isolated CNS relapse it was 40% at 3 years from relapse. In patients with relapse on treatment at more than one site, the overall prognosis appears to be that of the site which carries the worse prognosis. If a marrow relapse has occurred off treatment, survival is inversely proportional to the interval of time from discontinuation of therapy to relapse. Patients who have relapses <3 months from discontinuation have the worst prognosis, similar to patients who relapse while on chemotherapy. Those who relapse >12 months off chemotherapy have a 70% survival at four years after marrow relapse. Patients who are between 3 and 12 months off therapy at relapse have an intermediate prognosis. Recently, Rivera et al. reported results of intensive chemotherapy for children who had relapsed on therapy. Five of 31 (16%) were alive without disease 38 to 44 months after achieving a remission, and all 5 of these survivors had an initial marrow remission of more than 18 months [13].

Most, but not all, studies have shown superiority for marrow transplantation for patients in second remission as compared to chemotherapy. Chessells et al. reported 53 children in second remission, which included 40 treated with chemotherapy and 13 with a donor who were eligible for transplant, but only 10 of the 13 were actually transplanted. Actuarial analysis after a 1 to 5 year follow-up showed a disease-free 5 year survival of 30% for transplant patients and 20% disease free survival for the chemotherapy patients [14]. A Pediatric Oncology Group report described 198 patients who achieved a second remission who were treated with chemotherapy and 28 patients were transplanted from a matched sibling donor. Survival at 18 months was 24% for each of the groups [15].

Three single institution prospective studies of children in second remission of ALL compared results of marrow transplantation with chemotherapy. Of 14 children reported by Johnson et al., 4 are disease-free now 7 to 10 years after transplant while all 21 treated with chemotherapy relapsed and died by 3 years [16,17]. The University of Minnesota actuarial relapse-free survival for 15 children treated with a marrow transplant was 33% at 3 years compared to 5% for 23 children treated with chemotherapy [18]. The Genova group reported the actuarial probability of being in continuous remission at 2 years of 58% for 17 who received a marrow transplant compared to 18% for 19 children given chemotherapy [19]. Butturini et al. suggested that marrow transplantation was superior to chemotherapy for those children who relapsed within 18 months of first remission [20].

The probability of disease-free survival for 57 children with ALL transplanted in Seattle in second bone marrow remission shows a plateau at 40% extending from 2.5 to 10.4 years [21]. Overall disease-free survival from reports of other transplant centers range from 30% to 66% with the best survival reported from the Memorial Sloan-Kettering Cancer Center [22].

In conclusion, children who relapse more than 12 months off therapy should be given chemotherapy but those who have a marrow relapse while receiving chemotherapy are most likely to benefit from marrow transplantation from a matched sibling donor while in second marrow remission.

For adults with ALL a study of the type proposed for patients with ANL would be appropriate to determine if marrow transplantation in first remission is superior to combined chemotherapy cures plus cures from transplantation after elapse. In the absence of a study transplantation should be delayed till after 1st relapse.

<u>REFERENCES</u>

1. Clift RA, Buckner CD, Thomas ED, Kopecky KJ, Appelbaum FR, Tallman M, Storb R, Sanders J, Sullivan K, Banaji M, Beatty P, Bensinger W, Cheever, M, Deeg J, Doney K, Fefer, A, Greenberg P, Hansen JA, Hackman R, Hill R, Martin P, Meyers J, McGuffin R, Neiman P, Sale G, Shulman H, Singer J, Stewart P, Weiden P, Witherspoon R The treatment of acute non-lymphoblastic leukemia by allogeneic marrow transplantation. Bone Marrow Transplantation, in press.

2. Bortin MM, Gale RP (1986) Current Status of Allogeneic Marrow Transplantation: A Report From the International Bone Marrow Transplant Registry. In: Terasaki PI (ed) Clinical Transplant, UCLA Tissue Typing Laboratory, Los Angeles, CA pp 17-28, 219a
3. Appelbaum FR, Dahlberg S, Thomas ED, Buckner CD, Cheever MA, Clift RA, Crowley J, Deeg HJ, Fefer A, Greenberg P, Kadin M, Smith W, Stewart P, Sullivan K, Storb R, Weiden P (1984) Bone marrow transplant or chemotherapy after remission induction for adults with acute nonlymphoblastic leukemia - A prospective comparison. Ann Intern Med 101:581-588
4. Appelbaum FR, Clift RA, Buckner CD, Stewart P, Storb R, Sullivan KM, Thomas ED (1983) Allogeneic marrow transplantation for acute non-lymphoblastic leukemia after first relapse. Blood 61:949-953
5. Champlin RE, Ho WG, Gale RP, Winston D, Selch M, Mitsuyasu R, Lenarsky C, Elashoff R, Zighelboim J, Feig SA (1985) Treatment of acute myelogenous leukemia. A prospective controlled trial of bone marrow transplantation versus consolidation chemotherapy. Ann Int Med 102:285-291
6. Bleyer WA, Sather H, Coccia P, Lukens J, Siegel S, Hammond GD (1986) The staging of childhood acute lymphoblastic leukemia: Strategies of the Childrens Cancer Study Group and a three-dimensional technic of multivariate analysis. Med Pediatr Oncol 14:271-280
7. Steinherz PG, Gaynon P, Miller DR, Reaman G, Bleyer A, Finklestein J, Evans RG, Meyers P, Steinherz LJ, Sather H, Hammond D (1986) Improved disease-free survival of children with acute lymphoblastic leukemia at high risk for early relapse with the New York regimen- A new intensive therapy protocol: A report from the Childrens Cancer Study Group. J Clin Oncol 4:744-752
8. Niemeyer CM, Hitchcock-Bryan S, Sallan SE (1985) Comparative analysis of treatment programs for childhood acute lymphoblastic leukemia. Semin Oncol 12:122-130
9. Bloomfield CD, Goldman AI, Alimena G, Berger R, Borgström GH, Brandt L, Catovsky D, de la Chapelle A, Dewald GW, Garson OM, Garwicz S, Golomb HM, Hossfeld DK, Lawler SD, Mitelman F, Nilsson P, Pierre RV, Philip P, Prigogina E, Rowley JD, Sakurai M, Sandberg AA, Secker Walker LM, Tricot G, van Den Berghe H, Van Orshoven A, Vuopio P, Whang-Peng J (1986) Chromosomal abnormalities identify high-risk and low-risk patients with acute lymphoblastic leukemia. Blood 67:415-420
10. Pullen D, Jackson J, Crist W, Carroll A, Boyett J, Borowitz M, Brock B, Iyer R, Buchanan G, Head D, McWilliams N, Ragab A (1985) Philadelphia chromosome positive (Ph^+) acute lymphocytic leukemia (ALL) in children has clinical and biologic features that predict poor prognosis and is cytogenetically and immunophenotypically heterogeneous. Amer Soc Hematol (Abstract)
11. Bleyer WA, Sather H, Hammond GD (1986) Prognosis and treatment after relapse of acute lymphoblastic leukemia and non-Hodgkin's lymphoma: 1985. A report from the Childrens Cancer Study Group Cancer 58:590-594
12. Schauer P, Zalmen AA, Mertelsmann R, Cirrincione C, Friedman A, Gee TS, Dowling M, Sanford K, Straus DJ, Koziner B, McKenzie S, Thaler HT, Dufour P, Little C, Dellaquila C, Ellis S, Clarkson B (1983) Treatment of acute lymphoblastic leukemia in adults: Results of the L-10 and L-10M protocols. J Clin Oncol 1:462
13. Rivera GK, Buchanan G, Boyett JM, Camitta B, Ochs J, Kalwinsky D, Amylon M, Vietti TJ, Crist WM (1986) Intensive retreatment of childhood acute lymphoblastic leukemia in first bone marrow relapse. N Engl J Med 315:273-278
14. Chessells JM, Leiper AD, Plowman PN, Levinsky R, Rogers DW, Blacklock H, Richards S, Festenstein H (1986) Bone-marrow transplantation has a limited role in prolonging second marrow remission in childhood lymphoblastic leukaemia Lancet i:1239-1241
15. Buchanan GR, Boyett J, Rivera GK: (1986) Comparison of bone marrow transplantation and intensive chemotherapy for children with acute lymphoblastic leukemia in second marrow remission: A pediatric oncology group (POG) study. Blood 68:755 (abstract)
16. Johnson FL, Thomas ED, Clark BS, Chard RL, Hartmann JR, Storb R (1981) A comparison of marrow transplantation with chemotherapy for children with acute lymphoblastic leukemia in second or subsequent remission. N Engl J Med 305:846-851
17. Johnson FL, Thomas ED (1984) Treatment of relapsed acute lymphoblastic leukemia in childhood. (Letter to the Editor) N Engl J Med 310:263
18. Woods WG, Nesbit ME, Ramsay NKC, Krivit W, Kim TH, Goldman A, McGlave PB, Kersey JH (1983) Intensive therapy followed by bone marrow transplantation for patients

with acute lymphocytic leukemia in second or subsequent remission: Determination of prognostic factors (A report from the University of Minnesota Bone Marrow Transplantation Team). Blood 61:1182-1189

19. Bacigalupo A, Van Lint MT, Frassoni F, Occhini D, Pittaluga PA, Comelli A, Dini G, Massimo L, Marmont AM (1986) Allogeneic bone marrow transplantation versus chemotherapy for childhood acute lymphoblastic leukaemia in second remission. Bone Marrow Transplantation 1:75-80
20. Butturini A, Rivera GK, Bortin MM, Gale RP (1987) Occasional Survey: Which treatment for childhood acute lymphoblastic leukaemia in second remission? Lancet 1: 429-432
21. Sanders JE, Thomas ED, Buckner CD, Doney K Marrow transplantation for children with acute lymphoblastic leukemia in second remission. Blood (Concise Report), in press
22. Brochstein JA, Kernan N, Emanuel D, Laver J, Flomenberg N, Gulati S, Castro-Malaspina H, Cunningham I, Shank B, O'Reilly RJ (1986) Marrow transplantation for acute leukemia after hyperfractionated total body irradiation (HFTBI) and cyclophosphamide (CTX) Blood 68: Suppl 1, 962, p 271a (Abstract)

10: Perspectives in Treatment of Adult Leukemia with High Dose Cytoreductive Therapy and Autologous Bone Marrow Treated Ex Vivo

Leonard J. Horwitz, Karel A. Dicke, Sundar Jagannath, and Gary Spitzer

INTRODUCTION

Even with the advances in treating adult leukemia achieved in the last several decades, it still remains a disease which is fatal for the majority of people who acquire it. Modern chemotherapy regimens alone have been successful in getting more people into first remission, and many of these first remissions are prolonged. However, the majority relapse, and once this happens, hope for a complete cure becomes very low (1,2).

One attempt to change this natural history is the use of high dose chemotherapy, with or without total body irradiation, followed by bone marrow transplantation. The most favorable results have been with allogeneic bone marrow transplantations. Unfortunately, however, this modality cannot be available for all patients, either by virtue of age, performance status, or lack of a compatible bone marrow donor (3). To this end, methodologies have been developed which involve high dose chemotherapy followed by transplantation of autologous bone marrow and, most recently, treatment of bone marrow outside the body ex vivo before storage.

CHEMOTHERAPY OF ACUTE LEUKEMIA

The benchmark for any current studies done with high dose chemotherapy and transplantation, of course, is how well one can expect to do with standard levels of chemotherapy. The treatment of acute lymphocytic leukemia (ALL) has met with some success. In children, remission rates as high as 90% with simple vincristine and prednisone alone were seen in some studies. For adults, the addition of an anthracycline and possibly also L-asparaginase is necessary to attain remission rates of roughly 75-85%. Nevertheless, in all age groups, intensive post-remission chemotherapy is required to enjoy continuous remissions. A variety of these maintenance programs have been developed. The Sloan Kettering studies have been showing 5-year survivals of up to 51% in some of the younger patients. Other studies involving maintenance and intensification therapies which utilize drugs such as cytosine arabnoside, L-asparaginase, and methotrexate have been able to show similar results. Prophylactic intrathecal chemotherapy has also been useful in prolonging remission duration. These programs are reviewed in more detail elsewhere (1). In acute myelogenous leukemia (AML), modern chemotherapy, consisting of prolonged continuous infusions of standard doses of cytosine arabinoside combined with anthracyclines or related compounds and often also with 6-thioguanine, is able to produce remissions from 50 to 85% patients. Once in remission from AML, 25% will enjoy long-term freedom from disease (2).

The problem, both with ALL and AML, is that once relapse has occurred, the situation becomes much more grave. There are many chemotherapy regimens that have been used in attempts to reinduce remission. In AML, with m-AMSA, mitoxantrone, high dose cytosine arabinoside, 5-azacytidine, and others, remission reinduction can be obtained in roughly 30-50% of the patients (4), depending on time of relapse. Unfortunately, few of these remissions are long lived—generally fewer than 5% of the patients will enjoy freedom from disease for more than a year. In the case of ALL, the disease is diverse, with certain subgroups of patients, particularly those with B-cell ALL, unable to attain even a first remission; such patients are also more likely to relapse earlier (5).

The current problem to be approached in leukemia centers around prolonging the patients' remissions. Success in this matter would be more apparent in second or subsequent remissions, where the long-term survival is small. In addition, although effective therapy may not be able to provide a particular patient with indefinitely long freedom from disease, it may allow the length of a subsequent remission to go beyond the time seen for the first remission (6). Such an "inversion" of remission duration is unusual, seen in less than 10% of patients successfully reinduced by chemotherapy. A treatment able to do this in a significantly greater number of patients could well be assumed to have altered the natural history of leukemia. As such, it might be used in first remission in good conscience as part of a randomized study or for special risk patients (7).

SYNGENEIC BONE MARROW TRANSPLANTATION

One of the first approaches in dealing with acute leukemia, especially after relapse, has been to use higher doses of chemotherapy. Such doses generally require bone marrow support. The first group of patients to receive such attention were those with an identical twin, who could provide the bone marrow for the affected sibling. The conditioning regimens generally have consisted of cyclophosphamide with a single dose of total body irradiation of 10Gy. In refractory leukemia, of 46 patients reviewed by Fefer, close to 70% were able to attain a remission. Unfortunately, only 17% are enjoying long-term disease-free survival after treatment for relapsed or refractory leukemia (8).

The same review reported on results of the syngeneic approach in patients who have attained complete remissions; there was no distinction made between first and subsequent remissions in his analysis. With this approach, fully one half, both AML and ALL, are enjoying continuous complete remissions. Those who have relapsed generally have done so early on, the median time to relapse being about five months for ALL and ten months for AML. Furthermore, about 40% of these patients worldwide transplanted in second or later remission have had an "inversion" in their remission duration, being in post-transplant remission longer than first remission (8).

Many consider this 50% long term survival to be the ideal situation, the goal to be approached using autologous transplantation in remission. Any relapse which occurs after twin transplant in remission would have to be due to inadequacy of the preparative regimen in the face of residual disease, since the donated twin marrow is presumed to be free of disease. However, to use this as a standard is not totally realistic. First of all, these are results which combine both first remission and subsequent remission patients, whereas with autologous bone marrow transplants, these situations are studied separately. Second, there are probably host immunologic effects against the tumor, even with autologous bone marrow. Investigators have predicted, theoretically, both more and less antileukemic effect! In the first case, there is evidence that the T-lymphocytes in the autologous graft may be sensitized against the patient's own tumor; in the other, immune deficiency has been documented after autologous transplantation, although it is not as long lasting as that seen in allogeneic transplantation (9). Further confounding of the comparability comes from the tendency to do syngeneic transplants very soon after remission, versus autologous transplants being done at least several months later. Therefore, the simple statement, that the ideal long term survival for autologous bone marrow transplantation with current conditioning regimens should be 50%, may not be totally true. At this point, it is probably the best available benchmark for remission intensification. This is in contrast to the situation with relapsed or refractory leukemia being transplanted—the nearly 80% failure rate after syngeneic transplant would suggest that the problem in this instance lies in the need for a more effective antileukemic agent. The role of marrow contamination disappears in such a setting.

AUTOLOGOUS UNPURGED BONE MARROW TRANSPLANTATION — ACUTE LYMPHOBLASTIC LEUKEMIA

Gorin reported the experience in Europe with autologous bone marrow transplantation (ABMT) for leukemia with untreated bone marrow using a variety of conditioning regimens. For ALL treated in relapse, there is 10% survival at 20 months; for those treated in remission (CR), survival at 12 months is 60% (10). Data for second and subsequent CR in ALL treated with cyclophosphamide, BCNU, and VP-16, 213 (CBV) and ABMT shows a median remission duration of five months (range one to eight months) after transplant (11,12). For ALL in relapse, CBV conditioning with ABMT resulted in a 44% complete complete remission rate, but all patients relapsed within eight months (median three months) (11). Of three patients in third CR, one showed a 33 months disease-free survival, but developed leukoencephalopathy (13). Other small studies of ALL relapse compiled by Herve show similar results (14).

AUTOLOGOUS UNPURGED MARROW TRANSPLANTATION — ACUTE MYELOGENOUS LEUKEMIA (AML)

Lowenberg showed in four selected patients that long term remissions of 21 to 84 months were possible. These patients were treated with cyclophosphamide and total body irradiation (TBI) followed by autologous bone marrow stored five to ten months into first remission (15,16).

Burnett treated 23 adult patients with AML (M1, 2 or 3) in first CR with cyclophosphamide or melphalan, TBI, and infusion of bone marrow which had been refrigerated for 54 hours between the time of withdrawal and the time of infusion. Twelve are in CR 5 to 60 months after transplant (median 40 months); one died in CR at 36 months. The other 10 have relapsed from 3 to 11 months (median 5 1/2 months). Six of 10 patients treated 6 to 22 months into their remission are still in remission, versus 6 of 13 patients treated within the first five months of attaining remission (17,18,19). These authors present data showing a tendency for fewer relapses in patients autografted at least nine months after remission (20). They also note that the vast majority of relapses, both in their own studies and with other groups occur in the first year (17).

Thirteen patients, age 13 to 38, were given cyclophosphamide and TBI for AML in first CR by the Seattle group. Eight relapsed after two to 12 months (median nine months), one died early of septicemia, and one died at three and 1/2 months of cytomegalovirus pneumonitis. The other three (23%) continue to do well at 26, 46 and 51 months after transplant (21).

Of 14 patients in second or greater CR treated with CBV and ABMT, nine have relapsed at 1-12 months (median 5 months), two have died of infections, and three are well at 2, 3 and 30 months. With 13 patients transplanted in relapse, 54% achieved remission with CBV and ABMT, but all relapsed within eight monghs (two months median (11,12)). Piperazinedione and total body irradiation have afforded similar results, but with more toxicity

(22). Out of 22 total patients in these two studies (ALL and AML), two patients have had long-term remissions longer than their first remission, for an inversion rate of 9% (95% confidence interval, 0-21%) Also at M. D. Anderson Hospital, a study of AML first CR using CBV as part of a one-year maintenance program has not yet reached its median time to relapse in 15 patients followed at least ten months from transplant (12).

TANDEM HIGH-DOSE CHEMOTHERAPY WITH AUTOLOGOUS BONE MARROW TRANSPLANTATION — "IN VIVO PURGING"

The ultimate pretreatment of bone marrow with drugs occurs when the patient himself receives the chemotherapy and his own marrow, which regenerates subsequently, is harvested for use after a second course of high dose chemotherapy. One of the earliest studies of this type was attempted in our group. Fourteen ALL patients underwent bone marrow aspiration two to three months into first remission and subsequently received first intensification with cyclophosphamide 4.5 gm/m^2, BCNU 30 mg/m^2, and VP-16 600 mg/m^2 (low dose CBV). Three patients relapsed shortly after intensification. The other 11 patients had a second bone marrow withdrawn two months after the first procedure and were immediately reintensified and transplanted. Their overall remission duration was a median of 11 months, with four patients (28%) surviving over one year. The sub-optimal chemotherapy and early marrow storage before second transplantation may have affected the results adversely (23).

Another study of this type was done by Maraninchi and colleagues using high dose melphalan. Eleven patients were originally treated in relapse and 10 of these achieved CR; 11 other patients received this treatment protocol while already in CR. Only eight in total went on to receive a second course of high-dose melphalan and transplantation, and six of them still remain in CR (24).

Goldstone and colleagues also performed a double transplant procedure. The patients had either AML or ALL and were either in first or second CR. The preparative regimen included cyclophosphamide, Adriamycin, BCNU, cytarabine, and 6-thioguanine. After recovery, a second bone marrow was harvested and the protocol was repeated. Patients who had ALL were further given maintenance with 6-mercatopurine, methotrexate, vincrinstine, and prednisone. Of these patients, two died before reaching the second course and five relapsed before reaching the second course. Two patients relapsed 3 1/2 and 5 1/2 months after receiving the second course, while four are in remission, 3 1/2, 15 1/2, 18, and 23 months after the second transplant. All patients who made it to second transplant were in first CR. (25).

The problems with this approach, then, are remaining in remission between the two courses of chemotherapy, having sufficient marrow recovery to allow sufficient number of cells for harvest before the second transplant, and excess cumulative toxicity following the second course of therapy. According to Brun del Re (26), even patients whose marrow is harvested shortly after intensification with VP-16 plus high-dose Ara-C, hematologic recovery after transplant is delayed beyond the time expected for the amount of CFU-C infused.

BACKGROUND OF EX VIVO CHEMOTHERAPY

In vitro growth of granulocyte-macrophage colony forming cells (CFU-GM) from bone marrow after treatment with chemotherapeutic agents has already been used as a model for selecting drugs and doses with favorable in vitro therapeutic ratios for use against particular tumors (27). Similarly, in vitro growth of normal marrow cells and tumor cells can be compared in the same way. One such drug is 4-hydroperoxycyclophosphamide (4HC), which at doses causing reduction of over 95% of in vitro growth of CFU-GM, erythroid burst forming cells (BFU-e), and multilineage precursor cells (CFU-GMEM), still does not inhibit the ability of ex vivo treated autologous marrow to engraft (28,29,30). Long-term bone marrow cultures were examined in an attempt to elucidate this phenomenon. Doses of 4HC on fresh bone marrow which were able to inhibit CFU-GM, BFU-e and CFU-GMEM were considerably lower than the doses needed to depress the formation of fibroblastic colonies (CFU-F). At doses required to prevent new CFUs from forming in long term cultures, CFU-F were suppressed and the monolayer characteristic of such cultures did not form (31).

The IC90 of 4HC may vary markedly, depending on time of incubation, cell concentration, and whether bone marrow buffy coat or mononuclear cells were used. With both 4HC (31) and ASTA-Z (32), an inverse correlation could be demonstrated between cell concentration and IC90 drug dose (the drug dose found to cause a 90% reduction of CFU-GM growth of non-leukemic marrow) in humans. With 30 minute incubations of buffy coat cells, the IC90 of 4HC determined by Siena, et al. was 51.1 ug/ml for 2 x 10^7 cells/ml and 29.2 ug/ml for 1 x 10^7 cells/ml (31). Rowley et al., incubating 2 x 10 buffy coat cells/ml (packed red cell volume, 5%) for 30 minutes, found the IC90 of 4HC to be 97 ug/ml (28); one will note that this is just about the highest ex vivo 4HC dose (100/ug which regularly allowed engraftment (33). His co-workers, Zuehlsdorf, et al. (34), determined that a variation in sensitivities to ex vivo 4HC was due partly to the packed red cell volume of the treated marrow, with individual variations in sensitivity to 4HC also playing a large role. Because of our longer incubation time (60 minutes) and because the mononuclear cell fraction of marrow with a minimal amount of red cells was used, we find the IC90 of 4HC to be considerably lower.

A related cyclophosphamide derivative, ASTA-Z-7557 (ASTA-Z, or Mafosfamide) was used in vitro against a lymphoblastic leukemia cell line, a dose dependent kill of clonogenic leukemic cells of 3 to 4.7 logs was demonstrated (35,36).

Several drugs may be used ex-vivo at concentrations not achievable in vivo. For instance, vincristine was able to produce a cell kill of about 50% to 75% of that of 4HC, at a dose significantly below its IC 90. This was accomplished at an ex vivo concentration of vincristine that is 10-fold higher than that attainable in serum (37). The killing of hydrocortisone was superior even to 4HC in all tested leukemic cell lines, once concentrations of 7mg/ml were exceeded; these concentrations can be obtained only ex vivo (38). Furthermore, drugs which would have significant extramedullary toxicity may be tested ex vivo. Several lymphoblastic leukemia lines were sensitive in vitro to hydrocortisone doses which were above those obtainable clinically in man (39). A pre-T Cell malignant lymphoma cell line and a T-ALL line were 7.5 and 9.3 times more sensitive to vincristine than were CFU-GM and a B-Cell lymphoma was 94 times more sensitive to Vinblastine (40).

Other drugs with promise for in vitro use, showing large cell kills at doses not as toxic to bone marrow include VP-16 (41), Adriamycin, cisplatin, and 5-azacytidine (42). Adriamycin and mitoxantrone were mostly equivalent to 4HC at their IC90 doses on all cell lines. VP-16 kill in three lines was similar to 4HC, but inferior in a fourth. Methylprednisolone and taxol were ineffective, and their doses were limited by solubility problems (43).

Janowski-Wieczorek and colleagues have attempted to use verapamil with vincristine in an effort to potentiate tumor cell death of multiple drug-resistant cell lines; up to 40 uM verapamil did not potentiate toxicity towards normal hematopoietic cells. Its addition did not enhance the level of killing of multiple drug resistant variants of HL60 or CEM cell lines in a four hour exposure, although it did improve the uptake of vincristine by these cells (44).

Drugs specific for normal T-cells may be directed against T-cell leukemias. Russell, et al., have used a combination of deoxyadenosine and deoxycoformycin to rid peripheral blood totally of its ability to produce normal T-cell colonies while inhibiting marrow CFU-GM by only about 10% at the same dose (45). Actual studies against leukemic cells or T lymphoma cells have not been reported. However, Epstein, et al. successfully prevented graft-versus-host disease in mice with this regimen (46).

ANIMAL TUMOR MODELS

BN rat leukemia cells and normal mouse marrow were incubated with either ASTA-Z or 4HC. Treated cells were tested in a rat spleen colony forming assay for the number of leukemic colonies (LCFU-S) produced and these were compared to the number of spleen colony forming cells (CFU-S) derived from pretreated normal marrow. The tumor cells indeed were more sensitive, with their LD63 being 10.9 um versus 16.4 and 22 um respectively for CFU-C and CFU-S, using ASTA-Z. For 4HC, the respective dosage for LCFU-S, CFU-C, and CFU-S were 4.9, 9.6 and 16.7 mm. When ASTA-Z treated leukemic cells were mixed with untreated rat marrow and infused into syngeneic irradiated rats, these rats lived to a normal life span. However, when the leukemic cells and marrow were mixed first and then treated and infused, the life span of the recipient rats was 20% shorter (47).

Mice treated with total body radiation were infused with normal mouse marrow purposely contaminated with BN rat Leukemia cells with or without pretreatment in vitro with 4HC. Doses under 50 uM 4HC led to prolonged overall survival of the animals, while doses of 60 uM led to increased survival without the reappearance of leukemia (48).

IN VITRO CORRELATIONS

The question of the correlation between in vitro sensitivity of leukemia cells and clinical effect was explored in 22 patients who received cytosine arabinoside (Ara C) and Adriamycin for induction. The surviving fraction of clonogenic leukemia cells of untreated patients grown in agar after incubation with these drugs correlated with attainment of remission and was significant at the P=0.005 and the P=0.02 levels for Ara C and Adriamycin respectively (49). In another study, retrospective analysis showed a relationship between the drug sensitivity of established acute lymphoblastic leukemia cell lines and the responsiveness of the original tumor from which each line was derived in vivo (39). These correlations give some justification for the use of in vitro tumor cell sensitivity to determine appropriate drugs for ex vivo therapy. From these studies and the previously discussed in vitro murine studies, in vitro assays of tumor killing may correlate with the actual degree of tumor kill in ex vivo treated marrow.

BACKGROUND OF EX-VIVO MONOCLONAL ANTIBODY USE

Monoclonal antibodies (MCAs) are nonspecific immunological reagents produced by cloned hetero-karyons, or "hybridomas", which are produced by fusion of immune murine B lymphocytes with murine plasmacytoma cells (50). Hybridoma clones are selected on the basis of screening for production of antibodies which bind specific target antigens, with absence of reactivity with other targets (51). The cloned cell lines are capable of producing large amounts of the specific antibody in culture (10-100 ug/ml).

Although there are no "leukemia-specific" MCAs, there are a large number of antibodies which react with leukemic cells. For use in bone marrow transplantation, the antibodies must be tested for reactivity both with leukemia cells and with normal hematopoietic progenitors. Of the MCAs reactive with hematopoietic elements, at least 200 have been grouped into 26 "cluster designations" (CDs) through the efforts of three international workshops. These CDs are groupings of similar antibodies based on a large number of criteria of reactivity to hematopoietic cells of different maturities and lineages and which have been reviewed elsewhere (52-56).

With the advent of MCAs, efficient methods for their use with marrow were required. Three major avenues and a number of minor roads have been used.

Complement-mediated cell lysis is possible with certain subclasses of MCAs which can fix complement. Although this is the most popular method, many methodological problems have to be overcome. Its reproducibility is hampered by variations in the sera used as a source of complement (57-59), sometimes due to the presence of complement inhibitors such as "decay accelerating factor" (59,60). In addition, the generated complement fragments, which, besides being toxic, are powerful and poorly understood immuno-regulators, may have effects on hematopoietic elements (61). Furthermore, high cell densities (58) or interference by red cells can inhibit complement-mediated lysis (62,63), and even cells which bind complement-fixing MCAs might not be lysed. The latter phenomenon may occur when there is a low cell density of the recognized antigen; repeated purging with MCA plus complement may select for clones of such cells (64,65). These problems have lead to published discrepancies concerning the reactivitiy of at least 14 MCAs with CFU-GM (66-74). Using complement, it has been difficult to obtain two logs of MCA-reactive cell removal reproducibly, though this could be improved with the addition of pools of MCAs (75). Monitoring the effectiveness of purging may be done by either leukemic colony assays or chromium release assays (76).

A second approach has been to join MCAs and natural protein toxins (such as ricin) covalently to make "immunotoxins" (77,78). Their biochemical preparation is quite complicated, and this has limited the number and variety of reagents available. In addition, decreased recoveries were observed after freezing (79); although CFU-GM may not have been affected by immunotoxins initially, this may indicate that residual immunotoxins in treated autologous marrow might be toxic to progenitors after thawing cryopreserved marrow. Treatment of a B-ALL cell line by monoclonal antibody B-43 bound to another toxin, pokeweed antiviral protein, followed by Asta-Z chemopurging, resulted in up to 7 logs cell removal without significance loss of progenitors (80).

A third approach involves magnetic separation of the MCA-reactive cells. Jansen, et al., have shown that tumor cells with low levels of expressed tumor specific antigens may be removed using immunomagnetic separation, whereas complement lysis may not be possible. The model they used for this was a mixture of a cell line bearing low levels of tumor antigen mixed with whole peripheral blood (81). Kemshead, et al., used 4.5 micron polystyrene-coated magnetite beads produced by Ugelstad and coworkers (82), to treat marrows from neuroblastoma patients (83,84). Overall cell loss varies between 20 to 50%, depending on the monoclonal antibody used. Results were better using an indirect approach, i.e., coating the beads with high affinity sheep- or goat-anti-mouse antibodies, rather than with the actual mouse MCAs used.

Studies on MCA purging have been conducted in Lyon, France, comparing immunomagnetic beads with complement lysis. In vitro studies suggested that the choice of the particular MCA was paramount, that neither method was clearly superior, but that the methods could be complementary and combined. A similar study in Burkitt's lymphoma conducted by the same group was inconclusive, but the authors again alluded to a possible benefit from addition of the two methods; they feared that this combination would disrupt the hematopoietic stem cells also (85,86).

In our unit, Reading and his coworkers developed magnetic affinity separation based on magnetic colloidal cobalt rather than magnetic beads (87). This procedure allows a 4.3 to 4.5 log removal of antibody-reactive cells with a reasonable recovery (e.g., approximately 50-90%) of the hematopoietic progenitors. The colloid contains avidin, which in turn tightly binds the biotin which is covalently attached to the MCAs. It proved easier and more effective to use a "sandwich" procedure whereby the mouse MCAs binding the leukemic cell are themselves bound by biotinylated goat-anti-mouse immunoglobulins which in turn become attached to the avidin-containing magnetic colloid (88,89).

A novel variation of this procedure is to couple rat anti-mouse immunoglobulin to "floating beads"; the leukemic cell-immunobead conjugates are then decanted. This proved successful in a model mixing experiment and in a preclinical test on seven patients (90).

Other ways of removing cells with MCAs are being explored. A stable, circular tetramolecular complex of two antigen specific mouse MCA molecules linked with two rat anti-mouse antibodies proved capable of forming immune complexes, which could be removed by centrifugation (91, 92). The efficiency, however, is below 95%. Similarly, Rieber et al., have tried to use MCA-coated erythrocytes. Preliminary results show these may be effective in recognizing and removing cells even with low antigen densities (93). A technique using the tetrameric complexes discussed above but bound to human erythrocytes is also under investigation by Slaper-Cortenbach, et al., with encouraging preliminary results (94).

MCAs conjugated to mitomycin C has proven more effective in vitro against CEM and HI30 cells than free mitomycin C by a factor of 30. The effect on marrow is yet unknown (95).

CLINICAL STUDIES OF EX VIVO CHEMOTHERAPY PURGING OF BONE MARROW

Johns Hopkins reported results of phase I studies of ex vivo 4HC treatment of marrow. 2×10^7 bone marrow buffy coat cells per ml were incubated with between 40 and 120 ug/ml of 4HC before reinfusion into patients with leukemia or lymphoma. Approximately one-third of these patients were not in remission, with the others being in first to sixth remission. Engraftment occurred regularly with in vitro doses of up to 100 ug/ml. The overall results showed 50% survival at four months and 20% at eight months. There are two long-term remissions of over 17 and 30 months (33). It must be noted that despite the fact that patients often engrafted when CFU-GM were absent, it has been shown clinically that CFU-GM indeed can be correlated with the rapidity of engraftment (96). Furthermore, no other in vitro test, including long term cultures, has been shown to predict rapidity of engraftment in humans. Also, in support of using CFU-GM toxicity as the limit for purging is the fact that immune responsiveness, measured by mixed lymphocyte culture, shows inhibition in the presence of 4HC at doses comparable to those toxic to CFU-GM (97).

In a subsequent phase II trial, 40 AML patients in second or third remission received cyclophosphamide and either busulphan or TBI conditioning followed by infusion of marrow treated ex vivo with 100 ug/ml 4HC. Seven died early, one died of sepsis after failing to engraft at five months, 2 died of veno-occlusive disease of the liver, 3 died of interstitial pneumonitis, 15 relapsed at a median of six months, and 13 are free of disease seven to sixty months (median 19 months) after transplant. At the time of present analysis, eight had a second remission longer than the first, for an inversion rate of at least 20%. When compared to the 9% inversion rate of our patient population treated with unpurged bone marrow (95% confident interval 0-21%) this would be considered marginally positive (98-100).

Between the phase I and phase II studies, a total of 18 patients with ALL in second CR were treated in this way. Two still survive in first CR beyond one year after their bone marrow transplant (one beyond three years); two others relapsed at 15 and 17 months, one died in CR at 5 1/2 months, and the remaining patients relapsed at a median of 4 1/2 months (98-100). We cannot draw any further conclusions because specific data to determine the inversion rate are not available.

When Asta-Z was used as a marrow ex vivo pretreatment on 16 leukemic patients in relapse or remission, the median survival was 8.3 months, compared to 4 to 6 months in historical cases using untreated marrow (101). One small study shows continued disease-free survival without maintenance chemotherapy in three ALL patients four to eight months after grafting with marrow purged with Asta-Z (102). For AML, four of five survived at one to eight months disease-free, and the fifth relapsed at seven months. Of interest is that patients tranfused with Asta-Z purged bone marrow show an inversion of the T4:T8 ratio for up to 17 months (9); immunosuppression could become a problem with such patients and should be monitored.

Updated results from Gorin, et al., are available on 57 patients treated with cyclophosphamide 120 mg/kg and 10 Gy fractionated TBI. Bone marrow was treated with Asta-Z at a dose determined for each patient to produce an IC-95 against GM-CFC (103). Twenty-two of 31 AML CR1 patients are free of disease one at 42 months after transplant, with two graft failures, seven toxic deaths and three patients dying in remission; the median follow-up time is still less than one year. Of four patients with AML in CR2, two relapsed at one and four months, one died of a cytomegalovirus infection, and a fourth is still in remission at 26 months. For 18 ALL CR1, ten are disease-free with a median follow-up of 8.5 months. There have been two toxic deaths, and six have relapsed. In ALL CR2, only three patients have been transplanted; one relapsed at four months, but two continue in remission at four and five months (104). The Mafosfamide Italian Cooperative Group also used ASTA-Z (80 to 100 ug) to treat patients with ALL. Of 16 patients treated in CR1, six patients relapsed from 1-16 months (median 4 months), two died during the course of the transplant, and the remainder are in remission up to 54 months. This compares with six patients that were done by the same group in CR1 without purging; three relapsed at 2, 6 and 8 months, one died during the procedure and two are still in remission. For CR2, four patients relapsed between 1 and 7 months (median about 3 months). One died of sepsis and the remainder are doing well up to 21 months (105). It is too soon to draw a conclusion from either study group of patients. In addition, it is difficult to determine which patients had good prognostic factors at presentation and would be expected to do well in CR1. However, patients with poor prognosis seem to benefit the least (106).

A novel approach for AML purging was reported by Chang et al. He set up long-term bone marrow cultures on one patient in relapse. After 10 days in long-term culture, the cells were reinfused, after cyclophosphamide TBI preparation. The patient remained in remission for at least six months (107).

Our group explored the combination of 4HC, the drug deemed among the most effective against a battery of 4 ALL and 2 AML cell lines, with vincristine, a drug which has an appreciable kill against most cell lines at a dose relatively sparing of bone marrow (42). Other combinations which were tested in the laboratory include hydrocortisone, (5 to 10 mg/ml), plus 4HC, (5 ug/ml), vincristine with Adriamycin, and vincristine with hydrocortisone. However, combining 1 ug/ml or 5 ug/ml of vincristine to 5 ug/ml of 4HC, which result in an IC75 and IC90, respectively, enhanced the cell kill in some tested cell lines by up to 1.5 logs over that obtained with 5 ug/ml of 4HC alone. (A difference of 0.5 logs is significant in the limiting dilution system used.) To date, five patients have been conditioned with cyclophosphamide, BCNU and VP-16 and subsequently have been reinfused with bone marrow treated in this fashion. All have engrafted satisfactorily, including two at the higher dose level. One with acute lymphocytic leukemia relapsed after four months and subsequently died after being unable to achieve another remission. Two AML, one mixed lineage leukemia, and one lymphoblastic lymphoma are still in complete remission, but after no more than eight months follow-up for any.

CLINICAL STUDIES OF EX VIVO MONOCLONAL ANTIBODY PURGING OF BONE MARROW

CD10 monoclonal antibody J5 has been used clinically both with complement and magnetic colloid. Ritz et al. report 24 children (23 cALLA positive) with acute lymphoblastic leukemia who were transplanted in first to fourth CR using bone marrow treated with either J2 or J5 antibody and complement. The conditioning regimen was VM26, cytarabine, and cyclophosphamide with TBI. All patients who survived the transplant regimen recovered their granulocytes; nine patients never recovered to 25,000 platelets/ul. Four died of infection, one died of pneumonitis, and three died of hemorrhage. Eight relapsed from 2-8 months (median 3 months). The other eight patients remained in remission 4 to 44 months after transplant (median 22 months); one of these was in first remission originally when transplanted. Only one is known to have a current remission time longer than his first remission; the consequent "inversion" rate of 4.3% is not significantly different than that seen in unpurged marrow, though this may change as the data of mature (108-111).

In our group, patients in ALL second remission were intensified with cyclophosphamide, BCNU, and VP-16, followed by infusion of bone marrow depleted of J5 positive cells by immunomagnetic colloid. All engrafted fully and without toxicity. Immunoflourescence showed roughly one log reduction in J5 positive cells. All patients eventually relapsed at 3-11 months (87).

Leukemia cells are heterogeneous in their expression of antigens (112). To circumvent this, most recent studies have used pools of MCAs rather than single ones; this is based on in vitro data showing improvement of cell removal from two to five logs by combining MCAs (113). Ramsey, et al., reported 23 children with ALL in CR2 or later whose marrows were treated ex vivo with MCAs BA1, BA2 and BA3 plus complement. Conditioning was with cyclophosphamide and total body irradiation. Although one died of infection and 15 relapsed by 7.4 months (median 4.3 months), seven are in complete remission at one to 32 months. Inversion rate has been reported as 27%—a very encouraging number

(114-115). Nakamura et al., also show encouraging results with the same combination of antibodies, but full details are not yet available (116). Campana, et al., first conducted an extensive investigation of native cases of ALL and B cell non-Hodgkin's lymphoma in vitro to determine the best MCAs to use before preceding clinically. They concluded that a combination of CD10 and CD19 MCAs with rabbit complement will lyse 80% of null-cell ALL and cALL (117), a result corroborated elsewhere (118). Similarly, they found CD7 antibodies optimal for T-ALL. A clinical study still in its early stages reports good engraftment (117).

T-cell reactive MCAs from CD2, CD3, CD5, CD6, CDw18 have been used successfully for T-cell depletion with allogeneic transplantation (119-125), but there are some studies done in remission T-ALL or T cell lymphoma patients also. Appropriate reactivity to the target cells can be demonstrated (79,125,126). In one such study, Filipovich and colleagues treated three patients, one in first remission and one in second remission from T-cell ALL. Autologous bone marrows were pretreated with anti-TA-1 and anti-T101 antibodies linked to the cell toxin ricin. Granulocytes recovered in all these patients, but all relapsed within a short period of time (125). Larger studies with longer follow-up are awaited.

In these cases, where the monoclonal antibodies do not react with GM-CFC, normal hematopoietic recoveries have been observed. On the other hand, some of the MCAs used for AML purging are known to remove the majority if not all of the CFU-GM, BFU-E and CFU-GEMM (66,70,72,127-134). In long-term bone marrow cultures, some regeneration may be seen (74). Prolonged recoveries and/or infections have been observed with complement and anti-HLA DR monoclonal antibodies (118), though Maraninchi et al. were able to engraft two patients with HLA-DR positive ALL after marrow purging with a pool of anti-DR antibodies (132).

Because clonogenic leukemic cells may be antigenically different from the total leukemic population, it may be possible to "fine tune-in" the choice of antibodies to harm these cells and perhaps escape damage to normal cells (127,133). To this end, CDw16 monoclonal antibodies PM-81 and AML-2-23 were used by Ball et al., to purge the marrow of 16 patients with AML. Preparation was with cyclophosphamide and TBI. Of 11 patients transplanted in second CR, two never recovered platelets and died of subarachnoid hemorrhage. Five relapsed at 2 to 21 months (median 6 months) and 4 are in CR at 7, 15, 19, and 22 months; the length of first has not been presented, so inversion rate is unknown. Of two patients transplanted in first relapse, one relapsed again at 11 months and one died of pneumonitis. The results of three patients transplanted in first CR are still too early (134,135).

OTHER EXPERIMENTAL APPROACHES TO MARROW PURGING

Soybean agglutinin (SBA) has been used to remove T lymphocytes prior to allogeneic transplantation (136-139). Reading and coworkers of our group have found that soybean agglutinin binds to leukemic blast cells from most patients with ALL or AML. When conjugated with magnetic cobalt colloid, virtually all bone marrow cells reactive with biotinylated SBA were removed, with 50-90% recoveries of CFU-GM.

A number of studies have been done on alkyl-lysophospholipids (ALPL). These are compounds which take advantage of the absence of the enzyme by which they are metabolized and detoxified in many kinds of leukemic cells, including the murine Wehi-3 B line and the human HL60 cell line (140). A dose-related anti-tumor response of ALPL was demonstrated by Okamoto et al; also, the length of incubation improved its effect against HL60 cells. The CFU-GM BFU-E, and CFU-GEMM escaped virtually unscathed. No clinical studies have been reported, however (141).

Okamoto, et al., also studied several ether lipids, which damage cell membranes and are seemingly selective for leukemic cells. Cell kills of 0.5 to 2 logs were noted against a variety of AML and ALL lines, with sparing of normal hematopoietic progenitors. Fresh leukemic cells were similarly affected. The toxic effect is dose, time, and temperature dependent (142).

The light-activated compound merocyanine-540 has been investigated by Sieber and coworkers. By a mechanism not totally explained, in the presence of serum, it binds preferentially to the cell membranes of leukemic cells and, to a lesser extent, to those of normal immature marrow cells. The energy of applied white or green light is transferred to the cell membrane, which is disrupted; the dye then enters the cell and continues to damage cell components by virtue of generated oxygen radicals. Reductions in viable cells of the order of five logs or greater are noted with a number of established leukemic cell lines; yet, the concurrent loss of mouse pluripotent stem cells is only one log (143). Marrows of seven patients have been treated with this compound. All had advanced disease. One patient died before engraftment, another patient was too early for evaluation. Results of the anti-leukemic effect are not yet available. Other oxygen radical-producing systems have been tried in vitro, using differences in glutathoine-metabolizing enzymes (144).

Nucleoside transport systems in normal hematopoietic cells are more sensitive to nitrobenzylthioinosine (NBTI), and in its presence will not take up toxic 7-deazo-adenosine. Cass, et al., pretreated both marrow and leukemic cells with this NBTI for 16 hours before exposing the cells to 7-deazo-adenosine. The toxic compound entered and inhibited cell growth in HL60 and CEM cell lines, but spared 50 to 95% of the CFU-GM, BFU-E and CFU-GMEM. Unfortunately, most cell lines tested had both sensitive and insensitive nucleoside transport systems, and this method cannot be used on all of them (145).

In vitro treatment of B cell leukemia cell lines with combined chemotherapy and immunotherapy can reduce viable tumor cells by up to 6.1 logs compared to 3.5 logs with single drug treatment (146); clinical studies at the University of Minnesota are underway (personal communication).

SUMMARY

In acute leukemias in first remission, although transplantation studies are still early, preliminary results showing a significant proportion of patients with long-term disease-free survival. In this setting, it is impossible to determine the relative roles of the conditioning regimen and the purging method, which would be necessary if one wants the results in first remission to continue to improve. In second and subsequent remissions, however, the prognosis is so dismal that investigations on these patients should reveal any superior treatments readily. Evidence for success of a particular transplant intensification regimen could appear not only as improvements observed in disease-free survival at one year or longer, but also as prolongation of the transplantation remission time relative to the previous remission in a large proportion of patients, i.e., as an "inversion" in remission time. This parameter also would serve to eliminate any bias due to patients who relapsed after a long first remission, who may be expected to have long subsequent remissions. In addition, since treatment-related mortality is around 10% but can be as high as 33%, the relative risk to first remission patients may be too high. The safety of any regimen would best be tested on patients in second or subsequent CR who are at greater risk from their disease.

A number of novel approaches to purging bone marrow have been tried. Most of these are still too early to determine the clinical anti-leukemic effect. However, on the basis of inversion rates and long-term survival, there seems to be promise in AML with ex vivo chemotherapy and in ALL using monoclonal antibody pools. Using combinations of modalities, combinations of drugs ex vivo, or novel ways of separating cells may prove to be even more effective approaches in eradicating leukemia cells. A regimen which can demonstrate both improved "inversion" rates and significant one year disease-free survival in second and subsequent CR can be said to have changed the natural history of the disease. It could then be assumed that it might improve the length of first remission also. Therefore trials in first remission would be justified. If only an improved inversion rate, but not improvement in long-term survival, were to be seen, changes in the conditioning regimen would have to be considered.

With AML, even those patients presenting with the most favorable prognostic signs enjoy no more than 30% long-term disease-free survival with chemotherapy alone (147); therefore, any AML CR1 patient stands to benefit from intensification with ABMT in first remission. A randomized trial may even be necessary to determine relative efficacy of purged and unpurged marrow. With ALL, young patients presenting with WBC less than 10,000/mm^3 and having no extramedullary disease do well with chemotherapy alone; studies in ABMT in the CR1 should concentrate first on patients presenting with at least one of these risk factors. This approach could bring the most effective conditioning and purging methods into use in first remission, and patients with leukemia could hope for curative regimens early in their disease course.

REFERENCES

1 Prentice HG, Grob JP, (1986) Acute lymphoblastic leukaemia in adults. In: Gale RP, Hoffrand AV (eds) Clinics in haematology: acute leukaemia, Vol. 15, No. 3. W. B. Saunders Company: London, Philadelphia, Toronto

2 Gale RP, Foon KA (1986) Acute myeloid leukaemia: Recent advances in therapy. In: Gale RP, Hoffrand AV (eds) Clinics in haematology: acute leukaemia, Vol. 15, No. 3. W. B. Saunders Company: London, Philadelphia, Toronto

3 Gale RP, Champlin RE (1986) Bone marrow transplantation in acute leukaemia. In: Gale RP, Hoffrand AV (eds) Clinics in haematology: acute leukaemia, Vol. 15, No. 3. W. B. Saunders Company: London, Philadelphia, Toronto

4 Gale RP, Foon KA (1986) Acute myelogenous leukemia. In: Gale RP (ed) Leukemia therapy, Blackwell Scientific Publications: Boston, Oxford, London, Edinburgh, Palo Alto, Melbourne

5 Jacobs AD, Gale RP (1986) Acute lymphoblastic leukemia in adults. In: Gale RP (ed) Leukemia therapy, Blackwell Scientific Publications: Boston, Oxford, London Edinburgh, Palo Alto, Melbourne

6 Dicke KA, Spitzer G (1986) Clinical studies of autografting in acute lymphocytic leukaemia. In: Goldstone AH (ed) Clinics in haematology: autologous bone marrow transplantation, Vol. 15, No. 1 W. B. Saunders Company: London, Philadelphia, Toronto

7 Dicke KA, Jagannath S, Spitzer G, McCredie K (1986) A realistic study design to determine the role of autologous bone marrow transplantation in acute leukemia. In: Dicke KA, Spitzer G, Jagannath S (eds) Autologous Bone Marrow Transplantation: Proceedings of the Third International Symposium, The University of Texas M. D. Anderson and Tumor Institute: Houston, Texas (In press)

8 Fefer A (1986) Current status of syngeneic marrow transplantation and its relevance to autografting. In: Goldstone AH (ed) Clinics in haematology: autologous bone marrow transplantation, Vol. 15, No. 1 W. B. Saunders Company: London, Philadelphia, Toronto

9 Le Blanc G, Douay L, Laporte JP, Dominh A, Deloux J, Najman A, Duhamel G, Gorin NC (1986) Evaluation of lymphocyte subsets after autologous bone marrow transplantation with marrow treated by Asta-Z 7557 in acute leukemia: Incidence of the in vitro treatment. Exp Hematol 14:366-371

10 Gorin NC (1985) Autologous bone marrow transplantation for acute leukemia in Europe. In: Dicke KA, Spitzer G, Zander AR (eds) Autologous Bone Marrow Transplantation: Proceedings of the First International Symposium, The University of Texas M. D. Anderson Hospital and Tumor Institute: Houston, Texas

11 Vellekoop L, Jagannath S, Spitzer G, Zander AR, Horwitz LJ, Keating M, McCredie KB, Dicke KA (1986) High-dose cyclophosphamide,

BCNU, and etoposide followed by autologous bone marrow rescue as treatment for adult acute leukemia in relapse. Am J Clin Oncol (CCT)9:307-310

12 Dicke KA, Jagannath S, Estey EH, Horwitz LJ, Spitzer G (1987) Autologous bone marrow transplantation in acute leukemia: The Houston experience. In: Gale RP, Champlin (eds) Progress in bone marrow transplantation. Alan R. Liss, Inc: New York

13 Haas RJ, Netzel B, Kolb HJ, Rodt H, Meyer G, Helmig, Thierfelder, Munchen AK (1985) Autologous bone marrow transplantation in children with recurrent acute lymphoblastic leukemia: Summary of clinical results of the Munich cooperative group. In: Dicke KA, Spitzer G, Zander AR (eds) Autologous Bone Marrow Transplantation: Proceedings of the First International Symposium, The University of Texas M. D. Anderson Hospital and Tumor Institute: Houston, Texas

14 Herve P, Philip T, Flesch M, Rozenbaum A, Plouvier E, Cahn JY, Noir A, Peters A, Des Floris RL (1983) Intensive cytoreductive regimen and autologous bone marrow transplantation in leukemia. Present status and the future: A Review. Eur J Cancer Clin Oncol 19:1043-1052

15 Lowenberg B, Abels J, van Bekkum DW, Dzoljic G, Hagenbeek A, Hendriks WDH, van De Poel J, Sizoo W, Sintnicolaas K, and Wagemaker G (1984) Transplantation of non-purified autologous bone marrow in patients with AML in first remission. Cancer 54:2840-2843

16 Lowenberg B, Abels J, Van Bekkum DW, Dzoljic G, Hagenbeek A, Hendriks WDH, Van De Poel J, Sizoo W, Sintnicolaas K, Wagemaker G (1984) Autologous bone marrow transplantation in patients with AML without tumor cell purging and post transplant chemotherapy. In: Lowenberg B, Hagenbeek A (eds) Minimal residual disease in acute leukemia. Martinus Nijhoff Publishers: Boston, The Hague, Dordrecht, Lancaster

17 Burnett AK, Mackinnon S, Morrison A (1986) Autologous BMT for acute myeloid leukaemia in first remission using unpurged marrow. In: Dicke KA, Spitzer G, Jagannath S (eds) Autologous Bone Marrow Transplantation: Proceedings of The Third International Symposium, The University of Texas M. D. Anderson Hospital and Tumor Institute: Houston, Texas (In press)

18 Burnett AK, Watkins R, Maharaj D, McKinnon S, Tansey P, Alcorn M, Sincer CRJ, McDonald GA (1984) Transplantation of unpurged autologous bone marrow in acute myeloid leukaemia in first remission. Lancet 2:1568-9

19 Burnett AK, Tansey P, Alcorn M, Singer CRJ, McDonald GA, Robertson AG (1984) Autologous bone marrow transplantation in acute myeloid leukemia in first remission. In: Lowenberg B, Hagenbeek A (eds) Minimal residual disease in acute leukemia. Martinus Nijhoff Publishers: Boston, The Hague, Dordrecht, Lancaster

20 Linch DC, Burnett AK (1986) Clinical studies of ABMT in acute myeloid leukaemia. In: Goldstone AH (ed) Clinics in haematology: autologous bone marrow transplantation, Vol. 15, No. 1 W. B. Saunders Company: London, Philadelphia, Toronto

21 Stewart P, Buckner CD, Bensinger W, Appelbaum F, Fefer A, Clift R, Storb R, Sanders J, Meyers J, Hill R, Thomas ED (1985) Autologous marrow transplantation in patients with acute nonlymphocyte leukemia in first remission. Exp Hematology 13:267-272

22 Dicke KA, Spitzer G, Peters L, McCredie KB, Zander AR, Verma DS, Vellekoop L, Hester (1979) Autologous bone marrow transplantation in relapsed adult acute leukaemia. Lancet:i:514-516

23 Vellekoop L, Dicke KA, Zander AR, Spitzer G, Verma DS, Keating MM, McCredie KB (1984) Repeated high dose cyclophosphamide, BCNU and VP-16-213 and autologous bone marrow transplantation in adult leukemia in first remission. Eur J Cancer Clin Oncol 20:593-599

24 Maraninchi D, Mascret B, Gastaut JA, Sebahoun G, Perrimond H, Orsini A, Tubiana N, Novakovitch G, Lejeune C, Baume D, Carcassonne Y (1985) Single or repeated high-dose chemotherapy with melphalan and autologous marrow transplantation in acute leukemias: The Marseilles experience with 31 patients. In: Dicke KA, Spitzer G, Zander AR (eds) Autologous Bone Marrow Transplantation: Proceedings of the First International Symposium, The University of Texas M. D. Anderson Hospital and Tumor Institute: Houston, Texas

25 Goldstone AH, Linch DC, Anderson CC, Jones M, Closs SP, Cawley JC, Richards JDM (1984) Double ablative chemotherapy with autologous marrow rescue in the treatment of acute leukemia. In: Lowenberg B, Hagenbeek A (eds) Minimal residual disease in acute leukemia. Martinus Nijhoff Publishers: Boston, The Hague, Dordrecht, Lancaster

26 Brun del Re, GP (1987) In vivo and in vitro purging of bone marrow in autologous bone marrow transplantation? Abstracts from the First International Workshop On Bone Marrow Purging, Orlando, Florida (In press)

27 Ajani JA, Blaauw AA, Spitzer G, Baker FL, Tomasovic B, Umbach G, Thielvoldt D, Zander AR, Dicke KA (1985) differential cytotoxic activity of chemotherapy agents on colony-forming cells from human tumors and normal bone marrow in vitro. Exp Hematology 13:95-100

28 Rowley SD, Colvin OM, Stuart RK (1985) Human multilineage progenitor cell sensitivity to 4-Hydroperoxycyclophosphamide. Exp Hematology 13:295-298

29 Gordon MY, Goldman JM, Gordon-Smith EC (1985) 4-Hydroperoxycyclophosphamide inhibits proliferation by human granulocyte-macrophage colony-forming cells (GM-CFC) but spares more primitive progenitor cells. Leukemia Research 9:1017-1021

30 Gordon MY, Hibbin JA, Kearney LU, Gordon-Smith EC, Goldman JM (1985) Colony formation by primitive haemopoietic progenitors in cocultures of bone marrow cells and stromal cells. British Journal of Haematology 60:129-136

31 Siena S, Castro-Malaspina H, Gulati SC, Lu L, Colvin MO, Clarkson BD, O'Reilly RJ, Moore MAS (1985) Effects of in vitro purging with 4-Hydroperoxycyclophosphamide on the hematopoietic and microenvironmental elements of human bone marrow. Blood 65:655-662

32 Brock N (1983) Autologous stem cell grafting in acute myeloid leukaemia: Technical approach of marrow incubation in vitro with pharmacological agents (prerequisite for clinical applications). British Journal of Haematology 53:683-690

33 Kaizer H, Stuart RK, Brookmeyer R, Beschorner WE, Braine HG, Burns BW, Fuller DJ, Korbling M, Mangan KF, Saral R, Sensenbrenner L, Shadduck RK, Shende AC, Tutschka PJ, Yeager AM, Zinkham WH, Colvin OM, Santos GW (1985) Autologous bone marrow transplantation in acute leukemia: A phase I study of in vitro treatment of marrow with 4-hydroperoxycyclophosphamide to purge tumor cells. Blood 65:1504-1510

34 Zuehlsdorf M, Rowley S, Yeager A, Davis J, Jones R, Braine H, Colvin M, Saral R, Sensenbrenner L, Santos G (1987) Evaluation of parameters for purging of autologous bone marrow grafts with 4-hydroperoxycyclophosphamide. Abstracts from the First International Workshop On Bone Marrow Purging, Orlando, Florida (In press)

35 Uckun FM, Ramakrishnan S, Haag D, Houston LL (1985) Ex vivo elimination of lymphoblastic leukemia cells from human marrow by mafosfamid. Leukemia Research 9:83-95

36 Douay L, Gorin NC, Laporte JP, Lopez M, Najman A, Duhamel G (1984) Asta-Z 7557 (INN mafosfamide) for the in vitro treatment of human leukemic bone marrows. Investigational New Drugs 2:187-190

37 Auber M, Horwitz LJ, Spitzer G, Khorana S, Jagannath S, McCredie K, Dicke KA (1987) 4-Hydroperoxycyclophosphamide (4HC) and vincristine as ex vivo bone marrow treatment for acute leukemia in second remission. Abstracts from the First International Workshop On Bone Marrow Purging, Orlando, Florida (In press)

38 Horwitz LJ, Auber ML, Khorana S, Jagannath S, Dicke KA (1986) 4-hydroperoxyclyclophosphamide and vincristine as ex vivo bone marrow treatment for acute leukemia in second remission. In: Dicke KA, Spitzer, Jagannath S (eds) Autologous Bone Marrow Transplantation: Proceedings of the Third International Symposium, The University of Texas M. D. Anderson Hospital and Tumor Institute: Houston, Texas (In press)

39 Beranek JT, Ohnuma T, Takahashi I, Minowada J, Holland JF (1984) Chemotherapeutic sensitivity of acute lymphoblastic leukemia cells in culture: Correlation with clinical efficacy on donor patients. Cancer Drug Delivery 1:307-17

40 Smith SD, Trueworthy RC, Kisker SE, Noller LG, Lowman JT (1983) In vitro sensitivity of normal granulocytic and lymphoma colonies to vinca alkaloids. Cancer 51:417-422

41 Ciobanu N, Paietta E, Andreeff M, Papenhausen P, Wiernik PH (1986) Etoposide as an in vitro purging agent for the treatment of acute leukemias and lymphomas in conjunction with autologous bone marrow transplantation. Exp. Hematol. 14:626-635

42 Stiff PJ, Koester AR, Fassero JJ (1985) Chemopurification of bone marrow: Initial experience using combinations. Exp Hematology 13:Suppl:16:190

43 Auber ML, Horwitz LJ, Blaauw A, Khorana S, Tucker S, Woods T, Warmuth M, Dicke KA, Spitzer G (1987) Evaluation of drugs for elimination of leukemic cells from the bone marrow of patients with acute leukemia. (Manuscript submitted)

44 Janowska-Wieczorek A, Tupas J, Janmohamed N, McGann LE, Selner M, Lynch MA, Cass CE (1987) Investigation of modulation of resistance to vincristine by verapamil in clonogenic leukemic cell lines. Abstracts from the First International Workshop On Bone Marrow Purging, Orlando, Florida (In press)

45 Russell NH, Carron J, Hoffbrand AV, Bellingham AJ (1985) The relative sensitivity of peripheral blood T-lymphocyte colony forming cells and bone marrow CFU-GM to deoxyadenosine and 2 'deoxycoformycin. Leukemia Research 9:315-319

46 Epstein J, Bealmear PM, Kennedy DW, Herrmann MJ, Islam A, Wiedl SC (1986) Prevention of graft-versus-host disease in allogeneic bone marrow transplantation by pretreatment with 2'-deoxycoformycin. Exp Hematol 14:845-849

47 de Jong JP, Nikkels PGJ, Brockbank KGM, Ploemacher RE, Voerman JS (1985) Comparative in vitro effects of cyclophos-

phamide derivatives on murine bone marrow-derived stromal and hematopoietic progenitor cell classes. Cancer Research 45:4001-4005

48 Sharkis SJ, Santos GW, Colvin M (1980) Elimination of acute myelogenous leukemic cells from marrow and tumor suspensions in the rate with 4-hydroperoxyclophosphamide. Blood 55:521-3

49 Gustavsson A, Olofsson T (1984) Prediction of response to chemotherapy in acute leukemia by in vitro drug sensitivity testing on leukemic stem cells. Cancer Research 44:4648-4652

50 Reading CL (1982) Theory and methods for immunization in culture and moab production. J Immunol Methods 53:261-291

51 Nicolson GL, Neri A, Reading CL, Miner KM (1981) In vivo and in vitro selection of experimental metastatic variants of rodent melanoma, mammary carcinoma and lymphosarcoma. In: Hellman Kd, Hilgard, Eccles S (eds) Developments in oncology, A. Martinus and Nijhoff: The Hague

52 Bernard A, Boumsell L, Hill C (1984) Joint report of the First International workshop on human leucocyte differentiation antigens by the investigators of the participating laboratories. In: Bernard A, Boumsell L, Dausset J, Milstein C, Schlossman SF (eds) Leukocyte typing: human leukocyte differentiation antigens detected by monoclonal antibodies, Springer-Verlag: Berlin

53 Haynes BF (1986) Summary of T-cell studies performed during the second international workshop and conference on human leukocyte differentiation antigens. In: Reinherz EL, Haynes BF, Nadler LM, Bernstein ID (eds) Leukocyte Typing II, Vol 1, Springer-Verlag: New York

54 Nadler LM (1986) B cell/leukemia panel workshop: summary and comments. In: Reinherz EL, Haynes BF, Nadler LM, Bernstein ID (eds) Leukocyte Typing II, Vol 2, Springer-Verlag: New York

55 Bernstein ID, Self S (1986) Joint report on the myeloid section of the second international workshop on human leukocyte differentiation antigens. In: Reinherz EL, Haynes BF, Nadler LM, Bernstein ID (eds) Leukocyte Typing II, Vol 3, Springer-Verlag: New York

56 Macintyre EA (1986) The use of monoclonal antibodies for purging autologous bone marrow in the lymphoid malignancies. In: Goldstone AH (ed) Clinics in haematology: autologous bone marrow transplantation, Vol. 15, No. 1 W. B. Saunders Company: London, Philadelphia, Toronto

57 Jansen J, Falkenburg JHF, Stepan DF, LeBien TW (1984) Removal of neoplastic cells from autologous bone marrow grafts with monoclonal antibodies. Semin Hematol 21:164-181

58 Reading CL (1984) Carbohydrate structure, biological recognition, and immune function. In: Ivatt RJ (ed) The biology of glycoproteins. Plenum Press: New York

59 Boyle MDP, Gee AP (1987) Limitations to the use of antibody and complement for purging cells from bone marrow. Abstracts from the First International Workshop On Bone Marrow Purging, Orlando, Florida (In press)

60 Gee AP, Bruce KM, Morris TD, Boyle MDP (1985) Evidence for an anticomplementary factor associated with human bone marrow cells. JNCI. 75:441-445

61 Weiler JM, Ballas ZK, Needleman BW, Hobbs MV, Feldbush TL (1982) Complement fragments suppress lymphocyte immune responses. Immunol Today 3:238-243

62 Gorb JP, Campana D, Timms A, Coustan-Smith E, Janossy G, Pretince HG (1986) Immunologic purging in autologous bone marrow transplantation: relevance at target antigen density on blasts to the efficiency of complement-mediated cytolysis. J Cell Biochem Suppl 10D:217, (ABSTR)

63 Ball ED, Kadushin JM, Schacter B, Fanger MW (1982) Studies on the ability of monoclonal antibodies to selectively mediate complement-dependent cytotoxicity of human myelogenous leukemia blast cells. J Immunol 128:1476-1481

64 De Fabritiis P, Bregni M, Lipton J, Reynolds C, Nadler L, Ritz J, Bast RC Jr. (1986) Antigenic heterogeneity among Burkitt's lymphoma cells surviving treatment with monoclonal antibody and complement. Leukemia Research 10:35-42

65 Gee AP, Bruce KM, van Hilten J, Siden EJ, Braylan RC, Bauer PC, Boyle MDP (1987) Selective loss of expression of a tumor-associated antigen on a human leukemic cell line induced by treatment with monoclonal antibody and complement. JNCI 781:29-35

66 Alonso MC, Solana R, Torres A, Ramirez R, Navarrete C, Pena Y, Festenstein H (1986) Study of the antigenic profile of normal myelo-monocytic progenitors and leukemic cell lines using monoclonal antibodies. In: Reinherz EL, Haynes BF, Nadler LM, Bernstein ID (eds) Leukocyte typing II": human myeloid and hematopoietic cells, Springer-Verlag: New York

67 Janowska-Wieczorek A, Mannoni PJ, Krantz MJ, Turner AR, Turc JM (1986) Inhibition of CFU-GM, BFU-E, and CFU-GEMM colony formation by monoclonal antibodies selected from the myeloid panel. In: "Reinherz EL, Haynes BF, Nadler LM, Bernstein ID (eds) Leukocyte typing II: human myeloid and hematopoietic cells, Springer-Verlag: New York

68 Peschel C, Knowalinka G, Geisler D, Majdic O, Stockinger H, Braunsteiner H, Knapp W (1985) Studies on differentiation of committed hematopoietic progenitor cells with monoclonal antibodies directed aginst myeloid differentiation antigens. Exp Hematol 13:1211-1216

69 Mannoni P, Janowska-Wieczorek A, Fromont P, Weiblen B, Turner AR, Turc JM (1984) Human myeloid differentiation studied by monoclonal antibodies. In: Bernard A, Boumsell L, Dausset J, Milstein C, Schlossman SF (eds) Leukocyte typing: human leukocyte differentiation antigens detected by monoclonal antibodies, Springer-Verlag: New York

70 Peschel C, Konwalinka G, Geissler D, Grunwald K, Liszka K, Stockinger H, Majdic O, Braunsteiner H, Knapp W (1986) Reactivity of anti-myeloid monoclonal antibodies at committed hematopoietic precursor cells. In: Reinherz EL, Haynes BF, Nadler LM, Bernstein D (eds) Leukocyte typing II: human myeloid and hematopoietic cells, Springer-Verlag: New York

71 Andrews RG, Brentnall TA, Torok-Storb B, Bernstein ID (1984) Stages of myeloid differentiation identified by monoclonal antibodies. In: Bernard A, Boumsell L, Dausset J, Milstein C, Schlossman SF (eds), Leukocyte typing: human leukocyte differentiation antigens detected by monoclonal antibodies, Springer-Verlag: New York

72 Andrews RG, Torok-Storb B, Bernstein ID (1983) Myeloid associated differentiation antigens on stem cells and their progeny identified by monoclonal antibodies. Blood 62:124-132

73 Ball ED, Graziano RF, Fanger MW (1983) A unique antigen expressed on myeloid cells and acute leukemia blast cells defined by a monoclonal antibody. J Immunol 13:2937-2941

74 Greenberger JS, Rothstein L, DeFabritiis P, Bregni M, Bast R Jr., Ritz J, Nadler LM, Lipton JM, Sakakeeny MA (1985) Effects of monoclonal antibody and complement treatment of human marrow on hematopoiesis in continuous bone marrow culture. Cancer Research 45:758-767

75 Levitt L, Kipps TJ, Engleman EG, Greenberg PL (1985) Human bone marrow and peripheral blood T lymphocyte depletion: efficacy and effects of both T cells and monocytes on growth of hematopoietic progenitors. Blood 65:663-679

76 LeBien TW, Stepan DE, Bartholomew RM, Stong RC, Anderson JM (1985) Utilization of a colony assay to assess the variables influencing elilmination of leukemic cells from human bone marrow with monoclonal antibodies an complement. Blood 65:945-950

77 Vitetta ES, Uhr JW (1984) The use of immunotoxins to kill neoplastic B cells. In: Lowenberg B, Hagenbeek A (eds) Minimal residual disease in acute leukemia. Martinus Nijhoff Publishers: Boston, The Hague, Dordrecht, Lancaster

78 Jansen FK, Blythman HE, Bourrie B, Canat X, Carayon P, Casellas P, Carriere D, Deroco JM, Dussossoy D, Gros O, Gros P, Laurent G, Richer G, Vidal H (1987) Immunotoxins with therapeutic potential against cancer. Abstracts of the Satellite Symposium of the 18th International Leucocyte Culture Conference: Clinical Applications of Anti-Leucocyte Monoclonal Antibodies, La Grande Motte, France (In press)

79 Gorin NC, Douay L, Laporte JP, Lopez M, Zittoun R, Rio B, David R, Stachowiak J, Janssen J, Cazellas P, Poncelet P, Liance MC, Voisin GA, Salmon C, LeBlanc G, Delous J, Najman A, Duhamel G (1985) Autologous bone marrow transplantation with marrow decontaminated by immunotoxin T 101 in the treatment of leukemia and lymphoma: first clinical observations. Cancer Treatment Reports 69:953-959

80 Uckun FM, Ramakrishnan S, Houston LL (1985) Increased efficiency in selective elimination of leukemia cells by a combination of a stable derivative of cyclophosphamide and a human B-cell-specific immunotoxin containing pokeweek antiviral protein. Cancer Research 45:69-75

81 Janssen WE, Lee C, Bruce KM, Gee AP (1987) Low antigen density leukemia cells: Selection and resistance to antibody mediated marrow purging. Abstracts from the First International Workshop On Bone Marrow Purging, Orlando, Florida (In press)

82 Ugelstad J, Ellingsen T, Berge A (1987) Magnetic polymer particles for cell separation. Abstracts from the First International Workshop On Bone Marrow Purging, Orlando, Florida (In press)

83 Clavell LA, Lipton JM, Bast RC, Kudisch M, Pesando J, Schlossman SF, Ritz J (1981) Absence at common ALL antigen on normal bipotent myeloid, erythroid, and granulocyte progenitors. Blood 58:333-336

84 Kemshead JT, Gibson FM (1987) Monoclonal antibodies and magnetic microspheres used for the depletion of tumor cells from bone marrow. Abstracts from the First International Workshop On Bone Marrow Purging, Orlando, Florida (In press)

85 Philip T, Favrot M, Philip I (1987) Complement and magnetic purging: A comparison with the burkitt lymphoma model. Abstracts from the First International Workshop On Bone Marrow Purging, Orlando, Florida (In press)

86 Combaret V, Poncelet P, Philip T, Favrot MC (1987) Comparison of the immunomagnetic

depletion and the complement lysis to eliminate burkitt's cells from excess bone marrow. Abstracts of the Satellite Symposium of the 18th International Leucocyte Culture Conference: Clinical Applications of Anti-Leucocyte Monoclonal Antibodies, La Grande Motte, France (In press)

87 Poynton CH, Dicke KA, Culbert S, Frankel LS, Jagannath S, Reading CL (1983) Immunomagnetic removal of calla positive cells from human bone marrow. Lancet:i:524-526

88 Dicke KA, Poynton CH, Reading CL (1984) Elimination of leukemic cells from remission marrow suspensions by an immunomagnetic procedure. In: Lowenberg B, Hagenbeek A (eds) Minimal residual disease in acute leukemia. Martinus Nijhoff Publishers: Boston, The Hague, Dordrecht, Lancaster

89 Poynton CH, Reading CL, Dicke KA (1985) Colloidal immunomagnetic fluids for cell separation. In: Dicke KA, Spitzer G, Zander AR (eds) Autologous Bone Marrow Transplantation: Proceedings of the First International Symposium, The University of Texas M. D. Anderson Hospital and Tumor Institute: Houston, Texas

90 Hirn J, Brailly H, Maranchini D, Manoni P, Mawas C, Delaage M (1987) Elimination of leukemic cells from human bone marrow using floating immunobeads. Abstracts of the Satellite Symposium of the 18th International Leucocyte Culture Conference: Clinical Applications of Anti-Leucocyte Monoclonal Antibodies, La Grande Motte, France (In press)

91 Lansdorp PM, Thomas TE (1987) Tetramolecular complexes of monoclonal antibodies for antigen-specific cell separation procedures. Abstracts from the First International Workshop On Bone Marrow Purging, Orlando, Florida (In press)

92 Lansdorp PM, Aalberse RC, Bos R, Schutter WG, Van Bruggen EFJ (1986) Cyclic tetramolecular complexes of monoclonal antibodies: a new type of cross-linking reagent. Eur. J. Immunol. 16:679-683

93 Rieber EP, Wilhelm M, Pechumer H, Haas R, Reiter C, Rank G, Riethmuller G (1987) Direct monoclonal antibody rosetting technique (Dart): An effective method for bone marrow purging. Abstracts from the First International Workshop On Bone Marrow Purging, Orlando, Florida (In press)

94 Slaper-Cortenbach ICM, Admiraal LG, von dem Borne AEGK, van Leeuwen EF, Engelfriet CP, Tetteroo PAT (1987) A new immunorosette technique for the depletion of leukemic cells from autologous bone marrow grafts. Abstracts from the First International Workshop On Bone Marrow Purging, Orlando, Florida (In press)

95 Yang C-Z , Zhang C, Zhu Z-P, Sun T-Z (1987) Monoclonal antibody-mitomycin conjugate. Abstracts of the Satellite Symposium of the 18th International Leucocyte Culture Conference: Clinical Applications of Anti-Leucocyte Monoclonal Antibodies, La Grande Motte, France (In press)

96 Spitzer G, Verma DS, Fisher R, Zander AR, Vellekoop L, Litam J, McCredie KB and Dicke KA (1980) The myeloid progenitor cell—its value in predicting hematopoietic recovery after autologous bone marrow transplantation. Blood 55:317-23

97 Korbling M, Hess AD, Tutschka PJ, Kaizer H, Colvin MO, Santos GW (1982) 4-hydroperoxycyclophosphamide a model for eliminating residual human tumor cells and T-lymphocytes from the bone marrow graft. British Journal of Haematology 52:89-96

98 Yeager AM, Kaizer H, Colvin OM, Rowley SD, Braine HG, Stuart RK, Saral R, Santos GW (1986) Autologous bone marrow transplantation in acute nonlymphocytic leukemia using marrow treated with 4-hydroperoxycyclophosphamide. In: Dicke KA, Spitzer G, Jagannath S (eds) Autologous Bone Marrow Transplantation: Proceedings of The Third International Symposium, The University of Texas M. D. Anderson Hospital and Tumor Institute: Houston, Texas (In press)

99 Yeager AM, Kaizer H, Braine HG, Colvin M, Rowley SD, Saral R, Fuller DJ, Ambinder RF, Burns WH, May S, Sensenbrenner L, Stuart RK, Vogelsang GB, Wingard JR, Santos GW (1986) Autologous bone marrow transplantation in acute nonlymphocytic leukemia , a study of ex vivo marrow treatment with 4-hydroperoxycyclophosphamide. In: Hagenbeek A, Lowenberg B, (eds) Minimal residual disease in acute leukemia 1986. Martinus Nijhoff Publishers: Dordrecht, Boston, Lancaster

100 Yeager AM, Wiley JM, Jones R, Rowley SD, Zuehlsdorf M, Colvin OM, Santos GW (1987) Pharmacologic treatment of bone marrow to eliminate clonogenic tumor cells: Laboratory and clinical studies. Abstracts from the First International Workshop On Bone Marrow Purging, Orlando, Florida (In press)

101 Herve P, Cahn JY, Plouvier E, Flesch M, Rozenbaum A, Tamayo E, Noir A, Peters A (1984) Autologous bone marrow transplantation in acute leukemia using marrow cells chemopurified with a cyclophosphamide derivative (Asta-Z 7557) clinical results. Exp Hematology 12, Supp 15:133-134

102 LaPorte JP, Gorin NC, Douay L, Lopez M, Salmon CH, Najman A, Duhamel G (1984) Autologous bone marrow transplantation (ABMT) with marrow purged by Asta-Z 7557, as consolidation therapy for acute leukemias in first remission. Exp Hematology 12, Supp 15:132

103 Douay L, Laporte JP, Mary JY, Lopez M, Najman A, Gorin NC (1986) Chemopurging of

autologous bone marrow with mafosfamide (Asta-Z 7557) in adult leukemia. In: Dicke KA, Spitzer G, Jagannath S, (eds) Autologous Bone Marrow Transplantation: Proceedings of The Third International Symposium, The University of Texas M. D. Anderson Hospital and Tumor Institute: Houston, Texas (In press)

104 Gorin NC, Laporte JP, Douay L, Lopez M, Stachowiak J, Aegerter P, Deloux J, Marin JL, Duhamel G, Laugier A, Salmon Ch Najman A (1986) Autologous bone marrow transplantation using marrow incubated with Asta-Z 7557 in adult acute leukemia in remission: The experience of the Paris Saint Antoine transplant team on 57 patients. In: Dicke KA, Spitzer G, Jagannath S (eds) Autologous Bone Marrow Transplantation: Proceedings of The Third International Symposium, The University of Texas M. D. Anderson Hospital and Tumor Institute: Houston, Texas (In press)

105 Rizzoli V, Mangoni L, Degliantoni G, Porcellini A, Carella AM, Allessandrino EP, Aglietta M, Torlontano G, Coleselli P, Mozzana A, Madon E (1986) Autologous bone marrow transplantation for acute lymphocytic leukemia: Mafosfamide Italian Cooperative Group. In: Dicke KA, Spitzer G, Jagannath S (eds) Autologous Bone Marrow Transplantation: Proceedings of The Third International Symposium, The University of Texas M. D. Anderson Hospital and Tumor Institute: Houston, Texas (In press)

106 Gorin NC, Douay L, Laporte JP, Lopez M, Mary JY, Najman A, Salmon C, Aegerter P, Stachowiak J, David R, Pene F, Kantor G, Deloux J, Duhamel E, van den Akker J, Gerota J, Parlier Y, Duhamel G (1986) Autologous bone marrow transplantation using marrow incubated with Asta-Z 7557 in adult acute leukemia. Blood 67:1367-1376

107 Chang J, Morgenstern G, Deakin D, Testa NG, Coutinho L, Scarffe JH, Harrison C, Dexter TM (1986) Reconstitution of haemopoietic system with autologous marrow taken during relapse of acute myeloblastic leukaemia and grown in long-term culture. Lancet 1:294-295.

108 Ritz J, Bast RC Jr, Clavell LA, Hercend T, Sallan SE, Lipton JM,Feeney M, Nathan DG, Schlossman SF (1982) Autologous bone marrow transplantation in calla-positive acute lymphoblastic leukaemia after in-vitro treatment with j5 monoclonal antibody and complement. Lancet:ii:60-62

109 Sallan SE, Bast RC, Lipton JM, Ritz J (1984) Autologous bone marrow transplantation in CALLA positive acute lymphoblastic leukemia. In: Lowenberg B, Hagenbeek A (eds) Minimal residual disease in acute leukemia. Martinus Nijhoff Publishers: Boston, The Hague, Dordrecht, Lancaster

110 Bast Jr RC, Sallan SE, Reynolds C, Lipton J, Ritz J (1985) Autologous bone marrow transplantation for calla-positive acute lymphoblastic leukemia: An update. In: Dicke KA, Spitzer G, Zander AR (eds) Autologous Bone Marrow Transplantation: Proceedings of the First International Symposium, The University of Texas M. D. Anderson Hospital and Tumor Institute: Houston, Texas

111 Takvorian T, Sallan S, Ritz J (1986) Monoclonal antibody purged autologous bone marrow transplantation for relapsed non T-cell acute lymphoblastic leukemia. In: Hagenbeek A, Lowenberg B, (eds) Minimal residual disease in acute leukemia 1986. Martinus Nijhoff Publishers: Dordrecht, Boston, Lancaster

112 Lowenberg B, Bauman J (1984) AML cell heterogeneity. Implications for leukemia cell separation from autologous bone marrow grafts. In: Lowenberg B, Hagenbeek A (eds) Minimal residual disease in acute leukemia. Martinus Nijhoff Publishers: Boston, The Hague, Dordrecht, Lancaster

113 Kvalheim G, Funderud S, Fodstad O, Dorken B, Sorensen O, Nustad K, Ugelstad J, Pihl A (1987) An efficient procedure for immunomagnetic purgin of B-lymphoma cells from human bone marrow. Abstracts from the First International Workshop On Bone Marrow Purging, Orlando, Florida (In press)

114 Ramsay N, LeBien T, Nesbit M, McGlave P, Weisdorf D, Kenyon P, Hurd D, Goldman A, Kim T, Kersey J (1985) Autologous bone marrow transplantation for patients with acute lymphoblastic leukemia in second or subsequent remission: Results of bone marrow treated with monoclonal antibodies BA-1, BA-2, and BA-3 plus complement. Blood 66:508-513

115 Kersey J, LeBien T, Vallera D, Filipovich A, McGlave P, Kim T, Ramsay N (1986) Allogeneic and autologous marrow transplantation: Ex vivo purging with monoclonal antibody of immunotoxins to remove leukemic cells or to prevent graft versus host disease. In: Hagenbeek A, Lowenberg B (eds) Minimal residual disease in acute leukemia 1986. Martinus Nijhoff Publishers: Dordrecht, Boston, Lancaster

116 Nakamura H, Shibata, Masaoka T (1987) Autologous bone marrow transplantation utilizing monoclonal antibodies BA-1, BA-2, BA-3 plus complement: preliminary results. Abstracts from the First International Workshop On Bone Marrow Purging, Orlando, Florida (In press)

117 Campana D, Janossy G, Bouloux C (1987) MAbs for purging in bone marrow transplantation (BMT): A review. Abstracts of the Satellite Symposium of the 18th International Leucocyte Culture Conference: Clinical Applications of Anti-Leucocyte Monoclonal Antibodies, La Grande Motte, France (In press)

118 Wijdenes J, Herve P, Clement C, Lamy B, Peters A (1987) Monoclonal antibodies suitable for phenotyping and bone marrow purging in non-T acute lymphoblastic leukemia. Abstracts of the Satellite Symposium of the 18th International Leucocyte Culture Conference: Clinical Applications of Anti-Leucocyte Monoclonal Antibodies, La Grande Motte, France (In press)

119 Kersey JH, Vallera D, Ramsay N, Filipovich LF, Stong R, Lebien T, Youle R, Neville D, Beverley P (1984) Monoclonal antibodies for purging bone marrow of acute lymphoblastic leukemia or graft versus host producing cells: antibody plus complement or immunotoxins. In: Lowenberg B, Hagenbeek A (eds) Minimal residual disease in acute leukemia. Martinus Nijhoff Publishers: Boston, The Hague, Dordrecht, Lancaster

120 Reinherz EL, Geha R, Rappeport Jm, Wilson M, Penta AC, Hussey RE, Fitzgerald KA, Daley JF, Levine H, Rosen FS, Schlossman SF (1982) Reconstitution after transplantation with T-lymphocyte-depleted HLA haplotype-mismatched bone marrow for severe combined immunodeficiency. Proc Natl Acad Sci USA, 79:6047-6051

121 Mitsuyasu RT, Champlin RE, Ho WG, Winston D, Feig S, Wells J, Terasaki P, Billing R, Weaver M, Gale RP (1985) Prospective randomized controlled trial of ex vivo treatment of donor bone marrow with monoclonal antibodies anti-T cell antibody and complement for prevention of graft-versus host disease: a preliminary report. Transplant Proc 17:482-485

122 Herve P, Racadot E, Flesch M, Cahn JY, Plouvier E, Rozenbaum A, Lamy B, Noir A, Leconte des Floris R, Peters A (1984) T-cell depletion using Pan-T monoclonal antibodies combination and complement mediated cytolysis for prevention of acute graft-vs-host disease. Exp Hematol 12:59-60

123 Herve P, Cahn JY, Racadot E, Plouvier E, Flesch M, Lamy B, Rozenbaum A (1984) Prevention of acute graft-versus-host disease by removing T-cells in donor marrow using pan-T monoclonal antibodies and complement: pilot study in 10 patients. Exp Hematol 12:412 (ABSTR)

124 Trigg ME, Bozdech MJ, Sondel PM, Billing R, Finaly JL, Peterson AD, Stuiber M, Hong R (1984) Exp. Hematol. 12:412 (ABSTR)

125 Filipovich AH, Vallera DA, Youle RJ, Stong RC, Neville DM, Hersey JH (1985) Marrow purging with immunotoxins in allogeneic and autologous bone marrow transplantation: pilot clinical studies. In: Dicke KA, Spitzer, Zander AR (eds) Autologous Bone Marrow Transplantation: Proceedings of the First International Symposium, The University of Texas M. D. Anderson Hospital and Tumor Institute: Houston, Texas

126 Kaizer H, Levy R, Santos GW (1982) Autologous bone marrow transplantation in T-cell malignancies: use of in vitro monoclonal antibodies treatment of remission marrow to eliminate tumor cells. J Cell Biochem Suppl 6:41

127 Sabbath KD, Ball ED, Larcom P, Davis RB, Griffin JD (1985) Heterogeneity of clonogenic cells in acute myeloblastic leukemia. J Clin Invest 75:746-753

128 Robak T, Nolasco I, Hibbin J, Goldman JM (1985) Antigenic characteristics of circulating CFU-GM in chronic granulocytic leukaemia resemble those of CFU-GM in normal marrow and differ from those in normal blood. Leukemia Research 9:1023-1029

129 Pessano S, Palumbo A, Ferrero D, Pagliardi GL, Bottero L, Lai SK, Meo P, Carter G, Hubbell H, Lange G, Rovera G (1984) Subpopulation heterogeneity in human AML determined by monoclonal antibodies. Blood 64:275-281

130 Ferrero D, Gabbianelli M, Peschle C, Lange B, Rovera G (1985) Surface phenotypes of human hematopoietic progenitor cells defined by monoclonal antibodies. Blood 66:496-502

131 Fitchen JH, LeFevre C, Ferrone S, Cline MJ (1982) Expression of Ia-like and HLA-A, B antigens on human multipotential hematopoietic progenitor cells. Blood 59:188-190

132 Maraninchi D, Mawas C, Mascret B, Sebahoun G, Gastaut JA, Tublana N, Perrimond H, Schavennec J, Novakovitch G, Carcassonne Y (1985) In vitro marrow purging with anti-DR monoclonal antibodies and complement in high dose risk ALL: Preclinical studies and preliminary clinical experience. Exp Hematol (Suppl 17):13:28-29

133 Lange B, Ferrero D, Pessano S, Hubbell H, Palumbo SKL, Rovera G (1984) Discrimination between normal hematopoietic stem cells and myeloid leukemia cells using monoclonal antibodies. In: Lowenberg B, Hagenbeek A (eds) Minimal residual disease in acute leukemia. Martinus Nijhoff Publishers: Boston, The Hague, Dordrecht, Lancaster

134 Ball ED, Cornwell GG III, Mills LE, McMillan R, Miller W, Thompson LF (1986) A phase I/II trial of autologous bone marrow transplantation in patients with AML using marrow treated with anti-myeloid monoclonal antibodies and complement. In: Dicke KA, Spitzer G, Jagannath S (eds) Autologous Bone Marrow Transplantation: Proceedings of The Third International Symposium, The University of Texas M. D. Anderson Hospital and Tumor Institute: Houston, Texas (In press)

135 Ball ED, Thompson LF, Cornwell GG, Mills LE, Coughlin CT, Beck JR, Miller W, McMillan R (1987) Autologous bone marrow transplantation with monoclonal antibody-

treated marrow for patients with AML in remission: An update. Abstracts of the Satellite Symposium of the 18th International Leucocyte Culture Conference: Clinical Applications of Anti-Leucocyte Monoclonal Antibodies, La Grande Motte, France (In press)

136 Reisner Y, Kapoor N, O'Reilly RJ, Good RA (1980) Allogeneic bone marrow transplantation using stem cells fractionated by lectins: VI, in vitro analysis of human and monkey bone marrow cells fractionated by sheep red blood cells and soybean agglutinin. Lancet ii:1320-1323

137 Reisner Y, Kapoor N, Kirpatrick D, Pollack MS, Dupont B, Good RA, O'Reilly RJ (1981) Transplantation for acute leukaemia with HLA-A and B nonidentical parental marrow cells fractionated with soybean agglutinin and sheep red blood cells. Lancet ii:327-331

138 Reisner Y, Kapoor N, Kirpatrick D, Pollack MS, Cunningham-Rundles S, Dupont B, Hodes MZ, Good RA, O'Reilly RJ (1983) Transplantation for severe combined immunodeficiency with HLA-A, B, D, DR incompatible parental marrow cells fractionated by soybean agglutinin and sheep red blood cells. Blood 61:341-348

139 Friedrich W, Goldmann SF, Vetter U, Fliedner TM, Heymer B, Peter HH, Reisner Y, Kleihauer E (1984) Immunoreconstitution in severe combined immunodeficiency after transplantation of HLA-haploidentical, T-cell depleted bone marrow. Lancet i:761-764

140 Glasser L, Somberg LB, Vogler WR (1984) Purging murine leukemic marrow with alkyl-lysophospholipids. Blood 64:1288-1291

141 Okamoto S, Olson AC, Vogler WR, Winton EF (1987) Purging leukemic cells from simulated human remission marrow with alkyl-lysophospholipid. Blood 69:1381-1387

142 Okamoto S, Olson AC, Vogler WR (1987) Preclinical study for purging leukemic cells by ether lipids. Abstracts from the First International Workshop On Bone Marrow Purging, Orlando, Florida (In press)

143 Sieber F (1987) Marrow purging by merocyanine 540-mediated photolysis. Abstracts from the First International Workshop On Bone Marrow Purging, Orlando, Florida (In press)

144 Grygar G, Bruchelt G, Wolfart A, Handgretinger R, Niethammer D, Treuner J (1987) The efficiency of different reactive oxygen compounds for bone marrow purging from neuroblastoma cells. Abstracts from the First International Workshop On Bone Marrow Purging, Orlando, Florida (In press)

145 Cass CE, Peteya DJ, Lynch MA, Tupas J, Janmohamed N, Janowska-Wieczorek A (1987) Differential sensitivity of leukemic cell lines to nitrobenzylthioinosine. Abstracts from the First International Workshop On Bone Marrow Purging, Orlando, Florida (In press)

146 Uckun FM, Stong RC, Youle RJ, Vallera DA (1985) Combined ex=vivo treatment with immunotoxins and mafosfamid: A novel immunochemotherapeutic approach for elimination of neoplastic T cells from autologous marrow grafts. Journal of Immunology 134:3504-15

147 Keating MJ (1984) Factors influencing disease free interval after achieving complete remission in acute leukemia. In: Lowenberg B, Hagenbeek A (eds) Minimal residual disease in acute leukemia. Martinus Nijhoff Publishers: Boston, The Hague, Dordrecht, Lancaster

IV. Autologous and Allogenic Marrow Transplants in Leukemia and Lymphoma (Session A): G.W. Santos and J. Goldman, Chairpersons

11: Allogeneic and Autologous Marrow Transplants in Acute Nonlymphoblastic Leukemia (ANLL)

G.W. Santos, A.M. Yeager, R. Saral, W.H. Burns, J.R. Wingard, R. Jones, R.F. Ambinder, S.D. Rowley, W.S. May, G.B. Vogelsang, A.D. Donnenberg, W.E. Beschorner, J.E. Wagner, Jr., and A.D. Hess

A number of reports and reviews have presented the rationale, history, and results of bone marrow transplantation in the acute leukemias and lymphomas (1-4). Problems with marrow transplantation such as leukemia relapse, graft-versus-host disease (GVHD) and viral infections have been identified and solutions to these problems are being actively pursued in many centers around the world.

Below we will attempt to summarize our experience with allogeneic and autologous bone marrow transplants in acute non-lymphoblastic leukemia (ANLL) and summarize the current status of some of the remaining problems, ongoing studies designed to remedy some of them and what might be accomplished in the future.

ALLOGENEIC TRANSPLANTATION IN ANLL

We previously reported our initial results of HLA identical marrow transplantation in ANLL following preparation with busulfan (BU) and CY (5). As of June 2, 1987 we have transplanted a total of 99 patients, 48 in first remission, 28 in second remission, 2 in third remission, and 21 in early relapse (ER) (less than 50% tumor cells in the marrow) after their 1-3 remission. The results are found in Table 1.

Eight patients survive free of disease for less than 1 year; 7, between 1-2 years; 11, between 2-5 years; and 11, 5 to greater than 8 years following transplantation. Of the 11 relapses 6 occurred in the first 6 months, 4 between 1-2 years and 1 at 5 years. Three of these survive for 268, 288, and 296 days, one in remission after a second transplant.

Table 2 examines the effect of age of recipients at transplantation.

Table 3 compares patients transplanted in first remission versus in subsequent remission on early relapse.

Twelve patients were transplanted after preparation with CY (50 mg/kg i.v. daily x 4) followed by TBI 300 rad/day x 4 with lung shielding for the third dose. Except for two patients free of CNS leukemia in first remission who were part of a cooperative group study and two patients who entered the transplant protocol with active CNS disease all other patients had a history of prior CNS disease that was not present at transplantation. Results as of June 14, 1987 are recorded in Table 4.

AUTOLOGOUS MARROW TRANSPLANTATION IN ANLL

Sixty-two patients with ANLL in their first to third complete remission were given autologous bone marrow that had previously been incubated with 4-hydroperoxycyclophosphamide (4HC) as reported previously (6,7). All patients transplanted in their second and third remission were transplanted within three months of their induction treatment. Patients in their first remission were transplanted from 2-15 months (median, 4 months) after induction of remission. The results as of June 1, 1987 are displayed in Table 5.

It is of interest that of the 43 patients transplanted in second remission 9 have exceeded the length of their first remission, 22 have died or relapsed at a time shorter then their first remission, and 12 other patients who are disease free now have not yet exceeded their first remission. Relapses occurred between 60 and 453 days (median, 184 days).

CAUSES OF DEATH AFTER MARROW TRANSPLANTATION

Two-thirds of the deaths associated with allogeneic marrow transplantation have been related to graft-versus-host disease (GVHD) and viral infections. Cytomegalovirus (CMV) (primarily interstitial pneumonitis) and other enteroviral infections such as rotovirus, adenovirus, and coxsackie virus have been prominent offenders.

The other major contributing causes of death, each with about a 3-5% incidence of fatal outcome include sepsis, veno-occlusive disease of the liver, adult respiratory distress syndrome, renal failure, chronic pulmonary failure and other causes.

Of the 62 patients that received autologous transplants 28 are surviving in continuous remission and 3 after relapse of their leukemia. Sixteen patients died of recurrent leukemia, 8 of bacterial sepsis, 3 of fungal infection, and 2 each of veno-occlusive disease and interstitial pneumonitis.

DISCUSSION

ALLOGENEIC TRANSPLANTATION FOR ANLL

Most centers have reported excellent results following transplantation of patients with ANLL with genotypical HLA identical allogeneic donors in first remission, review of the results, however; (2-4) has indicated a high relapse rate in patients transplanted in second or subsequent remission. The Seattle Group, for instance has projected a relapse rate for these patients of 45% with an actuarial survival of 25% (8) a result not better than their experience in transplanting patients in first relapse (9).

The Memorial Sloan-Kettering Group has reported a series of allogeneic transplants in ANLL with somewhat better results than generally seen by others, particularly in patients transplanted in their second remission (10). This group prepares the patient with a regimen of hyperfractionated total body irradiation (TBI) for a total dose of 1320 rad delivered in 4 days followed by cyclophosphamide (CY) (60 mg/kg) given on each of 2 consecutive days. The actuarial disease-free survival of 30 patients transplanted in first remission was 55%. Only three patients relapsed. The actuarial disease-free survival of 11 patients transplanted in second remission was 64% (not statistically different from those transplanted in first remission). There were no relapses in this group.

A few statements can be made regarding our series of patients:

1. Long-term disease-free survival can result when patients with ANLL are transplanted in first or subsequent remission and early relapse following preparation with BU plus CY.

2. Patients age 20 or younger enjoy a significantly better survival than patients age 21-46.

3. Disease-free survival is significantly better for patients age 21-46 transplanted in their first remission as apposed to subsequent remissions or early relapse. This cannot, as yet, be concluded for patients 20 years and younger.

Although the results reported from the Sloan-Kettering Group appeared to have advantages over the preparative regimen employed in our patients final decision as to the relative merits of each preparative regimen must await further studies, ideally, a randomization of the two preparative regimens.

The series of 12 patients, 10 with poor risk factors, transplanted with CY and TBI is encouraging since 5 of 12 (42%) are in continuous remission from almost 2 years to 6 1/2 years. Initially we believed that CY and TBI might be a better preparative regimen because of the risk factor of CNS disease or history thereof. Subsequently we were presented with evidence that BU may penetrate the blood brain barrier and our present policy is to prepare all patients with ANLL with BU plus CY regardless of a history of CNS disease.

AUTOLOGOUS TRANSPLANTATION FOR ANLL

Increasing patient age is a negative factor for the outcome of allogeneic bone marrow transplantation. Further, there is interest and stated need in employing unrelated matched donors for those who do not have a related donor. The use of autologous marrow transplantation allows the procedure to be carried more easily in an older population at the same time fulfilling the need of an otherwise unavailable donor (7).

At present the question of whether a marrow should be "purged" of putative tumor even though the marrow is harvested in a remission is controversial. Elsewhere we have presented the rationale (11), phase 1 (6) and phase 2 studies (7) of the use of 4-HC in ANLL in CR2 and CR3. The present report with more patients including patients in first remission updates our experience since the last report. Although more time and perhaps more patients are required to establish the efficacy of autologous marrow transplants, the results so far, particularly in second and third remission, are very encouraging. The disease-free survivals and relapse rate are at this juncture not too dissimilar from several allogeneic series.

Two reports of patients transplanted in first remission suggest that the administration of untreated marrow may give excellent disease-free survivals (12,13). It should be noted that these patients had their marrow harvested and transplantation performed several months after remission induction and after having received a number of chemotherapy intensifications or consolidations. We, in contrast, have harvested, purged, and transplanted the autologous marrow much earlier after the induction of remission.

The Seattle Group gave untreated autologous marrow to 13 patients in first remission following preparation with CY and TBI. The duration of first remission before transplantation ranged from 1-13 months (median, 4 months). Two patients died of non-leukemic causes and 8 of recurrent leukemia. Three patients survived free of leukemia for 782, 1374, and 1526 days following transplantation. The actuarial survival was 22% and actuarial relapse rate 67% (14).

It has been estimated that syngeneic marrow transplantation in ANLL in remission will result in about a 50% actuarial relapse rate (11,15,16). This value is essentially the same we have found in the patients reported above in their second and third remission.

These observations as well as limited experience of others that the use of unpurged marrow "too" soon after induction of remission leads to a high relapse rate (17) has supported our prejudice that marrow "purging" is important in transplants when they are performed within 4 months of remission induction.

CAUSES OF DEATH

GVHD, viral infections, toxicity of preparative regimens, and leukemic relapse constitute problems that require at least partial solutions if marrow transplantation is to realize its full potential.

GVHD

Considerable progress has been made in the past several years that has resulted in a reduction in the incidence and severity of this complication. A number of different approaches have been employed with some success. They include: 1) Post.transplant immunosuppression; 2) T cell depletion of the marrow innoculum; and 3) earlier recognition and treatment of GVHD. In the past when CY or methotrexate (MTX) was used for prevention of GVHD there remained an incidence of overall stage 2 or greater GVHD of about 50%. In comparison, several studies (18-20) including that from our own center indicated that cyclosporine (CsA) decreased the incidence and severity of GVHD as compared to CY or MTX. Recent clinical trials suggest that CsA plus a short course of MTX is far superior in preventing serious GVHD than either agent used alone (21). Unfortunately GVHD was not totally eliminated and there was no change in the incidence of chronic GVHD. Patients failing this treatment showed a poor survival of 0-30% (22,23). Clearly new agents must be sought to prevent and control GVHD. Current animal studies suggest that thalidomide may offer considerable promise in this regard. Apart from its teratogenic effect in the first trimester of pregnancy, it has minimal toxicity and clearly no known renal toxicity (24,25).

T cell depletion of the marrow as prophylaxis for GVHD has been actively pursued with a variety of techniques that include monoclonal antibody purging (26,27), Lectin separation (28) and counterflow centrifugation elutriation (CCE) (29,30). This latter technique is of particular interest to our group since initial studies have indicated it to be a relatively simple, reproducible and rapid method for processing marrow.

In general, T cell depletion of marrow had been effective in preventing and/or reducing the severity of GVHD. Some problems, however, may limit this approach. Most monoclonal or lectin purging methods are complicated by a 10 to 25% rate of failure of sustained engraftment and an apparent increase in the relapse rate of leukemia (31).

In our trial of CCE, 25 patients ages 30-48 (median, 39 years with leukemia or lymphoma received elutriated marrow containing 1×10^6 lymphocytes (median, 60% T lymphocytes by limiting dilution analysis) following cytoreductive therapy. Post transplantation immunosuppression with CsA was given to all patients. One patient failed to show sustained engraftment. Thirteen of the remaining 23 (56%) showed no GVHD, 9 (39%) showed only stage 1 GVHD of the skin responsive to prednisone administration and 2 (9%) developed overall clinical stage 4 GVHD unresponsive to prednisone and subsequently died. Eighteen of 24 (75%) survive for 14-451 days (median, 322 days) following transplantation. One of these survivors transplanted in the accelerated phase of chronic myelogenous leukemia relapsed (cytogenetically) into the chronic phase of the disease. Three additional patients did not receive CsA. They all failed to show sustained engraftment. These initial results are of great interest to us. The true value of this approach must await an accumulation of more patients and a longer follow up time.

Chronic GVHD is a serious complication that is often refractory to standard immunosuppressive therapy with azathioprine and prednisone (32,33). We have found thalidomide an effective agent in treating this complication in an animal model of chronic GVHD that closely parellels the human disease. The first patient with resistant chronic GVHD (of 3 years duration) treated with thalidomide has responded with improved joint mobility, hair growth, resolution of erythema, and return of dermal appendages (sweat glands and hair follicles).

VIRAL INFECTIONS

Cytomegalovirus (CMV) infections particularly in the form of interstitial pneumonitis have until recently been a major problem with incidences as high as 15% in allogeneic transplants with attendant mortality of 85-90%. In the past few years this had been an uncommon occurence in our patients. Why has this occurred? CMV has often been associated with GVHD and its treatment. With new prophylaxis for GVHD we have seen a decrease in the incidence and severity of this complication. Secondly, about 30% of our patients and their donors are seronegative for CMV. These patients receive blood from seronegative donors. Our experience (unpublished) confirms the report of Bowden et al (34) that CMV infections are avoided in these patients with the use of seronegative blood products. Further, we and others (unpublished) are engaged in a study of the prophylactic use of acyclovir in seropositive CMV patients that currently demonstrates its effect in decreasing the incidence of CMV infection.

Herpes Zoster infections will occur in 30-40% of allogeneic transplants (35-37). We have essentially the same experience. Although prompt intravenous treatment with acyclovir has been shown to be effective in Zoster infections in the immunocompromised host (38), many of our patients develop Zoster infections after returning home where it is often not immediately recognized, resulting in delayed treatment. Furthermore, up to 16% of such patients may relapse (36). At present, we are developing methods whereby a Zoster vaccine might be given to the donor and subsequently adoptively transferred to the recipient.

TOXICITY OF PREPARATIVE REGIMENS

In the past, the major contributing causes of death, each with a 3-5% incidence, include sepsis, veno-occlusive disease of the liver, adult respiratory distress syndrome, renal failure, chronic pulmonary failure, and miscellaneous other causes. It is hoped that the development of predictive factors to these problems will assist us in reducing these problems. For instance patients with pulmonary function studies less than 70% of normal should probably not be done because of the high incidence of fatal pulmonary failure in such patients. Similarly, patients with marked hepatic enzyme abnormalities have a much higher incidence of fatal veno-occlusive disease. One should either defer such patients until liver function returns to normal or defer them altogether from transplantation. In general, the liver abnormalities are seen in the most heavily treated patients (i.e., patients with ANLL in their third or subsequent remission). Marrow transplantation early in their course should lessen this problem.

It is anticipated that studies with some of the newly genetically cloned hematopoietic stimulatory factors will be proven useful in lessening the period of aplasia following transplantation. Hopefully this will translate into a lower incidence of fatal aplasia.

RELAPSE OF LEUKEMIA

Relapse of leukemia following allogeneic transplantation in first remission has not been a major problem. The relapse of 18% in patients transplanted later in their course is troublesome, however. Clearly relapse has been a major problem in the syngeneic and autologous transplants.

In order to decrease the relapse rate, one might devise a chemotherapy maintenance program or devise another preparative regimen. Since BU plus CY are relatively effective in allogeneic transplantation but still reasonably toxic, we are examining in an animal model system of acute leukemia whether or not the systemic administration of an appropriate anti-ANLL monoclonal antibody will reduce the relapse rate without causing toxicity additive to the organ toxicity induced by the primary preparative regimen. Preliminary results to date are encouraging and suggest that this therapeutic approach may be effective and eventually practical.

ACKNOWLEDGMENTS

We wish to thank Lisa Butzner for editing and typing several drafts of this manuscript.

REFERENCES

1. Santos GW (1983) History of bone marrow transplantation. Clin Haematol 12:611-639

2. Santos GW (1984) Bone marrow transplantation in leukemia - Current Status. Cancer 54:2732-2740

3. O'Reilly R (1983) Review: Allogeneic bone marrow transplantation: Current Status and Future Directions. Blood 62:941-964

4. Thomas E (1983) Marrow transplantation for malignant diseases (Karnofsky Lecture). J Clin Oncol 1:517-531

5. Santos GW, Tutschka PJ, Brookmeyer R, Saral R, Beschorner WE, Bias WB, Braine HG, Burns WH, Elfenbein GJ, Kaizer H, Mellits D, Sensenbrenner LL, Stuart RK, Yeager AM (1983) Marrow transplantation for acute nonlymphocytic leukemia after treatment with busulfan and cyclophosphamide. N Engl J Med 309:1347-1353

6. Kaizer H, Stuart R, Brookmeyer R, Beschorner W, Braine H, Burns W, Fuller D, Korbling M, Managan K, Saral R, Sensenbrenner L, Shadduck R, Shende A, Tutschka P, Yeager A, Zinkham W, Colvin O, Santos G (1985) Autologous bone marrow transplantation (BMT) in acute leukemia: A phase I study of in vitro treatment of marrow with 4-hydroperoxycyclophosphamide (4HC) to purge tumor cells. Blood 65:1504-1510

7. Yeager A, Kaizer H, Santos G, Saral R, Colvin O, Stuart R, Braine H, Burke P, Ambinder R, Burns W, Fuller D, Davis J, Karp J, May W, Rowley S, Sensenbrenner L, Vogelsang G, Wingard J (1986) Autologous bone marrow transplantation in patients with acute non-lymphocytic leukemia: A phase II study of ex vivo marrow treatment with 4-hydroperoxycyclophosphamide. N Engl J Med 315:141-147

8. Buckner C, Clift R, Thomas E, Sanders G, Hackman R, Stewart P, Storb R, Sullivan K (1982) Allogeneic marrow transplantation for patients with acute nonlymphoblastic leukemia in second remission. Leuk Res 6:395-399

9. Appelbaum P, Clift R, Buckner C, Stewart P, Storb R, Sullivan K, Thomas E (1983) Allogeneic marrow transplantation for acute nonlymphoblastic leukemia after first relapse. Blood 61:949-953

10. Dinsmore R, Kirkpatrick D, Flomenberg N, Gulati S, Kapoor N, Brochstein J, Shank B, Reid A, Groshen S, O'Reilly J (1984) Allogeneic bone marrow transplantation for patients with acute non-lymphocytic leukemia. Blood 63:649-656

11. Santos GW, Colvin M (1986) Pharmacological purging of bone marrow with reference to autografting. Clinics in Haematology 15:67-83

12. Burnett A, Watkins R, Maharaj D, McKinnon S, Tansey P, Alcorn M, Singer C, McDonald G, Robertson A (1984) Transplantation of unpurged autologous bone marrow in acute myeloid leukemia in first remission. Lancet 2:1068-1070

13. Lowenberg B, Abels J, VanBekkum D, Dzoljic G, Hagenbeek A, Hendricks W, Von De Poel J, Sizoo W, Sintnicolaas K, Wagenater G. (1984) Transplantation of nonpurified autologous bone marrow in patients with AML in first remission. Cancer 54:2840-2843

14. Stewart P, Buckner DC, Bensinger W, Appelbaum F, Fefer A, Clift R, Storb R, Sanders J, Meyers J, Hill R, Thomas ED (1985) Autologous marrow transplantation in patients with acute non-lymphocytic leukemia in first remission. Exp Hematol 13:267-272

15. Gale RP, Champlin RE (1984) How does bone marrow transplantation cure leukemia? Lancet 2:28-30

16. Fefer A (1986) Current status of syngeneic marrow transplantation and its relevance to autografting. Clinics in Haematology 15:49-65.

17. Burnett A. Personal communication.

18. Powles RL, Clink HM, Spence D, Morgenstern G, Watson JG, Selby PJ, Woods M, Barret A, Jameson B, Lawlar SD, Kay HEM, Laudson D, McElwain TS, Alexander P (1980) Cyclosporine A to prevent graft-versus-host disease in man after allogeneic bone marrow transplantation. Lancet 1:327-329.

19. Santos GW, Tutschka PJ, Brookmeyer R, Saral R, Beschorner WE, Bias WB, Braine HG, Burns WH, Farmer ER, Hess AD, Kaizer H, Mellits D, Sensenbrenner LL, Stuart R, Yeager AM (1987) Cyclosporine plus methylprednisolone versus cyclophosphamide plus methylprednisolone as prophylaxis for graft-versus-host disease: A randomized double blind study in patients undergoing allogeneic marrow transplantation. Clin Transplantation 1:21-28

20. Gluckman E, Davergie A, Poisies O, Lokiec F (1983) Use of cyclosporine as prophylaxis of graft-versus-host disease after human allogeneic bone marrow transplantation. Transplant Proc 15:2628-2632

21. Storb R, Deeg JH, Whitehead J, Appelbaum F, Beatty P, Bensinger W, Buckner CD, Clift R, Doney K, Farewell V, Hansen J, Hill R, Lum L, Martin P, McGuffin R, Sanders J, Stewart P, Sullivan K, Witherspoon R, Yee G, Thomas ED (1986) Methotrexate and cyclosporine compared with cyclosporine alone for prophylaxis of acute graft-versus-host disease after marrow transplantation for leukemia. N Engl J Med 314:729-735

22. Remlinger K, Martin PJ, Hansen JA, Doney KC, Smith A, Deeg HJ, Sullivan K, Storb R, Thomas ED (1984) Murine monoclonal anti-T cell antibodies for treatment of steroid resistant acute graft-versus-host-disease. Human Immunol 9:21-35

23. Kennedy MS, Deeg HJ, Storb R, Doney K, Sullivan KM, Witherspoon RP, Appelbaum FR, Stewart P, Sanders J, Buckner CD, Martin P, Weiden P, Thomas ED (1985) Treatment of acute graft-versus-host disease after allogeneic marrow transplantation. Randomized study comparing corticosteroids and cyclosporine. Am J Med 78:978-983

24. Vogelsang GB, Hess AD, Gordon G, Santos GW (1986) Treatment and prevention of acute graft-versus-host disease. Transplantation 41:644-647

25. Vogelsang GB, Taylor S, Gordon G, Hess AD (1986) Thalidomide, A potent agent for the treatment of graft-versus-host disease. Transplant Proc 18:904-907

26. Mitsuyasu RT, Champlin RE, Gale RP, How G, Lenarksy G, Sinston D, Selch M, Elashoff R, Giorgi J, Wells J, Terasaki P, Billing R, Feig S (1986) Treatment of donor marrow with monoclonal anti-T cell antibody and complement for the prevention of graft-versus-host disease. Ann Int Med 105:20-26

27. Prentice HG, Blalock HA, Janossy G, Skegg D (1983) Use of anti-T cell monoclonal antibody OKT3 to prevent acute graft-versus-host disease in allogeneic bone marrow transplantation for acute leukemia. Lancet 1:700-703.

28. O'Reilly RJ, Kernan N, Collins N, Brochstein J, Cunningham H, Castro-Malaspina H, Lauer J, Emanuel D, Gulati S, Flomberg N, Keever C (1986) Abrogation of both acute and chronic GVHD following transplants of lectin agglutinated, E-rosette depleted (SBA-E) marrow for leukemia. Blood 68:1041

29. Noga SJ, Donnenberg AD, Schwartz CL, Civin CL, Santos GW (1986) Development of a simplified counterflow centrifugation elutriation procedure for depletion of lymphocytes from human marrow. Transplantation 41:226-229

30. DeWitte T, Hoogenhout J, dePauw B, Holdrine TR, Janseen J, Wessels J, VanDaul W, Hustinx T, Hannen C (1986) Depletion of donor lymphocytes by counterflow centrifugation successfully prevents acute graft-versus-host disease in matched allogeneic marrow transplants. Blood 67:1302-1308

31. Apperly JF, Jones J, Arthur G, Guo AP, Russol F, Hale G, Waldmann H, Goldman JM (1986) Incidence of relapse after T-cell depleted marrow transplant for chronic granulocytic leukemia in first chronic phase. Blood 68:957

32. Sullivan KM, Shulman HM, Storb R, Weiden PL, Witherspoon RP, McDonald GB, Schubert MM, Atkinson K, Thomas ED (1981) Chronic graft-versus-host disease in 52 patients: Adverse natural course and successful treatment with combination immunosuppression. Blood 57:267-276

33. Santos GW, Hess AD, Vogelsang GB (1985) Graft-versus-host reaction and disease. Immunol Reviews 88:169-192

34. Bowden RA, Sayers M, Flournoy N, Newton B, Nanaji M, Thomas ED, Meyers JD (1986) Cytomegalovirus immunoglobulin and sero-negative blood products to prevent primary cytomegalovirus infections after marrow transplantation. N Engl J Med 314:1006-1010

35. Atkinson K, Meyers JD, Storb R, Prentice RL, Thomas ED (1980) Varicella-Zoster infection after bone marrow transplantation for aplastic anemia or leukemia. Transplantation 29:47-50

36. Locksley RM, Fluornoy N, Sullivan KM, Meyers JD (1985) Infection with Varicella-Zoster virus after marrow transplantation. J Infect Dis 152:1172-1180

37. Ljungman P, Lonnqvist B, Gahrton G, Ringden A, Sundquist V, Wahren B (1986) Clinical and subclinical reactivations of Varicella-Zoster virus in immunocompromised patients. J Infect Dis 153:840-847

38. Meyers JD, Wade JC, Shepp DH, Newton B (1984) Acyclovir treatment of Varicella-Zoster virus infection in the immunocompromised host. Transplantation 37:571-574

Table 1: Allogeneic Marrow Transplantation in ANLL

Remission	Number	Median (Range) Age in years	Relapses*	Disease-free** Survival	Median (Range) Disease-Free survivors in days
First	48	24 (1-46)	2 (4%)	22 (46%)	830 (1-2983)
Second	28	27 (5-41)	4 (14%)	9 (32%)	400 (29-2561)
Third	2	36 (35-37)	1 (50%)	0 (0%)	--
ER 1-3	21	23 (3-46)	4 (19%)	6 (29%)	1586 (611-2346)
	99	25 (1-46)	11 (11%)	37 (37%)	1148 (1-2983)

*Actual number relapses (% relapse).
**Actual number surviving (% surviving).

Table 2: Allogeneic Marrow Transplantation in ANLL
Effect of Age

Remission	≤20 years Number	Disease free Survival*	Median (Range) Survivors in days	>20 years Number	Disease free survival*	Median (Range) Survivors in days
First	16	9 (56%)	1148 (386-2983)	32	13 (41%)	715 (1-2694)
Second	6	2 (33%)	1188 (57-2318)	22	7 (32%)	400 (29-2561)
Third	--	--	--	2	0 (0%)	--
ER 1-3	6	4 (67%)	1586 (611-2346)	15	2 (13%)	1816 (1303-2329)
	28	15 (54%)	1548 (57-2983)	71	22 (31%)	708 (1-2694

*Actual number of patients (% survival).

Table 3: Allogeneic Transplants in ANLL First Remission Versus Subsequent Remission and Early Relapse

Remission	Number	Median (Range) Age in years	Relapses*	Disease-free** Survival	Median (Range) Disease-Free Survivors in days
First	48	24 (1-46)	2 (4%)	22 (46%)	830 (1-2983)
Subsequent	51	26 (5-46)	9 (18%)	15 (29%)	1338 (29-2561)
	99	25 (1-46)	11 (11%)	37 (37%)	1148 (1-2983)

**Actual number surviving (% surviving).
* Actual number relapsing (% relapsing).

Table 4: Allogeneic Transplantation in ANLL with CY and TBI

Remission	Number	Median (Range) Age in years	Relapses	DFS Survival*	Disease-free Survivors** in months
CR1	5	14 (12-39)	0	3 (60%)	32.3,73.0,78.3
CR2	3	25 (23-35)	0	0 (0%)	--
ER1	2	22 (15-28)	0	1 (50%)	32.3
Rel	2	25 (21-29)	0	1 (50%)	23.4
	12	22 (12-39)	0	5 (42%)	Median 32.3

*Actual, not actuarial **. One of 2 patients transplanted without a history of CNS disease survives.

Table 5: Autologous Marrow Transplantation for ANLL

Remission	Number Patients	Median Age (Range) years	Number Non-leukemic Deaths	Number of Relapses	Number of Disease-free Survivors	Median duration (Range) Disease-free Survival in days
CR1	9	17 (12-37)	1	1 (14%)*	7 (76%)**	185 (181-2285)
CR2	43	22 (2-54)	10	15 (57%)	18 (31%)	256 (24-1484)
CR3	10	31 (19-54)	4	3 (49%)	3 (30%)	811 (766-2064)
CR 1-3	62	22 (2-54)	15 (29%)	19 (52%)	28 (35%)	339 (24-2285)

*Actuarial relapse rate.
**Actuarial disease-free survival.

12: Allogeneic Transplantation for Acute Lymphoblastic Leukemia

A.J. Barrett

There is now a large body of data on marrow allografts and autografts in acute lymphoblastic leukaemia (ALL) estimated from international registries to exceed 2000 allografts and possibly up to 1000 autografts.(1) It is therefore possible to define the success of transplant procedures in some detail and to determine the best treatment option for the individual patient with ALL. This becomes increasingly important with the emergence of improved chemotherapy treatment for children and adults with the disease. This review summarizes current indications for bone marrow transplantation (BMT) in ALL and recent BMT results. It focuses on the major problem of relapse after BMT identifying predisposing factors and treatment approaches and describes attempts to reduce relapse.

INDICATIONS FOR BMT IN ALL

Children

Improved chemotherapy for childhood ALL can now achieve a global long term disease free survival of up to 80%.(2) Intensified induction and consolidation programmes have eliminated many of the high relapse features that might previously have been considered as indications for BMT in first remission. However, there is general agreement that about 15% of childhood ALL is incurable by chemotherapy alone and BMT should be further evaluated in this group. Ultra poor prognostic features include ALL with chromosome translocations(3); true null cell or B cell subtype; presentation below the age of 2; leucocyte count over 200 x 10^9/l; and CNS or mediastinal involvement at presentation.(4,5) There has been some controversy over the value of BMT as a salvage procedure for ALL that has relapsed but has achieved a further remission. (6,7) Again, improved chemotherapy approaches have increased the likelihood of long term survival and possible cure, particularly for children who relapse after maintenance chemotherapy has ceased. A careful review by Butterini et al of chemotherapy and BMT data shows that BMT in remission is the preferred option, salvaging 20% of early relapses and 35% of late relapses, compared to reported figures for chemotherapy of less than 5% and 30% respectively.(8)

Adults

Above the age of 15 the cure rate for patients presenting with ALL falls drastically. Despite increased intensification of chemotherapy, the overall disease free survival for adults has not exceeded 40%. There is, however, evidence that new approaches to intensified consolidation may have improved adult ALL treatment further.(9,10) It has also become possible to identify prognostic features which, while not universally agreed, may help to determine risk. For example, standard risk features of age, sex, cell type and presenting leucocyte count applicable in childhood ALL appear to reliable predictors of outcome in adults. Notably prognosis is much poorer in patients over 35 years.(10,11) The high proportion of null cell sub-type in adults may account for the generally poorer results in adults. In an ongoing multicentre study Hoelzer reports 2 year disease free survivals of 57% broken down to 78% for good risk and 40% for poor risk patients.(12) With results for first remission BMT in the region of 50% or more most BMT teams will continue to accept all adults with ALL as candidates for BMT. As comparative studies continue it may in future be possible to select the best prognostic group for chemotherapy alone.

RECENT RESULTS OF BMT IN ALL

Data from two multicentre analyses, the International Bone Marrow Transplant Registry (IBMTR) and the European Bone Marrow Transplant Group (EBMT) is reviewed here alongside selected recent data from individual centres. With important exceptions, discussed further, there is close concordance for relapse and survival figures between groups. The multicentre data from international registries gives lower but possibly more representative figures which may be explained by the disinclination of centres with a small series of poor survivors to report their data. Disappointingly, a cohort review of leukaemia BMT results in Europe shows no improvement in graft outcome in the last five years.(13)

Bone marrow transplantation in first complete remission (Table 1)

Several groups have reported long term disease free survivals in the region of 45-65%. The data largely concerns adult transplants but where BMT has been used for children for childhood ALL the results are superior with 60-100% patients achieving long term survival. Relapse rates after first remission BMT range between 13-30%. This high figure reflects the selection of poor risk patients for BMT.(13,14,15,16,17,18,19,20)

TABLE 1

Recent results of BMT for high risk ALL in first complete remission*

Centre **	No.	Age++	% Actuarial DFS (years)	Rel.	Ref.
IBMTR M	236	A+C(22)	45 (4)	26	14
EBMT M	260	A+C	48 (7)	27	13
France+ M	59	A(24)	64 (1.5)	13	15
City of Hope	39	A(23)	63 (6)	16	17
Westminster	29	A+C(22)	55 (8)	20	19
		C(12)	100 (7)	0	
Baltimore+	18	A+C(24)	56 (2.5)	5	18
Seattle	14	C -	60 (3)	30	20

* Some adult series include a small proportion of "standard risk" features but all children were transplanted because of high risk or very high risk features.

** M=Multicentre data

\+ Actual, not actuarial figures used. Median survivals quoted

++ A=Adult, C=Children
Median age of group in years in parenthesis

BMT in second or subsequent remission (Table 2)

BMT in second complete remission represents the largest group of ALL recipients. Large multicentre series indicate that BMT in third or fourth remission has an outcome comparable to BMT in second remission. It is therefore possible to analyse second and subsequent remission transplants together.(13) The data from individual and multiple centres shows a long term survival between 22% and 62%. Better prognosis groups are children, patients with standard risk features or with slow disease, and in two series patients transplanted in second remission. The concept of slow and fast disease is considered further below.

TABLE 2

Recent results for 2nd or subsequent remission BMT for ALL

Centre	No.	Disease type*	Rem. status	% act. DFS (years)	% Rel.	Ref
IBMTR	208	H	CR2	22(3)	56	14
M	97	S	>CR2	36(3)	49	
EBMT	271	H+S	CR2	34(8)	54	13
M	83	H+S	>CR2	30(8)	50	
Seattle	94	H+S	CR2 >CR2	40(3)	40	20
Westminster	61	Fast	CR2 >CR2	10(7)	80	19
		Slow	CR2 >CR2	55(7)	27	
		Total	CR2 >CR2	36(7)	-	
Baltimore+	47	H+S	CR2	53(2)	3	18
			>CR2	24(3+)	35	
Memorial			CR2 H	62.5(2)	5	
Sloane	37	C	S		23	23
Kettering			>CR2	27(2)	58	
Minneapolis	15	C	CR2	33(3)	57	22

* H=High risk, S=Standard risk,
C= only children < 14 yrs transplanted
CR=Complete remission

\+ actual not actuarial figures used
median survivals quoted
++ median survivals quoted

BMT in relapse

Formerly BMT in relapse for ALL was an endstage experimental procedure and the 10% overall survival achieved appears commensurate with the selection of a highly resistant disease group.(25) More recent data for ALL BMT in relapse probably reflects attempts at early transplantation in patients who have not achieved a second remission induction, or who fail to achieve a complete first remission of their disease. It is therefore disappointing that there has been no improvement in the results for relapsed patients which still give an overall survival of 15% and a relapse rate of over 70%. (26,27)

COMPARISON OF ALLOGENEIC BMT WITH OTHER TREATMENTS

Only relatively small numbers of patients with ALL have received autologous transplants. The available data indicates three year disease free survivals for first remission transplants in the region of 35-56%. Lower figures are quoted for second remission transplants.(28,29) A strictly comparative study at the Westminster Hospital of 18 autologous and 25 allografts for ALL in first, second and third remission showed no statistical difference in outcome for the two treatment approaches. Better evaluation awaits the outcome of several multicentre national co-operative studies now underway and an EBMT "registration study" which will evaluate the outcome of a cohort of over 400 leukaemia patients subjected to HLA typing in order to find a donor, according to the treatment they receive, be it allograft, autograft or chemotherapy. These new studies will make available for the first time truly comparable and contemporaneous data on the three treatment options available to the patient with ALL who achieves the remission.

RELAPSE AFTER BMT

Relapse is the particular complication that confronts transplantation attempts in ALL. It occurs from any stage in the early post-transplant period up to three years after BMT and may arise either in the bone marrow, extramedullary sites or lymph nodes. With rare exceptions relapse occurs in recipient cells that have failed to be eradiacted by the transplant procedure. Reports of ALL relapse in donor cells are exceptional.(30) Ultimately, patients who relapse after BMT die of recurrent disease but nevertheless, several long term survivors have been reported whose current remission exceeds the interval between the BMT and the relapse. Such cases have created interest in identifying prognostic features for survival and optimum treatment approaches. We reported a series of 21 relapses after BMT for ALL, 19 of whom received further antileukaemia treatment.(31) 5 became long term survivors after remission induction and in 3 patients the survival has exceeded the interval between the bone marrow transplant and the relapse. We showed that remission induction was more likely to be achieved in patients who had relapsed beyond two years from BMT and in patients where the relapse occurred in extramedullary sites. In 2 patients BMT was attempted in remission but both patients died early from procedural complications. The question of further BMT in these patients has not been completely resolved. Second bone marrow transplants have a high relapse rate and a high incidence of BMT complications.(32) Clearly, treatment of relapse after BMT has to be considered as a form of salvage treatment and should not divert attention from efforts to prevent relapse occurring.

PREDICTION OF RELAPSE

The recognition of specific disease characteristics highly predictive of prognosis after chemotherapy has encouraged a number of analyses of prognostic features for relapse of ALL after BMT. There is evidence that many of the standard prognostic features applicable for chemotherapy and ALL are also predictive for relapse after BMT. Multicentre analyses and individual studies have identified presenting leucocyte count, cell subtype, presenting age and karyotype as useful predictors of relapse risk (14,8). In a single centre study of 63 patients we showed that presenting leucocyte count was the most important standard risk feature with counts of over 30 x 10^9/l conferring a significantly higher relapse risk. A further powerful predictor which appeared to be independent of other factors was the interval between diagnosis and relapse for patients who were transplanted in second or subsequent remission. Patients with an interval greater than two years (slow disease) showed a 29% relapse risk while patients who relapsed within two years from diagnosis (fast disease) had a 74% relapse rate.(33) This concept of slow and fast disease is therefore a useful and easily applicable predictor of outcome after BMT for patients grafted in second and subsequent remission.

EFFECT OF THE ALLOGRAFT ON LEUKAEMIC RELAPSE

While transplantation models in animals can be made to show significant graft versus leukaemia (GVL) effects, the importance of GVL in ALL transplants is harder to establish.(34) Evidence for an allograft effect comes from a number of clinical models:

1. Relationship between Graft versus host disease (GVHD) and relapse
   The concept that the presence or absence of GVHD and its severity and duration might be related to a GVL action has been supported by data from Seattle which identify a decreased relapse risk for patients with acute and chronic GVHD.(35,36) Graft versus host disease exerts a highly significant and important effect on relapse. For example, in the study by Saunders presence of GVHD confers a 20% relapse risk compared with a 40% relapse risk for patients without acute GVHD. These findings should not be accepted uncritically: patients with severe GVHD may die of this complication before relapse can occur and the treatment given for acute and chronic GVHD includes agents such as steroids, methotrexate and azathioprine which may in their own right exert an antileukaemia effect.
2. Comparison of allograft with autologous BMT or syngeneic BMT
   The heterogeneity of ALL in terms of relapse probability, the differing results obtained in first remission BMT compared with later transplants, the relative paucity of data and the diversity of conditioning regimens used in autotransplants for ALL make it difficult to make meaningful comparisons of relapse in the presence or absence of an allograft effect. In the small series of BMT from identical twins in refractory ALL Johnson and Mauer identified a significantly higher relapse risk with syngeneic BMT (78% vs. 33% allogeneic).(37) Fefer reported 11 syngeneic BMT in ALL in first, second or third remission recipients. 5 survived disease free, 5 relapsed.(38) The small available data therefore supports a high relapse rate for syngeneic BMT.

   Large numbers of ALL patients have now received autologous BMT (ABMT) (39) and some patients have received bone marrow purged of leukaemia cells with a variety of monoclonal antibodies. In terms of identifying an allograft effect the results are conflicting. Firstly, there appears to be a beneficial effect of bone marrow purging on relapse incidence, suggesting that some of the relapses occurring after autologous BMT may result from retransfusion of residual leukaemia. Secondly, some series show identical relapse rates to allogeneic transplants while others show a higher relapse rate. For example, Gorin et al reported in a multicentre study of 77 autologous transplants in ALL that the relapse probability was 44% and 45% for first and second remission transplants respectively. In this series purging did not affect the relapse rate.(29) In our single centre comparative study of 18 autografts compared with 25 allografts, we did not identify a difference in relapse risk, either for the whole group or for patients in the three different relapse categories, first remission or fast or slow disease in second and subsequent remission.(40) Conversely, the Minnesota group identify a beneficial effect of purging for second and further remission transplants and relapse rates of 48% purged and 60% unpurged for second and further remission transplants.(41)

3. T lymphocyte depletion of donor marrow
   The relationship between T depletion and subsequent relapse demonstrated in animal experiments is now emerging in clinical practice. The strongest association and the biggest effect on relapse occurs in BMT for chronic myeloid leukaemia.(42) However, the same effect is demonstrable in smaller series of acute myeloblastic leukaemia and ALL transplants.(43) The mechanism whereby T depletion predisposes to leukaemic relapse is not known. Apart from removing GVL reacting lymphocytes with T depletion, there is the possibility that immune reconstitution is compromised or that the grafted bone marrow is unstable and favours the emergence of a residual leukaemia clone. Gale has drawn attention to the reciprocal relationship between GVHD and graft rejection which may parallel a similar relationship between GVL and relapse.(44) Until more is known about the precise nature of the allogeneic antileukaemic effect, however, it is not clear how best the immune system could be manipulated to deter leukaemia recurrence, nor whether improved graft conditioning regimens can transcend any benefits from GVL effects.

In conclusion, there is considerable evidence that an allograft effect exists which diminishes relapse after BMT for ALL but because of small numbers of patients and lack of comparative studies the case is not completely proven.

PREVENTION OF RELAPSE

The numerous attempts to reduce ALL relapse after BMT can be classified into treatment attempts before, during or after the transplant.

Influence of treatment pregraft

Clearly, elective BMT for ALL in first remission confers the best survival and highest cure rate. Optimum selection for first remission BMT is therefore important. However, there is no data indicating the best time in first remission to carry out the transplant. In our experience prior cranial irradiation is not necessary to prevent later CNS relapse and increasingly BMT is being carried out earlier in first remission with the avoidance of cranial irradiation. The question of intensive consolidation before BMT has been considered by the Basle group who used high dose Ara-C and VP16 6-8 weeks before BMT as additional cytoreduction. Disappointingly, while not affecting transplant complications, this procedure did not decreased the ultimate relapse probability.(45) In an attempt to decrease the severity of intensive consolidation before BMT, we have used high dose VP16 and Ara-C with autologous bone marrow rescue in 5 patients 6 weeks before BMT using total body irradiation (TBI). 3 patients have died from pulmonary complications, suggesting that such double transplant procedures may be limited by unacceptable toxicity. There is therefore at present little indication that pretransplant intensification offers hope of improving leukaemia cytoreduction.

Variations in the conditioning regimen.

The majority of patients transplanted for ALL have received the Seattle conditioning schedule of cyclophosphamide and TBI with minor modifications. The possibility that other agents with more specificity for ALL could be substituted for cyclophosphamide led us and other groups to investigate alternative regimes. Blume has reported promising results with a combination of high dose Ara-C and VP16 given immediately prior to TBI for a series of relapsed leukaemia patients which may prove to be superior to the standard conditioning schedules.(46) After extensive evaluation of standard dose combinations of VM26, Ara-C, daunorubicin, vincristine and prednisolone (VVRAPID) we conclude that such regimens did not significantly reduce the relapse risk for fast or slow disease patients.(47) Interestingly, Santos has reported extremely favourable results using a 4 day cyclophosphamide induction schedule in conjunction with TBI which merits further study.(18) There has been much interest in optimising TBI schedules to reduce relapse while minimising normal tissue damage. There is, however, no clear evidence that fractionated TBI as opposed to single dose TBI has a particular antileukaemic effect in ALL(48) and increase in the total biological dose of radiation received is limited to about 14Gy when using fractionated TBI. An important exception is the hyperfractionated TBI schedule used by the Memorial Sloan Kettering group which produces improved disease free survival in second remission transplants (23). These isolated but significantly improved results from centres using modified or novel conditioning regimens indicate that the search for optimum conditioning schedules for ALL transplant recipients is worthwhile actively pursuing.

Treatment after BMT

The value of maintenance treatment in reducing and elimination minimal disease after chemotherapy, remission induction, and consolidation suggests that it may also be effective following BMT for ALL. Maintenance chemotherapy after BMT employing methotrexate and mercaptopurine has been used by a number of transplant teams. The tolerance of the transplanted marrow to chemotherapy is the limiting factor in applying such schedules. The Minnesota group have not shown a significant reduction in relapse but this treatment requires further evaluation.(49)

Another interesting possibility is the application of immunotherapy after BMT. The availability of recombinant growth factors such as interleukin 2 opens up the possibility of using powerful stimulators to activate natural killer cell populations, and antigen specific T cell clones which may play a regulatory role in the elimination of residual leukaemia.(50) The toxicity of interleukin 2, the risk of induction of GVHD and the difficulty of knowing how long to continue with such treatment are daunting problems which may curb initial enthusiasm for modern immunotherapy approaches.

CONCLUSIONS

Bone marrow transplantation for ALL could be considered to have reached an impasse with no major improvement in relapse and survival in recent years. With improvements in chemotherapy patients selected for BMT represent a group with increasingly resistant disease in whom poorer outcomes can be anticipated. However, the relatively good results for first remission transplants and the possibility that some teams are using considerably superior conditioning regimens, together with the prospects for intelligent immunotherapy to prevent relapse and GVHD may ultimately improve the outlook for this poor risk group of patients.

REFERENCES

1. Gale RP (1986) Analysis of bone marrow transplantation data in man. Bone Marrow Transplantation 1:3-9

2. Mauer AM (1986) New directions in the treatment of acute lymphoblastic leukaemia in children. New Engl J Med 315:316-7

3. Williams DL, Harber J, Murphy SB et al (1986) Chromosomal translocations play a unique role in influencing prognosis in childhood acute lymphoblastic leukaemia. Blood 68:205-212

4. Greaves MF, Janossy G, Peto J, Kay H (1981) Immunologically defined subclasses of acute lymphoblastic leukaemia in children: their relationship to presentation features and prognosis. Brit J Haematol 48:179-97

5. Hann HWL, Lustbader ED, Evans AE et al (1981) Lack of influence of T cell marker and importance of mediastinal mass on prognosis of acute lymphoblastic leukaemia of childhood. J Nat Cancer Inst 66:285-90

6. Chessells JM, Rogers DW, Leiper AD (1986) Bone marrow transplantation has a limited role in prolonging second marrow remission in childhood lymphoblastic leukaemia. Lancet 1:1239-41

7. Poynton CH, Barrett AJ (1986) Bone marrow transplantation for childhood acute lymphoblastic leukaemia. Lancet 2:395

8. Butturini A, Rivera GK, Bortin MM, Gale RP (1986) Which treatment for childhood acute lymphoblastic leukaemia in second remission ? Lancet 1:429-33

9. Hoelzer D, Thiel E, Löffler H (1984) Intensified therapy in acute lymphoblastic and acute undifferentiated leukaemia in adults. Blood 64:38-47

10. Clarkson B, Ellis S, Little C (1985) Acute lymphoblastic leukaemia in adults. Semin Oncol 15:755-80

11. Marcus RE, Catovsky D, Johnson SA (1986) Adult acute lymphoblastic leukaemia: A study of prognostic features and response to treatment over a ten year period. Brit J Cancer 53:175-180

12. Hoelzer D, Thiel E, Löffler H (1987) Risk adapted therapy in adult ALL: Experience in the German multicentre trial 02/84. 4th International Symposium on therapy of acute leukaemias, Rome 1987, Abstracts p175

13. Gratwohl A, Hermans J, Lyklema A, Zwaan FE (1987) Bone marrow transplantation for leukaemia in Europe. Report from the Leukaemia Working Party 1987. Bone Marrow Transplantation 2, Supp.1:15-19

14. Herzig RH, Bortin MM, Barrett AJ et al (1987) Bone marrow transplantation in high risk acute lymphoblastic leukaemia in first and second remission. Lancet 1:786-789

15. Vernant JP, Maraninchi D, Guyotat D et al (1987) Allogeneic bone marrow transplantation in adults with acute lymphoblastic leukaemia in first complete remission. Bone Marrow Transplantation 2, Supp.1:23

16. Proctor SJ, Hamilton PJ, Reed MM et al (1987) A comparative study of combination chemotherapy vs. marrow transplantation in first remission acute lymphoblastic leukaemia. Bone Marrow Transplantation 2, Supp.1:21

17. Blume KG, Forman SJ, Snyder DS et al (1987) Allogeneic bone marrow transplantation for acute lymphoblastic leukaemia during first complete remission. Transplantation 43:389-92

18. Santos GW (1987) Allogeneic bone marrow transplantation in acute leukaemia. 4th International Symposium on therapy of acute leukaemias, Rome 1987, Abstracts p295

19. Barrett AJ, Poynton CH, McCarthy DM et al (1987) Allogeneic bone marrow transplantation for poor risk acute lymphoblastic leukaemia. 4th International Symposium on therapy of acute leukaemias, Rome 1987, Abstracts p287

20.Downey J, Martin P, Beatty P, Thomas ED (1987) Allogeneic marrow transplantation for patients with acute lymphoblastic leukaemia. 4th International Symposium on therapy of acute leukaemias, Rome 1987, Abstracts p292

21.Bacigalupo A, Van Lint MT, Frassoni F et al (1986) Allogeneic bone marrow transplantation vs. chemotherapy for childhood acute lymphoblastic leukaemia in second remission. Bone Marrow Transplantation 1:75-80

22.Woods WG, Nesbit NE, Ramsay NKC, Kersey J (1983). Intensive therapy followed by bone marrow transplantation for patients with acute lymphoblastic leukaemia in second or subsequent remission: determination of prognostic factors. Blood 61:1182-89

23.Dinsmore R, Kirkpatrick D, Flomenberg N et al (1983) Allogeneic bone marrow transplantation for patients with acute lymphoblastic leukaemia. Blood 62:381-88

24.Coccia PF, Shandjord SE, Gordon GM (1984) High dose cytosine arabinoside and fractionated total body irradiation: an improved preparative regimen for bone marrow transplantation in children with acute lymphoblastic leukaemia in second remission. Blood 64, Supp.1, 213a

25.Thomas ED, Buckner CD, Banaji M et al (1977) One hundred patients with acute leukaemia treated by chemotherapy, total body irradiation and allogeneic marrow transplantation. Blood 49:511-533

26.Clift RA, Buckner CD, Thomas ED et al (1982) Allogeneic marrow transplantation using fractionated TBI in patients with acute leukaemia in relapse. Leukaemia Research 6:401-407

27.Zwaan FE, Hermans J, Barrett AJ, Speck B (1983) Bone marrow transplantation for acute lymphoblastic leukaemia: a survey of the European Group for Bone Marrow Transplantation. Brit J Haematol 58:33-42

28.O'Reilly RJ (1986) New promise for autologous marrow transplantation in leukaemia. New Engl J Med 315:186-188

29.Gorin NC, Herve P, Aegerter P et al (1986) Autologous bone marrow transplantation for acute leukaemia in remission. Brit J Haematol 64:385-95

30.Boyd CN, Ramberg RC, Thomas ED (1982) The incidence of recurrence of leukaemia in donor cells after allogeneic bone marrow transplantation. Leukaemia Research 6:833-37

31.Barrett AJ, Joshi R, Tew C (1985) How should acute lymphoblastic leukaemia relapsing after bone marrow transplantation be treated. Lancet 1:1188-92

32.Atkinson K, Biggs J, Concannon A, Dodds A, Dale B, Norman J (1986) Second marrow transplantation for recurrence of haematological malignancy. Bone Marrow Transplantation 1:159-166

33.Barrett AJ, Joshi R, Kendra JR et al (1986) Prediction and Prevention of relapse of acute lymphoblastic leukaemia after bone marrow transplantation. Brit J Haematol 64:179-86

34.Truitt RL, Shih C, Kaehler DA, Le Fever AV, Bortin M M (1983) Graft versus leukaemia and graft versus host reactivity following alloimmunisation of MHC-compatible donor mice. In: Recent advances in Bone Marrow Transplantation, (ed) RP Gale. Alan R Liss: New York 243-253

35.Weiden PL, Sullivan KM, Flournoy N et al (1981) Antileukaemic effects of chronic GVHD: contribution to improved survival of allogeneic marrow transplantation. New Engl J Med 304:1529

36.Sanders JE, Flournoy N, Thomas ED et al (1985) Marrow transplantation experience in children with acute lymphoblastic leukaemia: an analysis of factors associated with survival, relapse and graft versus host disease. Medical and Paediatric Oncol (in press)

37.Johnson FL, Mauer AM (1983) Marrow transplantation in childhood acute lympho lastic leukaemia. In: Recent advances in Bone marrow transplantation. (ed) R P Gale. Alan R Liss: New York 123-139

38.Fefer A (1986) Current status of syngeneic marrow transplantation and its relevance to autografting. In: Autologous Bone Marrow Transplantation, Clinics in Haematology 15,1:49-65

39.Dicke KA, Spitzer G (1986) Clinical studies for autologous grafts in acute lymphoblastic leukaemia. In: Autologous Bone Marrow Transplantation, Clinics in Haematology 15, 1:85-103

40.Barrett AJ, Poynton CH, McCarthy D et al (1987) Allogeneic bone marrow transplantation for high risk acute lymphoblastic leukaemia. 4th International Symposium on therapy of acute leukaemias, Abstracts p294

41.Ramsay N, Lebien T, Nesbit M et al (1985) Autologous marrow transplantation for acute lymphoblastic leukaemia following marrow treatment with Ba-1, Ba-2, Ba-3 and rabbit complement. Blood 66:508

42.Apperley JF, Jones L, Hale G et al 91986) Bone marrow transplantation for patients with chronic myeloid leukaemia: T cell depletion reduces the incidence of graft versus host disease but may increase the risk of leukaemic relapse. Bone Marrow Transplantation 1:53-66

43. Arthur CK (1987) Bone marrow transplantation for leukaemia. Meeting Report. Bone Marrow Transplantation 1:329-38

44. Gale RP, Reisner Y (1986) Graft rejection and graft versus host disease: Mirror images. Lancet 1468-1470

45. Gratwohl A, Osterwalde E, Lori A, Nissen C, Speck B (1985) High dose Ara-C and VP16 as preconditioning for marrow transplantation before cyclophosphamide and total body irradiation for patients with acute lymphoblastic leukaemia. Experimental Haematol 13, Supp.17, 11

46. Blume KG, Forman SJ, O'Donnell MR (1987) Total body irradiation and high dose etoposide: a new preparatory regimen for bone marrow transplantation in patients with advanced haematologic malignancies. Blood 69:1015-1020

47. Barrett AJ, Davis HP, Revell P et al (1987) Is there an optimum conditioning regimen to prevent relapse after bone marrow transplantation for acute lymphoblastic leukaemia ? Bone Marrow Transplantation 2, Supp.1, 235

48. Clift RA, Buckner CD, Thomas ED et al (1982) Allogeneic marrow transplantation using fractionated total body irradiation in patients with acute lymphoblastic leukaemia in relapse. Leuk Res 6:401

49. Woods WG, Nesbit ME, Ramsay NKC et al (1982) Improved disease free survival and determination of prognostic factors for patients with acute lymphoblastic leukaemia in remission receiving intensive therapy followed by bone marrow transplantation. Blood 60, Supp.1:175a

50. Rosenberg SA, Lotze MT, Muul LM (1987) A progress report on the treatment of 157 patients with advanced cancer using lymphokine activated killer cells and interleukin-2 or high dose interleukin-2 alone. New Engl J Med 316:889-97

13: Autologous Bone Marrow Transplantation in Acute Lymphoblastic Leukemia—Mafosfamide Italian Study Group

V. Rizzoli, L. Mangoni, A.M. Carella, G. Torlontano, M. Aglietta, L. Resegotti, E. Madon, R. Mozzana, A. Porcellini, and P. Coleselli

INTRODUCTION

Clinical experience demonstrates that a number of human tumors show a high response rate to aggressive chemotherapy regimens (1-2).

Dose responsiveness of cytoreductive therapy has been proved in hematological malignancies, so in recent years an increasing number of "mega" dose ablative protocols utilizing bone marrow reinfusion have been used in an attempt to cure acute leukemias and lymphomas or prolong disease-free survival of patients (3-6).

Autologous graft was started as an alternative approach for patients lacking a matched donor; nevertheless, the most recent data on clinical results are similar to those obtained with allogeneic marrow and encourage us to consider autologous transplantation as a therapy of choice in selected subjects (7-9).

In acute leukemia, however, it is clearly demonstrated that about 10^6- 10^8 malignant clonogenic cells are present in marrow harvested in the complete remission phase, so one of the major limits of this technique may be that residual leukemic cells could be reinfused with normal marrow suspension. Therefore, it would seem reasonable to attempt "ex vivo" methods for bone marrow purging prior to transplantation. To date, various techniques have been proposed by several investigators to eliminate malignant cells.

From the clinical viewpoint, the optimal method should kill all clonogenic tumor cells by sparing enough normal stem cells for successful engraftment. As of now, none of the technical approaches are able to satisfy both requirements: Physical methods are not quite selective; Immunological methods employing monoclonal antibodies are strongly toxic to normal hemopoietic progenitors, and; Chemical methods are not highly selective on malignant cells (10-13).

The pharmacological technique, however, appears to be the most promising approach, showing moderate toxicity on normal stem cells and a good killing ability on leukemic cells as clearly demonstrated in animal experimental models (14-16).

In humans, with currently available techniques, we are not able to perform predictive studies of tumor cell sensitivity using clonogenic assays in vitro. Thus, we cannot easily demonstrate the efficacy of chemical purging. (17-21). Data showing that cleansed graft marrow is able to cure acute leukemias are derived only from clinical trials giving purged and unpurged marrow (22).

Other factors affecting the success of autologous bone marrow transplantation (ABMT) are the quality of remission, the first or subsequent remission as the optimal time to perform the graft, and the potential benefit of "in vivo" pretransplant ablative therapy (23-28).

Based on these considerations, we report using ABMT on 58 acute lymphoblastic leukemias (ALL), comparing the data from transplants performed in the first and the second complete remission and evaluating the efficacy of "ex vivo" marrow purging with mafosfamide.

MATERIALS AND METHODS

PATIENTS

Seven Italian teams participated in the Cooperative Mafosfamide Study Group, which reported data on 58 acute lymphoblastic leukemias (ALL) in first and second complete remissions (CR) treated with autologous bone marrow transplantation (ABMT) from June 1982 to June 1987. Forty-three patients were grafted with mafosfamide-purged marrow, and fifteen with unpurged marrow; thirty-nine patients were male and nineteen were female. The median age of the patients was 20 years (range 2-57 years).

Fifty-five percent of the patients were classified as "poor risk" on the basis of these characteristics: 1) leucocyte number $\geq$ $50x10^9/1$; 2) T or B phenotype; 3) CNS involvement; 4) large involvement of nodes or spleen; 5) mediastinal mass; 6) disease not responding to first-line therapy. Thirty percent of patients were defined as "standard risk," and 15% of the patients were unclassified.

MARROW PURGING

Twenty-eight patients were autografted in CR1: 23 of them received marrow "ex vivo" treated with mafosfamide, and 5 were transplanted with unpurged marrow.

Of the thirty CR2 patients, purging was performed in 20 cases.

The purging approach was the "ex vivo" treatment of bone marrow with mafosfamide (ASTA Werke, Bielefeld, F.R.G.), a cyclophosphamide derivative that is directly active "in vitro."

The mafosfamide concentration used was between 80 to $100\mu g/2x10^7$ nucleated cells. The bone marrow cells at the concentration of $2x10^7/ml$, with a final hematocrit of 5-10%, were incubated with the drug in a water bath with frequent agitation for 30 minutes at 37°C; the cells then were centrifuged at 2,800 RPM for 10 minutes. The supernatant was removed and mononuclear cells were resuspended at a concentration of $4x10^7/ml$ in 10% DMSO, 35% autologous plasma, 55% TC 199 solution for cryopreservation using a programmed biological freezer to ensure a constant cooling rate.

In six percent of patients, the sensitivity of hemopoietic tissue to the drug was previously tested by determining feeder layer colony growth (Gordon technique), defining optimal dose for each subject as the mafosfamide concentration able to spare 50% of the undifferentiated type 1 colonies at days 6-7 of culture (29-32).

PRE-TRANSPLANT HIGH-DOSE THERAPY
Seventy percent of the patients received total body irradiation (TBI: 10Gy) or fractionated TBI (cumulative dose: 12Gy) plus cyclophosphamide (Cy) 50μg/kg ideal body weight for 4 days or 60mg/kg for 2 days. Other regimens used were: busulphan (BU), 4mg/kg for 4 days plus Cy, 50mg/kg for 4 days (8#pts: 14%); BAVC, ARA-C-CY-TBI were used in the remaining 16% of patients. The patients did not receive any therapy after their discharge from the centers.

ANALYSIS OF RESULTS
The probability of remaining in remission (DFP: disease-free probability), the disease-free survival (DFS), and survival (S) were calculated by the KAPLAN-MEIER method (33).

ENGRAFTMENT
The parameters of engraftment were evaluated in all patients by daily count up to the mean recovery time of neutrophils over $0.5x10^9/l$ and platelets over $50x10^9/l$.

RESULTS
The survival, the disease free survival (DFS), and the disease-free probability (DFP) for all transplanted ALL patients are 36.7%, 34.4%, and 38.4% respectively, with a median follow up of 12.5, 10.7, and 11 months (range 1-61) (Fig.#1).

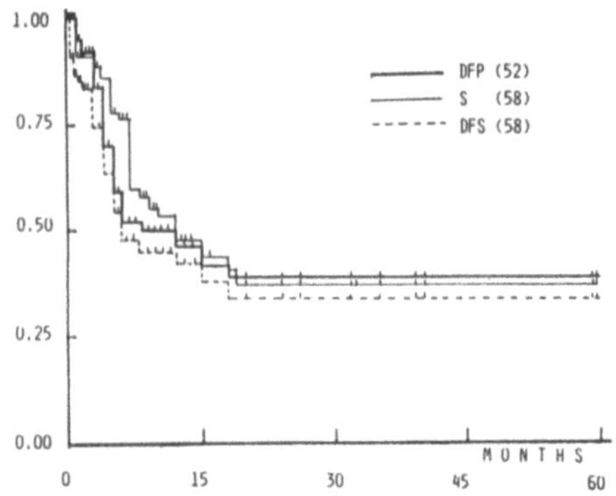

Fig.#1. Disease-free probability (DFP), survival (S) and disease free survival (DFS) after autologous bone marrow transplantation with INN-Mafosfamide-purged and non-purged marrow for acute lymphoblastic leukemia in remission. The heavy line represents a DFP of 38.4% of 52 patients transplanted in 1st and 2nd complete remission (CR). The light line represents a S of 36.7% of 58 patients grafted in 1st and 2nd CR. The dotted line represents a DFS of 34.4% of 58 patients transplanted in 1st and 2nd CR. The vertical ticks indicate patients surviving at the date of analysis.

The evaluation of DFP in ALL patients transplanted with purged and unpurged marrow demonstrates 46.4% vs. 22.2% with a trend in favor of the mafosfamide-treated group (p=NS). When we compare the results of purged ABMT performed in CR1 versus CR2, the DFP are 60.6% versus 32%, respectively (p=0.05). In the group of patients transplanted with the unpurged marrow, we observed a DFP of 40% in CR1 and 15% in CR2; the results are not statistically significant (Fig.#2).

In the patients grafted in CR1, the DFP were 60.6% and 40% at 61 months in groups receiving purged and unpurged marrow, respectively (p=0.5). For patients autografted in CR2, we observed a DFP of 32% in the mafosfamide-treated group, and 15% in patients treated with unpurged marrow (p=NS).

If we evaluate the difference between all patients transplanted with purged and non-purged marrow, comparing CR1 versus CR2, we demonstrate a significant difference in favor of ABMT performed in CR1 (54.4% in CR1, 24.2% in CR2, p=0.05) (Fig.#3).

LEUKEMIA RELAPSE
In ALL patients transplanted with purged marrow, leukemic relapse occurred in six cases of CR1 (30%): Four of them died of leukemia, and two obtained complete remission with conventional subsequent therapy. For CR2 patients the percentage of relapse was 47% (8 cases): Seven patients died from leukemia and only one is living in complete remission after conventional therapy.

The study of unpurged ABMT shows that 3 of 5 patients transplanted in CR1 relapsed and died from leukemia; eight of 10 patients grafted in CR2 relapsed; seven of them died from leukemia; and one patient is in complete remission after conventional therapy.

CAUSES OF DEATH
Seven of 58 patients developed complications during ABMT before discharge from the centers; five of them died from severe septicemia (four Gram positive, one Gram negative), one patient from veno-occlusive disease, and one from acute renal failure. Twenty-one patients died from recurrent leukemia (36.2%) (Table 1.).

KINETICS OF ENGRAFTMENT
The evaluation of marrow engraftment by daily count of neutrophils and platelets shows that hematologic reconstitution occurred in all patients (pts.) without any significant difference between the groups of mafosfamide-treated and untreated marrow. The recovery of $0.5x10^9/l$ granulocytes was at 18 days (range 14-23 days) and of $50x10^9/l$ platelets was at a median of 65 days post-transplant (range 33-91 days).

DISCUSSION
Since 1982, seven centers in Italy have consolidated data on "poor risk" or "standard risk" non-responder ALL patients in first and second remissions treated with mafosfamide-treated or untreated marrow (34-36).

We report the data here with several limitations and some critical points: The results are not derived from controlled clinical trials; the pre-transplant regimens and the time between marrow consolidation and harvest are heterogeneous.

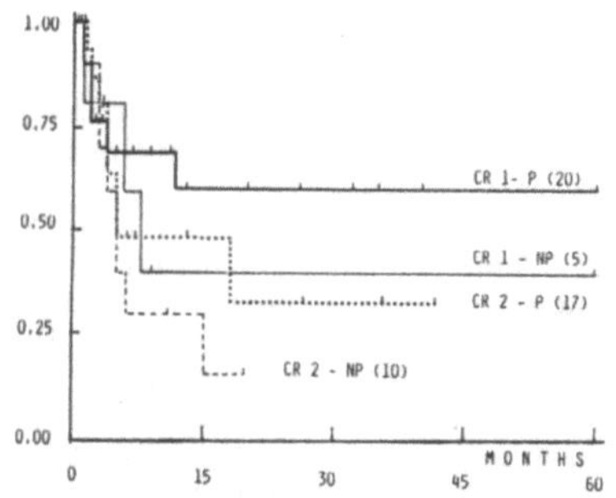

Fig.#2. Disease-free probability (DFP) after autologous bone marrow transplantation in patients grafted in 1st complete remission (CR1) and 2nd complete remission (CR2) with INN-Mafosfamide-purged (P) and non-purged (NP) marrow. The DFP of the analyzed groups are as follows: CR1 P (n=20): 60.6%; CR1 NP (n=5): 40%; CR2 P (n=17): 32%; CR2 NP (n=10): 15%. The statistical analysis is significant for the group CR1 P vs. CR2 P (P=0.05). The difference between CR1 NP and CR2 NP, CR1 P and CR1 NP, and CR2 P and CR2 NP are not significant. The vertical ticks indicate patients surviving at the date of analysis.

On the other hand, the seven groups participating in the study used a similar technical approach for the pharmacological "ex vivo" cleansing of marrow: The cell suspension was incubated with doses higher than 80μg/2x10⁷ cells.

The "in vitro" marrow treatment does not prevent the graft or the hematologic recovery; a delay of engraftment is observed essentially on platelet recovery, which reaches $50x10^9$/l at the 65th day.

Our rationale is to reduce the residual leukemic clone contaminating the remission marrow. The patients with ALL in complete remission have clonogenic cell involvement of the marrow (minimal residual disease); therefore, it appears to be appropriate to purge hemopoietic tissue for the graft. However, more sophisticated techniques for "in vitro" cloning and studying leukemic cells in culture are rapidly developing to clarify the unresolved problems and to verify the purging efficacy of mafosfamide.

Despite the limitations discussed above, the analysis of our clinical results gives interesting information at this time. If we evaluate the DFP of ALL at 60 months, we observe that the rate of relapse in this study in patients treated with ABMT (DFP=38.4%) was significantly less than that observed with current conventional therapy. Likewise, we obtained 60% of DFP at 60 months for 20 patients transplanted with treated marrow in CR1 with a plateau from 12 to 60 months. The analysis of clinical results of patients transplanted in CR1 with purged-unpurged marrow (DFP 54.8%) compared with those obtained in CR2 (purged-unpurged: DFP 24.2%) indicates that ABMT in "poor risk" or "standard risk" unresponder ALL is a consolidation therapy of high efficacy when performed in CR1 (p=0.05).

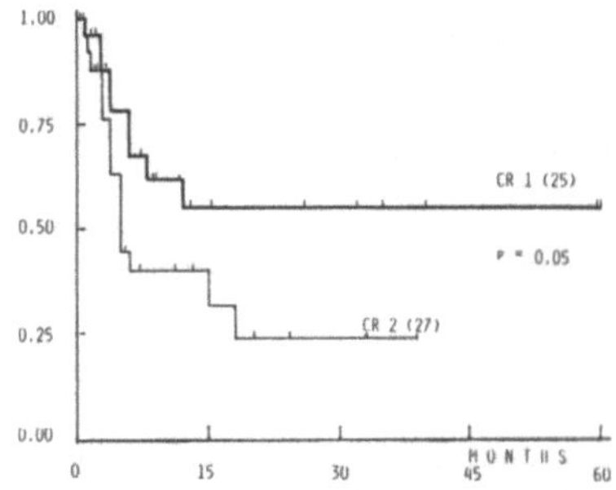

Fig.#3. Disease-free probability (DFP) of all acute lymphoblastic leukemia patients grafted with autologous INN-mafosfamide-purged and non-purged marrow in 1st complete remission (CR1) at 60 months and in 2nd complete remission (CR2) at 39 months. The DFP of the groups are as follows: CR1 (n=25): 54.8%; CR2 (n=27): 24.2% (P=0.05). The vertical ticks indicate patients surviving at the date of analysis.

Table #1. Autologous bone marrow transplantation for acute lymphoblastic leukemia in 1st and 2nd complete remission. Institutions contributing patients from June 1982 to June 1987.

TEAM	NO. OF PATIENTS	DEATHS FROM TOXICITY	DEATHS FROM LEUKEMIA	DISEASE-FREE (MONTHS)
PARMA	10	2	1	7(3+-60+)
GENOVA	12	2	9	1(39+)
TORINO	8	2	2	4(3.5+-20+)
PESARO	6	-	2	4(1+-61+)
PESCARA	10	1	3	6(1.5+-26+)
PADOVA	4		1	3(1+-12+)
MILANO	8	-	3	5(9+-32+)
	58	7(12.1%)	21(36.2%)	30(51.7%)

Median: 12.5 Mo+
Range: 1+-61+

In conclusion as of 1982, seven Italian Centers (INN-Mafosfamide Study Group) have reported data on 58 ABMT of patients with ALL, showing encouraging results, which are better than those reported and obtained with allograft or with conventional chemotherapy.

The fourth European Bone Marrow Transplantation Group survey (Interlaken 1987) demonstrated that there is no statistically significant advantage for mafosfamide-treated marrow in terms of disease-free survival; there is a trend in favor of "ex vivo" purging (37). Our results are in favor of purging in all groups of ALL transplanted in clinical complete remission phase. A longer median follow up is necessary to clarify if ABMT cures the leukemia. At this time, the autologous graft in our study appears better for purged groups in ALL CR1 and CR2.

Finally, the present survey at 5 years indicates that for a large number of "poor risk" ALL patients the probability of remaining in remission is 38.4%, with a long plateau between 12 to 60 months.

These results show that ABMT is an important and alternative therapeutic approach for ALL (38).

SUMMARY

Fifty-eight patients (pts.) with acute lymphoblastic leukemia were treated with autologous bone marrow transplantation (ABMT) using chemotherapy plus total body irradiation (TBI) or combination chemotherapy as high-dose ablative regimens. Forty-three patients were grafted with INN-mafosfamide-purged marrow. We compared the results obtained in 28 patients autografted in first complete remission (CR1) vs. 30 cases autografted in second complete remission (CR2) and purged vs. unpurged grafts.

The results demonstrate that the disease-free survival (DFS) and disease-free probability (DFP) are 34.4% and 38.4%, respectively, at 61 months. The ABMT performed in CR1 obtained a DFP of 60.6% vs 32% when the graft was performed in CF2. The results with purged marrow vs. non-purged marrow favor purged CFI. The most frequent causes of death were relapses of leukemia (21 pts.)and septicemia (5 pts.).

The kinetics of engraftment demonstrate a delay in platelet recovery. The data reported from seven Italian centers show encouraging results with ABMT in acute lymphoblastic leukemia with a significant advantage for mafosfamide-purged marrow and graft performed in CR1.

ACKNOWLEDGEMENTS

The Authors thank Dr. A. Malice for technical assistance and Mrs. A. Leporati for preparing this manuscript.

This work was supported in part by PFO 86.00553.44, 8600465.04, AIRC 1987, R.E.R. grant 1986, CNR 86.00703.44, 86.00280.44, 86.00463.44, 86.00559.44.

REFERENCES

1. Herzig GP (1981): Autologous marrow transplantation in cancer therapy. Prog. Hematol. 12:1
2. Gehan EA (1984): Dose-response relationship in clinical oncology. Cancer, 54 (suppl.):1204
3. Barret AJ, Kendra JR, Lucas CF, Joss DV, Joshi R, Desai M, Hugh Jones K, Phillips RH, Rogers TR, Tabara Z, Williamson S, Hobbs J (1982): Bone marrow transplantation for acute lymphoblastic leukemia. Br. J. Haematol. 52:181
4. Thomas ED, Buckner CD, Banaji M (1977). One hundred patients with acute leukemia treated by chemotherapy, total body irradiation and allogeneic marrow transplantation. Blood 49:511
5. Hagenbeeck A, Martens ACM (1984): Toxicity of asta Z 7557 (INN-mafosfamide) to normal and leukemic stem cells: Implications for autologous bone marrow transplantation. Invest. new drugs 2:237
6. Bortin MM, Gale RP, Kay HEM, Rimm AA (1983): Bone marrow transplantation for acute myelogenous leukemia. JAMA 249:1166
7. Gorin NC, Aegerter P, Parlier Y, for the working party on autologous bone marrow transplantation of the European Bone Marrow Transplantation Group (1985): Autologous bone marrow transplantation for acute leukemia in remission: Second European Survey. Exp. Hematol. B, suppl. 17:18
8. Mandelli F (1986): Autologous bone marrow transplantation (ABMT) in leukemia. Proc. of third int. symp. ABMT, Houston, in press.
9. Marmont AM, Carella AM (1986): Autologous bone marrow transplantation in haematologic malignancies. Haematologica, 71:1
10. Treleaven JG, Kemshead JT (1985): Removal of tumor cells from bone marrow: An evaluation of the available techniques. Haematol. Oncol., 3:6511
11. Bast RC JR, DeFabritiis P, Bregni M, Raso V, Reynolds C, Lipton JM, Grenberger JS, Nadler LM, Sallan SE, Ritz J (1984): Removal of malignant cells from human bone marrow using monoclonal antibodies and complement. In: Dicke K, Spitzer G, Zander A (eds): Proc. First Int. Symp. on Autologous Bone Marrow Transplantation, p.373
12. Bast RC, Ritz J, Lipton JM, Feeney M, Sallan SC, Nathan DG, Schlossman SF (1983): Elimination of leukemic cells from human bone marrow using monoclonal antibody and complement. Cancer Res. 43:1389
13. Hagenbeek A, Martens ACM: Toxicity of ASTA-Z 7557 (INN mafosfamide) to normal and leukemic stem cells: Implications for autologous bone marrow transplantation. Investigational New Drugs, 2:237
14. Sharkis SJ, Santos GW, Colvin M (1980):Elimination of acute myelogenous leukemic cells from marrow and tumor suspensions in the rat with 4-hydroperoxycyclophosphamide. Blood 55:521
15. Porcellini A, Manna A, Sparaventi G,Talevi N, Rizzoli V (1983):The selective effect of 4-hydroperoxycyclophosphamide. (ASTA -Z) on pluripotent and committed stem cell compartment in mice. Exp. Hematol. 11 (suppl.14): 133a
16. Zeller WJ, Berger MR, Matys R, Schmacher J (1984): Antineoplastic of ASTA Z 7557 (INN-mafosfamide) in transplant and autochthonous experimental rodent tumors. Investigational New Drugs 2:175
17. Hagenbeek A,Martens ACM (1985): Preclinical studies on detection of minimal residual disease in acute leukemia. In: Dicke DA, Spitzer G

Zander AR (eds): Proc. of the First Int. Symp. of Autologous Bone Marrow Transplantation, p.329
18. Philip I, Favrot MC, Philip T (1985): Detection of Burkitt's cells in remission marrow by a cell culture monitoring system: Implications for autologous bone marrow transplantation. In: Dicke KA, Zander AD (eds): Proc. of the First Int. Symp. of Autologous Bone Marrow Transplantation, p.341
19. Reynolds CP, Black AT, Woody JN (1985): Use of Hoechst 3342 for sensitive detection of viable cells seeded into bone marrow. In: Dicke KA, Spitzer G, Zander R (eds): Proc. of the First Int. Symp. of Autologous Bone Marrow Transplantation, 365
20. Douay L (1985): Cyclophosphamide derivatives for in vitro cleansing of leukemic bone marrow. Blood transfusion and immunohaematology, Tome 27, 5:427
21. Defabritiis P, Bregni M, Lipton J, Greenberger JS, Nadler LM, Rochstein L, Korbling M, Ritz J, Bast RC, Jr. (1985): Elimination of clonogenic Burkitt's lymphoma cells from human bone marrow using 4-hydroperoxycyclophosphamide in combination with monoclonal antibodies and complement. Blood 65:1064
22. Santos GW, Kaiser H (1984): In vitro chemotherapy as a prelude to autologous marrow transplantation in hematology malignancy. In: Lowemberg B, Hagenbeek A (eds): Minimal Residual Disease in Acute Leukemia, Boston, Martinus Nijhoff, Ed. 165
23. Rizzoli V, Mangoni L, Degliantoni G, Caramatti C, Costi D, Quaini P (1985): Autologous bone marrow transplantation in acute leukemia and lymphoma. Dicke KA, Spritzer G, Zander AR (eds): Proc. of the First Int. Symp. of Autologous Bone Marrow Transpl., 45
24. Rizzoli V, Mangoni L, Degliantoni G, Caramatti C, Costi D, Craviotto L (1985): Autologous bone marrow transplantation for acute leukemia in remission. Parma experience. Int. J. of Cell Cloning, 3:4, 246
25. Armitage J (1986) Report of an international cooperative study: Bone marrow autotransplantation in man. The Lancet, 960
26. Yeager AM, Kaizer H, Santos GW, et al (1986): Autologous bone marrow transplantation in patients with acute nonlymphocytic leukemia, using ex vivo marrow treatment with 4-hydroperoxycyclophosphamide. New Engl. Journal of Medicine, 3:141
27. Tura S (1983): Simposio sull'autotrapianto di midollo osseo. Haematologica 6 (suppl.1):25
28. Carella AM, Santini G, Santoro A, et al (1985): Massive chemotherapy with non-frozen autologous bone marrow transplantation in 13 cases of refractory Hodgkin's disease. Eur. J. cancer clin. oncol. 5:607-13
29. Gordon MY, Hibbin JA, Kearney V, Gordon-Smith EC, Goldman JM (1985): Colony formation by primitive haemopoietic progenitors in cocultures of bone marrow cells and stromal cells. Br. J. Haematol. 60:129
30. Siena S, Castro-Malaspina H, Gulati SC, et al (1985): Effects of in vitro purging with 4-hydroperoxycyclophosphamide on the hematopoietic and microenvironmental elements of human bone marrow. Blood 65:655
31. Degliantoni G, Mangoni L, Rizzoli V (1986): Normal blast colony formation : An in vitro tool for monitoring human bone marrow purging. Bone Marrow Transpl., 1:209
32. Hilton J, Colvin M (1984): The role of aldehyde dehydrogenase activity in cylophosphamide sensitivity of hematopoietic and leukemic cell populations. Proc. of the Am. Assoc. of Cancer Research, 25:1343 (abstr)
33. Kaplan EL, Meier P (1958): Nonparametric estimation from incomplete observations. J. Am. Stat. Assoc. 53:45734.
34. Rizzoli V, Mangoni L, Porcellini A, Carelli AM, Alessandrino EP, Aglietta M, Torlontano G, Coleselli P, Mozzana A, Madon E (1986): Autologous Bone Marrow Transplantation for acute lymphocytic leukemia. In: Proc. of Third Int. Symp. on Autologous Bone Marrow Transplantation (in press)
35. Rizzoli V, Mangoni L, Degliantoni G, Porellini A, Carella AM, Alessandrino EP, Mozzana A, Aglietta M, Coleselli P, Torlontano G, Italian Cooperative Group (1986): Mafosfamide bone marrow purging autologous transplantation in acute leukemia. Acta Hematologica (in press)
36. Mangoni L, Porcellini A, Carella AM, Alessandrino EP, Mozzana A, Aglietta M, Coleselli P, Torlontano G, Rizzoli V Italian Cooperative Group (1986): Autologous bone marrow transplantation in acute leukemia using marrow treated with mafosfamide. Blood, 68 (suppl.1):5, 276a
37. Gorin NC, Aegerter P, for the Working Party on Autologous Bone Marrow Transplantation of the European Bone Marrow Transplantion Group (1987): Autologous bone marrow transplantation for acute leukemia in remission: 4th European Bone Marrow Transplantation Group Survey. Bone Marrow Transplantation 2 (suppl.#1): 320
38. Gorin NC, Herve P, Aegerter P, Goldstone A, Linch D, Maraninchi D, Burnett A, Helbig W, Meloni G, Verdonck LF, De Witte T, Rizzoli V, Carella A, Parlier Y, Auvert B, Goldman J, for the Working Party on Autologous Bone Marrow Transplantation of the European Bone Marrow Transplantation Group (1986): Autologous bone marrow transplantation for acute leukemia in remission. Br.J. of Hematol., 64:385

14: Allogeneic Bone Marrow Transplantation for Chronic Myeloid Leukemia

John M. Goldman

A number of attempts were made in the 1970s to treat patients with chronic myeloid leukaemia (CML) in blastic transformation by allogeneic bone marrow transplantation (BMT) using HLA identical sibling donors. These efforts were unsuccessful in almost every case. Thus patients died either of transplant-related complications or of relapse of leukaemia. A small number of such patients became long term survivors but in general the prospects for treating CML by allogeneic BMT looked poor. In 1979 Fefer and his colleagues in Seattle reported the preliminary results of treating a small series of patients with CML by syngeneic BMT while their disease remained in chronic phase. These results were very much more encouraging (1). Three of the four patients in the original series became longterm survivors. Thus the possibility of curing CML by BMT became a reality and a number of specialist centres began in the early 1980s to treat selected patients with HLA-identical siblings donors by BMT in CP.

In 1987 the results of this worldwide experience can be summarized to some extent (Table 1). Thus approximately 45% of the patients who have been transplanted in chronic phase can expect to be alive and free of evidence of leukaemia 4 year post-transplant. In contrast during this decade the results of transplant for patients with more advanced stages of disease have not improved to any great extent. Thus one may reasonably conclude that a patient with an HLA-identical sibling should be offered the chance of treatment by BMT before the onset of transformation. If however this offer is accepted, a number of distinct problems remain. For example, the timing of the transplant within the chronic phase is still a matter for debate. The details of the actual transplant procedure cannot yet be standardized. What schedule of chemoradiotherapy should be employed? How should the spleen be managed pre-transplant and what method should be used to minimize the risk of graft-versus-host disease (GVHD)? An important question that has emerged in the last two years is the precise definition of cure. It has become apparent that the finding of a small number of Ph-positive metaphases in the marrow post-transplant does not automatically indicate impending relapse. Finally there are important questions that relate to the possibility of extending the use of transplant to patients not yet considered eligible: what should be the maximal age for patients submitted to transplant and what donors can be used in the absence of an HLA-identical sibling? Some of these questions are addressed in more detail in this chapter.

RESULTS OF BMT BY PHASE OF DISEASE

For the purpose of most analyses patients were classified at the time of BMT as being in chronic or stable phase, in accelerated phase or in blastic transformation. The definition of accelerated disease in not universally agreed and indeed it is likely that some features no longer consistent with uncomplicated chronic phase, such as a platelet count exceeding 1000 x $10^9/l$ or the finding of a second Ph chromosome, are intrinsically less ominous than others, such as the finding in the marrow of 20% blasts plus promyelocytes or the finding of trisomy for chromosome no. 8. These points notwithstanding, it seems clear on the basis of the relatively large series of patients reported from Seattle (2) and the results collected and analysed by the International Bone Marrow Transplant Registry (3) that the actuarial probabilities of survival, of relapse and of relapse-free survival at 3 years for patients in chronic phase are each significantly better than the corresponding values for patients transplanted in the accelerated phase or blastic transformation (Table 1).

Table 1. Actuarial results of allogeneic BMT using HLA-identical sibling donors according to phase of CML at time of transplant

	Actuarial probability (%) at 4 years		
Phase of CML	Survival	Relapse	Leukaemia free survival
Chronic phase	55±10	12±10	45±10
Accelerated phase	25±15	40±20	20±15
Blastic transformation	12±15	60±20	12±15

Results are based in part on data analysed by IBMTR. Values are means ±95 per cent confidence intervals.

RESULTS OF TREATMENT IN CHRONIC PHASE

The IBMTR has recently reported an analysis of results of BMT performed in 405 patients transplanted with marrow from HLA-identical sibling donors (4). A minority of the patients in this analysis had received marrow that had been depleted of T-lymphocytes ex vivo by incubation with monoclonal antibodies or by counterflow elutriation; the majority however had received unmanipulated marrow cells. The actuarial probability of survival at four years was 55±5%. The various causes of death are shown in Fig 1. The actuarial probability of relapse for all patients including the 89 who had received T-depleted marrow, was 19±8%, a figure that contrasts starkly with the figure of 9±5% for patients who received donor marrow that had not been depleted of T-lymphocytes ex vivo (see below).

In this analysis there were two major factors related to an increased probability of survival post-transplant - the absence of moderate or severe GVHD and younger age (4). It was interesting to note however that over the age of 20 there was no further increment is risk; in other words there was no significant difference in survival between patients in the third and those in the fifth decade of life. The duration of disease pre-transplant did not appear to predict for the probability of survival, a finding that conflicts with the observation reported from Seattle that patients submitted to transplant within one year of diagnosis have a survival superior to those with longer histories of chronic phase disease (2). The probability of relapse was greater in patients who received T-depleted marrow (as mentioned above) and in patients who did not develop chronic GVHD; there was apparently no influence of acute GVHD on relapse.

TIMING OF BMT WITHIN THE CHRONIC PHASE

Once it is accepted that the only approach to cure is treatment by BMT, one may logically conclude that every patient must be treated by BMT provided that the estimated mortality of the procedure is relatively low. This last consideration may for the present exclude patients older than 50 years and those who lack HLA-identical sibling donors. It also means that the transplant must be performed while the patient remains in the chronic phase. Since there is no clear evidence that the duration of chronic phase before transplant influences the probability of survival, it would be logical to delay the transplant until shortly before transformation to minimize the degree to which his life might be curtailed by a transplant that failed. The problem here is that the duration of chronic phase cannot be predicted with any accuracy for an individual patient. The optimal timing of transplant must therefore be decided in other ways.

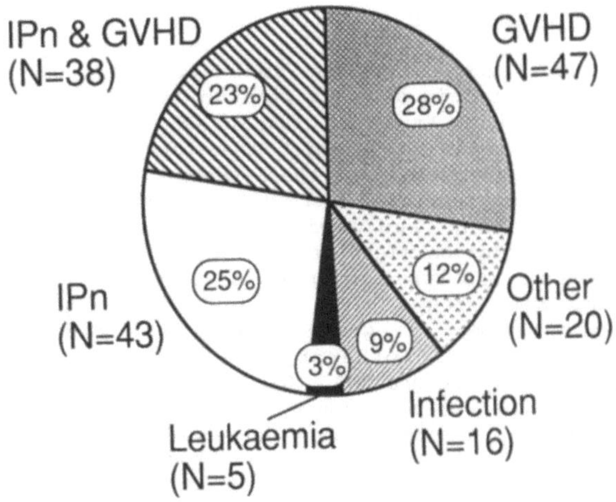

Figure 1. Principal causes of death for 169 patients who have died of the 409 patients treated by BMT for CML in chronic phase. IPn = interstitial pneumonitis. GVHD = graft-versus-host disease. Data collected and reproduced here by permission of the International Bone Marrow Transplant Registry.

Segel and his colleagues have recently reported the development of a mathematical model that attempts to balance for an individual patient the probability of transformation in any one year against the probability of death as a result of the transplant procedure (5). Application of such a model might then lead to the conclusion that a patient with a series of poor prognostic features (6), such as a man with a greatly enlarged spleen and a very high leucocyte count at diagnosis, might best be transplanted as soon as possible. Conversely a female patient whose disease was diagnosed incidentally when her spleen was still impalpable and her leucocyte count comparatively low might fall in a sub-category of patients whose median survival is 6 years. For such a patient the recommendation that she should undergo BMT immediately after diagnosis might be erroneous.

In practice these sorts of calculations are a valuable guide for the clinician but the patient will frequently base his or her decision about whether and when to undergo BMT on other more practical considerations. Thus some patients find the uncertainty of knowing they have CML intolerable and will opt to undergo transplantation as soon as possible. Others may wish to be reasonably certain of survival until a particular date one or two years in the future and will only wish to be subjected to the risk of transplantation thereafter.

HOW TO MANAGE THE SPLEEN

The spleen seems to be a site of preferential involvement both in the chronic phase and in transformation of CML. It may also be the site at which transformation is first recognized. For these reasons a number of workers have speculated that the chance of eradicating leukaemia at the time of transplantation might be enhanced if especial measures are taken to treat the spleen (7-9). Thus some groups have routinely performed splenectomy (9) while others have given additonal radiotherapy to the spleen immediately before BMT (10). The majority of transplant centres however take no additional measures. A recent survey performed by the European Bone Marrow Transplant Group showed a trend favouring survival in patients who had received splenic irradiation but the numbers of patients included in the analysis was relatively small and the differences not significant (11). The same group is now undertaking a prospectively randomized comparison of survival and relapse rate in patients who receive and patient who do not receive additional splenic irradiation.

T-CELL DEPLETION

A number of experimental studies using a variety of animal models have provided clear evidence that removal from donor marrow of T-lymphocytes reduces the incidence of GVHD. Such T-cell depletion also reduces the probability of engraftment and may increase the risk of relapse. These last two problems notwithstanding, a number of groups began about 4 years ago to deplete donor marrow of T-cells for prevention of GVHD before BMT for CML and acute leukaemia. It became rapidly clear that the incidence of GVHD was indeed reduced to a significant extent (10,12-14). It soon became clear also that the incidence of graft failure, normally less than 2% in recipients of HLA-matched donor marrow, rose to 10-15% in recipients of analogous marrow that had previously been depleted of T-cells in vitro. The group at the Royal Free Hospital in London proposed that graft failure in this setting was mediated by a relatively radioresistant lymphoid cell and that a modest increase in the dosage of radiotherapy for the patient might reduce the risk (15). In practice this seems to be true. Preliminary evidence suggests that increasing the number of 2 Gy fractions of total body irradiation (TBI) to 7 (total 14 Gy) or adding total lymphoid irradiation (6 or 8 Gy) to standard dose TBI (10 or 12 Gy) has indeed largely solved the problem of graft failure.

The problem of relapse is much more intractable. The actuarial probability of relapse in the series of patients reported from the Hammersmith Hospital in London was 29% at 2 years, which contrasted with a figure of 7% in a historical control group of patients who had received unmanipulated marrow cells (16). Similarly a multi-centre analysis of patients who received marrow depleted of T-cells with the monoclonal antibodies Campath-1 or CT-2 showed actuarial relapse rates of 3% and 33% for test and historical control groups respectively, a difference that was of course highly significant (17). In neither the Hammersmith study nor in the multi-centre analysis is there yet any significant difference in survival between recipients of T-depleted marrow cells and controls. Because many of the patients who received T-depleted marrow have relapsed, such a difference must inevitably emerge at some time in the future.

The observation in CML that recipients of T-depleted donor marrow cells have a significantly increased risk of relapse implies that the T cells that were removed would have played a crucial role in eradicating the leukaemia. This observation is therefore compatible with the existence of an important graft-versus-leukaemia effect in CML and such effect may be important also in transplantatoin for other types of leukaemia. This interpretation casts some doubt on the notion that the increased risk of relapse associated with T-depletion can be offset merely by increasing the dosage of chemoradiotherapy. It is more likely that further immunological manipulations, such as re-transfusion of selected T-cells of donor origin or of appropriate lymphokines or haemopoietic growth factors, could be effective.

DEFINITION OF CURE

For recipients of unmanipulated marrow the relapse rate is remarkably low (5 to 10%) and such relapses that do occur appear mainly within the first two years after transplant. Occasional relapses have been seen at longer intervals but the general pattern of the disease-free survival curve and the longer experience with follow-up of recipients of syngeneic transplants point firmly to the conclusion that the chance of later relapse for patients who survive 3 years may be exceedingly small. The majority of such patients may thus expect to be cured.

In a number of centres cytogenetic analysis of bone marrow within a few weeks of transplant has shown a minority population of Ph-positive metaphases (18, 19). These cells are presumed to be the remnants of a leukaemic population doomed to extinction and indeed their number has frequently dwindled or disappeared entirely on subsequent examination. However a small number of patients have been identified with Ph-positive marrow metaphases more than one year from diagnosis. Some of these patients with cytogenetic evidence of relapse will eventually proceed to show haematological features of relapse but in other cases the proportion of Ph-positive metaphases found in the marrow has dwindled in subsequent cytogenetic studies and they have perhaps disappeared entirely (20). Thus it appears that cure may not depend on the complete and permanent eradication of all Ph-positive cells at the time of transplant. Instead cure may still be a clinical reality in the presence of small number of Ph-positive cells which may persist in the marrow for months or possibly years. The nature of this Ph-positive population is of course not yet defined. The sequence of events would be readily explained if routine cytogenetic methods were for example on occasion revealing the presence of a long-lived Ph-positive cell committed to the lymphoid lineage.

USE OF MATCHED UNRELATED DONORS

CML is the disease par excellence in which it is logical to test the potential value of identifying and using suitably matched unrelated donors for allogeneic BMT. Thus far a relatively small number of transplants have been performed using unrelated donors who were HLA-identical with the patient at all six major HLA loci and were in most cases also mutually non-reactive in mixed lymphocyte culture. Preliminary results suggest that the use of such matched unrelated donors′ may be no less valuable than use of HLA-identical siblings. The advent of matching methods that exploit DNA restriction fragment length polymorphisms at HLA DR loci may greatly simplify and thereby expedite the recognition of suitable unrelated donors.

CONCLUSIONS

There has been major progress in the last eight years in defining more precisely the contribution of BMT to cure for patients with CML. Further progress will now depend both on success in combating the problems common to all transplant procedures, notably GVHD, interstitial pneumonitis and viral infections, and on success defining more precisely the way in which the details of a standard transplant procedure must be modified for a patient with CML.

REFERENCES

1. Fefer A, Cheever M, Thomas ED et al (1979) Disappearance of Ph-positive cells in four patients with chronic granulocytic leukemia after chemotherapy, irradiation and bone marrow transplantation from an identical twin. New Engl J Med 300:333-337

2. Thomas ED, Clift RA, Fefer A et al (1986) Marrow transplantation for the treatment of chronic myelogenous leukemia. Ann Intern Med 104:155-163

3. Speck B, Bortin M, Champlin RE et al (1984) Bone marrow transplantation for chronic myelogenous leukaemia. Lancet i:665-668

4. Goldman JM, Biggs JC, Bortin MM et al. Bone marrow transplantation for chronic myelogenous leukemia in chronic phase: increased risk of relapse associated with T-cell depletion. Submitted for publication

5. Segal GB, Simon W, Lichtman MA (1986) Variables influencing the timing of marrow transplantation in patients with chronic myelogenous leukaemia. Blood 68:1055-1064

6. Sokal JE, Baccarani M, Tura S et al (1985) Prognostic discrimination among younger patients with chronic granulocytic leukemia: relevance to bone marrow transplantation. Blood 66:1352-1357

7. Gluckman E, Devergie A, Bernheim A, Berger R (1983) Splenectomy and bone marrow transplantation in chronic granulocytic leukaemia. Lancet i:1392-1393(letter)

8. Lehn P, Devergie A, Benbunan M, et al (1986) Bone marrow transplantation for chronic granulocytic leukemia. J Nat Cancer Inst 314:202-207

9. Speck B, Gratwohl A, Nissen C (1982) Allogeneic marrow transplantation for chronic granulocytic leukemia. Blut 45:237-242

10. Goldman JM, Apperley JF, Jones L et al (1986) Bone marrow transplantation for patients with chronic myeloid leukemia. New Engl J Med 314:202-207

11. Gratwohl A, Goldman J, Gluckman E, Zwaan F (1985) Effect of splenectomy before bone-marrow transplantation on survival in chronic granulocytic leukaemia. Lancet ii:1290-1291

12. Prentice HG, Blacklock HA Janossy G et al (1984) Depletion of T lymphocytes in donor marrow prevents significant graft-versus-host disease in matched allogeneic leukaemic marrow transplant recipients. Lancet i:472-6

13. Waldmann H, Polliak A, Hale G et al (1984) Elimination of graft-versus-host disease by in-vitro depletion of alloreactive lymphocytes with a monoclonal rat anti-human lymphocyte antibody (Campath-1). Lancet ii:483-6

14. Mitsuyasu RT, Champlin RE, Gale RP et al (1986) Treatment of donor bone marrow with monoclonal anti-T-cell antibody and complement for the prevention of graft-versus-host disease: a prospective randomized double-blind trial. Ann Intern Med 105:20-25

15. Patterson J, Prentice HG, Brenner MK et al (1986) Graft rejection following HLA-matched T-lymphocyte depleted bone marrow transplantation. Br J Haematol 63:221-230

16. Apperley JF, Jones L, Hale G et al (1986) Bone marrow transplantation for patients with chronic myeloid leukaemia: T-cell depletion with Campath-1 reduces the incidence of graft-versus-host disease but may increase the risk of leukaemic relapse. Bone Marrow Transplant 1:53-68

17. Apperley JF, Mauro FR, Goldman JM et al. BMT for chronic myeloid leukemia in first chronic phase: importance of a graft-versus-leukemia effect. Submitted for publication

18. Zaccaria A, Rosti G, Testoni N et al (1987) Chromosome studies in patients with Philadelphia chromosome-positive chronic myeloid leukemia submitted to bone marrow transplantation: results of a European cooperative study. Cancer Genet Cytogenet 26:5-13

19. Arthur CK, Apperley JF, Guo AP et al. Cytogenetic events after bone marrow transplantation for chronic myeloid leukemia in chronic phase. Submitted for publication

20. Apperley JF, Rassool F, Parreira A et al (1986) Philadelphia positive metaphases in the marrow after bone marrow transplantation for chronic granulocytic leukemia. Amer J Hematol 22:199-204

V. Autologous and Allogeneic Marrow Transplants in Leukemia and Lymphoma (Session B): Roger H. Herzig and Shigetaku Asano, Chairpersons

15: Autologous Marrow Transplantation for Hodgkin's and Non-Hodgkin's Lymphoma: Preliminary Results Using New Conditioning Regimens

Roger H. Herzig, Gordon L. Phillips, Steven N. Wolff, Joseph W. Fay, C. Frederick LeMaistre, Donna E. Reece, D. Frei-Lahr, James N. Lowder, and Geoffrey P. Herzig

INTRODUCTION

Current combination chemotherapy regimens can produce durable remission in many patients with Hodgkin's disease (1) and certain intermediate- and high-grade non-Hodgkin's lymphomas (2). However, patients who do not achieve durable remission after these therapies usually respond poorly to salvage chemotherapies (3,4).

Intensive chemoradiotherapy and allogeneic bone marrow transplantation are curative in certain hematologic malignancies (5), including malignant lymphoma (6,9,10). However, only a minority of otherwise eligible patients have suitable donors available for syngeneic or histocompatible allogeneic transplantation. Moreover, the complications of graft-versus-host disease account for a substantial morbidity and mortality in the latter group. Autologous marrow offers the advantages of an expanded number of "donors" and the avoidance of the immunologic problems of allogeneic transplants. A potential limiting problem of autologous transplantation is a possible increased relapse rate due to the reinfusion of occult lymphoma cells in the marrow inoculum. However, the significance of this problem has not been clearly delineated, since most of the relapses occur in areas of previously-known disease and probably result from inadequate therapy (11).

We have previously reported a Phase I-II study of cyclophosphamide, total body irradiation, and cryopreserved but otherwise unmanipulated autologous bone marrow transplantation in 27 patients with progressive lymphoma (11). We have subsequently employed alternative preparative regimens to improve the therapeutic response and to hopefully decrease the treatment-related toxicity. We now report the preliminary results of these trials.

METHODS

Eligibility Criteria and Study Design

Since 1985, 122 patients with malignant lymphoma underwent intensive chemoradiotherapy and autologous bone marrow transplantation using four newer protocols. Eligibility criteria included: (1) progression of life-threatening lymphoma after primary or salvage chemotherapy; (2) age no greater than 65 years; (3) the presence of a remission bone marrow by conventional histology immediately before marrow harvest (specifically, a history of prior marrow involvement did not exclude patients); (4) absence of severe co-morbid medical illness that would preclude the use of protocol therapy; (5) no potentially curative salvage regimen was available.

The studies were performed with the approval of the respective Human Investigations Committees at Baylor University; Cleveland Clinic; the University of British Columbia; the University of Texas, San Antonio; and Washington University. Informed consent was obtained in all patients both at the time of bone marrow harvest and subsequent transplantation.

Remission bone marrow was harvested during either systemic remission or relapse. Intensive chemoradiotherapy or intensive chemotherapy with or without involved-field radiotherapy and autologous bone marrow transplantation was used after the failure of potentially curative chemotherapy. No further therapy was given after the transplant to maintain remission.

Bone Marrow Harvest, Cryopreservation, and Reinfusion

All patients underwent diagnostic bone marrow biopsies within two weeks of bone marrow harvest; bilateral specimens were obtained in most cases. The techniques of marrow harvest, cryopreservation, and reinfusion have been reported previously (11,12). The median dose of marrow cells was 2.0×10^8/kg ideal body weight (range, 0.4 - 7.7). Marrow was stored at $-196^\circ C$ in the liquid phase of a liquid nitrogen refrigerator for a median of 35 (range, 6-547) days. Marrow progenitor cell assays were not routinely performed.

Cyclophosphamide and Total Body Irradiation Regimens (CY/TBI)

The details of this regimen have been

published (11). Briefly, cyclophosphamide 60 mg/kg, calculated using ideal body weight, was infused on the fifth and fourth days before transplantation; total body irradiation (TBI) was given as a single fraction (1000 cGy, at a dose rate of 6-15 cGy per minute) or as fractionated total body irradiation (fTBI) (1200-1600 cGy). All patients who received involved-field radiotherapy (IFR) received the fTBI dose of 1200 cGy. The fTBI was given as 200 cGy fractions twice daily at dose rates of 10-45 cGy per minute. The experience with CY/TBI preparative regimens by the original investigators has expanded to 96 patients. The data obtained from this study is used for comparison purposes for the new conditioning regimens. Future studies and detailed analyses are planned for the 96 patients studied to date.

Etoposide, Cyclophosphamide, and Total Body Irradiation Regimen (VP/CY/TBI)

In January 1986, we explored the addition of etoposide (VP-16) to the preparative regimen. In addition, we wanted to maximize the cyclophosphamide and fTBI. Patients with refractory lymphomas and other hematologic malignancies were eligible, following the general criteria above and in reference 11. Of the 54 patients entered who are evaluable for toxicity, 38 had non-Hodgkin's lymphoma. The VP-16, 1800-2250 mg/m^2, given by continuous intravenous infusion over 26-32 hours on the first day of treatment. Cyclophosphamide, 50 mg/kg, was administered as a 2-hour infusion daily for the next 3 or 4 days (total 150-200 mg/kg). TBI was fractionated with 200 cGy fractions twice daily at dose rates of 10-45 cGy per minute to total doses of 1000 cGy in 17 patients and 1200 cGy in 37 patients.

Cyclophosphamide, Nitrosourea (BCNU), Etoposide (CBV)

In February 1985, we began treating patients with recurrent Hodgkin's disease with cyclophosphamide 1.8 g/m^2 daily for 4 days (day -7, -6, -5, -4), BCNU 600 mg/m^2 once (day -3), and VP-16 400 mg/m^2 every 12 hours for 3 days (6 doses) on days -7, -6, -5; bone marrow was infused 2 days after the BCNU. Cytoreductive therapy with 1-4 cycles of nitrogen mustard, Velban, procarbazine, prednisone (MVPP) alone (5 patients), IFR alone (8 patients), both MVPP and IFR (9 patients), or neither (20 patients). Preliminary experience with this regimen has been presented (15).

Etoposide, Triethylene Thiophosphoramide (Thiotepa), Cyclophosphamide (VP/TT; VP/TT/CY)

Patients who were not eligible for TBI because of previous radiotherapy were given VP-16, 800 mg/m^2 every other day (day -10, -8, -6) and thiotepa 135-300 mg/m^2 daily for 3 days (day -5, -4, -3); autologous marrow was given 2 days after the thiotepa. Because the preliminary results of the VP/CY/TBI regimen described above demonstrated only mild toxicity, the protocol was modified to include cyclophosphamide. A further modification of VP-16 administration was accomplished to ease administration: the VP-16 was given as a continuous infusion of the total dose of 1000 mg/m^2 (day -8); thiotepa 300 mg/m^2/day given for 3 days (day -7, -6, -5); cyclophosphamide 50 mg/kg/day on days -4, -3, -2 -1. Since February 1985, 26 patients were treated, 6 on the former protocol and 20 on the latter regimen.

Involved-Field Radiotherapy

Patients with "bulky" disease received involved-field radiotherapy (IFR), 1500-2400 cGy, over 10-14 days immediately before the preparative regimen whenever possible. The requirements for the use of the involved-field radiotherapy were as follows: (1) ninety percent of active lymphoma, excluding the bone marrow and/or central nervous system, could be encompassed in one or two standard radiotherapy ports; (2) rapidly progressive systemic disease was not present; and (3) cumulative radiotherapy doses were not excessive.

Supportive Care

All blood components were irradiated to at least 1500 cGy and given as needed after transplant to maintain the hemoglobin level above 9 gm% and a platelet count above 10-20 x 10^9/L. Empiric broad-spectrum antibiotics, Amphotericin B, and parenteral hyperalimentation were used as indicated.

Evaluation

Immediately before treatment patients were assessed with a toxicity profile for the lungs, heart, liver, and kidneys. Also, patients were clinically restaged, and repeat biopsies were performed if tissue was relatively easy to obtain or if this information would potentially influence therapy. Staging studies were repeated at days +30 and +90 and then at least every six months for two years in patients who achieved complete remission. Patients were studied only for recurrent symptoms or signs thereafter. Toxicity profiles were repeated only if clinically indicated. Patients were considered evaluable for antitumor response if they survived beyond day 30 post-transplant. Disease progression was considered evaluable at any time post-transplant. Death before day 30 without disease progression was evaluable for toxicity only.

Definitions

Complete remission was defined as the complete disappearance of tumor and survival at least to day +30. Patients who died before day +30 were not considered evaluable for hematologic recovery. Relapse-free survival and total survival were calculated from the day of marrow transplantation (day 0).

Statistical Methods

Comparison of proportions was performed with chi-square analysis and Fisher's exact test (13). Relapse-free survival was computed on those patients obtaining complete remission post-transplant. Resulting relapse-free and survival curves from all patients were compared using the method of Kaplan and Meier (14).

RESULTS

Transplant-Related Toxicity

Twenty-five (26%) patients of the 96 who received the CY/TBI regimen died due to treatment-related or miscellaneous causes. By comparison, 20% of patients on subsequent protocols had treatment-related mortality: 7 of 54 (13%)

VP/CY/TBI patients, 8 of 42 (19%) CBV patients, 2 of 6 (33%) VP/TT patients, and 8 of 20 (40%) VP/TT/CY patients. Table 1 summarizes the fatal toxicities encountered.

Complications due to pancytopenia account for about half the fatalities encountered. Of the 218 patients, 24 patients (11%) died of bleeding and/or infection before marrow recovery. Patients who received VP/TT or VP/TT/CY had a statistically significant higher incidence of fatal hemorrhage and/or infection (8/26, 31%) compared to CY/TBI (8/96, $p < 0.005$), VP/CY/TBI (2/54, $p < 0.005$), and CBV (5/42, $p < 0.02$). In patients who survived at least to day +30, the median time to recovery was not affected by the preparative regimen. The median (range in parentheses) for recovery of granulocytes to >500/µl was +20 (+12 to +140); for platelets >20,000 µl untransfused was +24 (+7 to +180). Most of the patients (nearly 90%) recover adequate granulocytes by day +30, and virtually all patients have more than 500 granulocytes/µl by day +45. Platelet recovery is somewhat delayed, with about 10-20% patients still requiring some platelet support at day +45.

The initial trials with CY/TBI explored the effect of dose escalation of TBI and the effect of IFR. Pulmonary toxicity (diffuse interstitial pneumonitis documented by antemortem invasive procedure or by autopsy) was dose-limiting. Exposure of the thoracic region to a cumulative dose of radiation in excess of 1400 cGy, either as prior mediastinal radiation, IFR, or fTBI of 1600 cGy, was associated with an increased incidence of interstitial pneumonitis. Table 1 includes the results of CY/TBI patients (11/96, 11%) for comparison. Overall, VP/CY/TBI protocol had nearly the same incidence of pulmonary toxicity (5/54, 9%). In the VP/CY/TBI protocol there was a trend for less interstitial pneumonitis comparing 1000 cGy fTBI and 1200 cGy fTBI, but the differences were not statistically significant (see Table 2). There was generally a lack of pulmonary toxicity with the non-TBI containing regimens: 3/68, 4% which is significantly lower than the two TBI-containing regimens (16/150, 11%), $p < 0.05$.

Veno-occlusive disease (VOD) of the liver only occurred in three patients and did not appear to be regimen-related. However, in the VP/CY/TBI protocol, the dose escalation of VP-16 was stopped partly because of VOD (see Table 2). The VP-16 dose which was considered maximal in this regimen was therefore 1800 mg/m^2. Escalations of either cyclophosphamide from 150 to 200 mg/kg or fTBI from 1000 to 1200 cGy were well tolerated. The final regimen of VP-16 1800 mg/m^2, cyclophosphamide 150 mg/kg, and fTBI 1000-1200 cGy was considered the maximally-tolerated regimen.

Other miscellaneous causes of fatal toxicity included isolated episodes perforated duodenal ulcer, asthma, congestive heart failure, and organic brain syndrome.

Antitumor Response and Survival

In Tables 3 and 4 the results of the protocols are presented. The updated results from CY/TBI (11) are shown for comparison purposes. VP/CY/TBI at the maximally-tolerated dose regimen (see above) had a comparable complete response rate (16/24, 67%) in patients with advanced non-Hodgkin's lymphoma (Table 3). Twelve of 16 patients remain in continuous complete remission a median of 9 months. Although this preliminary data appears favorable, it is too early to make conclusions about the durability of the responses. The regimens without TBI, VP/TT and VP/TT/CY, had more patients die within the first 30 days post-transplant (see above), but of the 11 patients evaluable for antilymphoma response, nine (82%) achieved a complete response. Of note, five of nine patients remain in continuous unmaintained complete remission a median of 14 months (range 8-26 months). It is also premature to conclude that the durability of the responses is superior to the other regimens. Additional follow-up is needed. In all protocols, partial responses were only temporary, with disease progression eventuating in all patients.

The results of autografting for patients with Hodgkin's disease are presented in Table 4. The CBV regimen, which was reasonably well tolerated, resulted in a somewhat higher complete response rate (29/34, 85%). The difference compared to CY/TBI was not statistically significant. Follow-up is still relatively brief, but 22 of 29 (76%) of the patients remain in unmaintained complete remission a median of 7 months (range: 1-23 months). Similar results for VP/TT/CY were obtained.

Patients receiving CY/TBI and IFR had a better response rate than patients receiving CY/TBI alone. Patients with Hodgkin's disease demonstrated a more marked benefit from the addition of IFR. Of the nine patients with Hodgkin's disease who had long-term responses, eight of the patients had IFR as part of the CY/TBI. Some of the patients who received the CBV regimen also had pre-transplant therapy with MVPP alone (5 patients), IFR alone (8 patients), or both (9 patients). Of these 22 patients, 20 were evaluable for antitumor response, of whom 18 (90%) achieved CR, and 15 of these patients remain in continuous remission a median of 10 months (range: 2-25 months). The three relapses occurred at 6, 9, and 9 months. By comparison, 16 of 20 patients received only the CBV (no pre-transplant therapy) and were evaluable for antitumor activity. The complete response rate of 69% (11/16) approached statistical significance compared to the complete responses obtained in patients given pre-transplant therapy. Of the 11 complete responders, three patients relapsed early (2, 3, and 5 months), while eight patients remain in continuous complete remission a median of 7 months (range 4-17 months).

Regardless of protocol, relapses occurred predominantly at sites of prior lymphomatous involvement and within 12 months of transplantation. The follow-up overall for the newer conditioning regimens is not long enough to determine whether fewer relapses will occur. The results to date, however, are promising. The pattern of relapses, so far, still will not permit a statement about potential marrow contamination as a source of relapse.

Survival using the newer protocols was quite good: of 100 patients entered for transplant, 43 remain in complete remission. Although the longest follow-up is only approaching two years, the median is approaching one year. The patient factors associated with improved survival for the

CY/TBI protocols and these newer protocols will be part of future publications.

DISCUSSION

The results of the protocols--VP/CY/TBI, CBV, VP/TT, and VP/TT/CY--are presented and compared to the previously-presented, but updated CY/TBI. It is not surprising that overall improved efficacy (antilymphoma activity) could not be demonstrated. Analysis of subgroups of patients that are comparable will have to be made. Even when segregating the patients by major histologic categories, Hodgkin's and non-Hodgkin's lymphoma, there is still great diagnostic heterogeneity. In addition, not all patients enter at the same point of their disease; i.e., some patients may be more sensitive or more resistant than others. It was our general feeling that patients treated on the VP/TT and VP/TT/CY protocols were sicker and more heavily pretreated (otherwise they would have been eligible for TBI regimens). Indeed, their acute toxicity was greater. However, if the patient survived the therapy, there was an excellent response rate (12/15 evaluable, 80%) and continuous response rate (8/12, median 11 months). The specific patient factors that predict outcome, survival, and disease-free survival need to be applied to this heterogenous group of patients to help clarify the optimal use of high-dose therapy and autologous bone marrow transplantation.

The results of the present studies obtained for patients with refractory lymphomas are comparable to other reports (16-20). Yet, the role of marrow purging is still not answerable, since the relapse pattern in sites of previously-known disease made the failures more likely due to inadequate therapy rather than reinoculation of clonogenic lymphoma cells. As improved preparative regimens evolve and/or patients are treated earlier in the course of the disease, the potential reinfusion of "contaminated" marrow may become an important question. Of interest, in the CY/TBI protocol, patients with bone marrow involvement who achieved a remission marrow that could be harvested for future relapse did quite well. Thirteen such patients were so treated, and at the time of treatment at progression, eight achieved complete remission. Five patients remain in remission 16, 28, 37, 51, and 94 months after transplant. This finding confirms the previous observation in patients with Burkitt's lymphoma who underwent autologous marrow transplantation with unpurged marrow (17). The question of purging remains unanswered.

Finally, the toxicities encountered with the new protocols were not significantly different from previous experience with CY/TBI. The protocols confirm a 10% pulmonary toxicity with TBI-containing regimens. Hepatic disease (VOD) was dose-limiting for the combination of VP/CY/TBI. At the maximally-tolerated dose, the radiation toxicity was minimal. The VP/TT/CY regimen still has not reached dose-limiting toxicity. These preparative regimens need further analysis and follow-up to determine their place in autografting for lymphoma.

The preliminary results of the newer regimens are promising. Future analyses will be needed to establish more optimum preparative regimens that permit maximum antilymphoma activity with minimal toxicity. Some of these analyses are currently in progress. The current results at least indicate that the regimens can be tolerated with acceptable toxicity. The durability of the responses remains to be tested. Further follow-up is needed.

ACKNOWLEDGEMENTS

The authors wish to acknowledge the support of referring physicians, colleagues, and staff at each of the institutions, without whose assistance these studies could not have been performed.

REFERENCES

1. Klimo P, Connors JM (1985) MOPP/ABV hybrid program: combination chemotherapy based on early introduction of seven effective drugs for advanced Hodgkin's disease. J Clin Oncol 3:1174-1182.
2. Klimo P, Connors JM (1985) MACOP-B chemotherapy for the treatment of diffuse large-cell lymphoma. Ann Intern Med 102:596-602.
3. Bergsagel DE (1987) Salvage treatment for Hodgkin's disease in relapse. J Clin Oncol 5:525-526.
4. Cabanillas F, Hagemeister FB, McLaughlin P, et al (1987) Results of MIME salvage regimen for recurrent or refractory lymphoma. J Clin Oncol 5:407-412.
5. Thomas ED (1983) Marrow transplantation for malignant disease. J Clin Oncol 1:517-531.
6. Hurd DD, Ramsey NKC, Nesbit ME, et al (1983) Allogeneic bone marrow transplantation for non-Hodgkin's lymphoma. Blood (Suppl 1) 62:223.
7. Appelbaum FR, Thomas ED (1983) Review of the use of marrow transplantation in the treatment of non-Hodgkin's lymphoma. J Clin Oncol 1:440-447.
8. Phillips GL, Herzig RH, Lazarus HM, Fay JW, Griffith R, Herzig GP (1986) High-dose chemotherapy, fractionated total-body irradiation, and allogeneic marrow transplantation for malignant lymphoma. J Clin Oncol 4:480.
9. Appelbaum FR, Sullivan KM, Thomas ED, Buckner CD, Clift RA, Deeg HJ, Neiman PE, Sanders JE, Stewart P, Storb R (1985) Allogeneic marrow transplantation in the treatment of MOPP-resistant Hodgkin's disease. J Clin Oncol 3:1490-1494.
10. Appelbaum FR, Fefer A, Cheever MA, et al (1981) Treatment of non-Hodgkin's lymphoma with marrow transplantation in identical twins. Blood 58:509-513.
11. Phillips GL, Herzig RH, Lazarus HM, Fay JW, Wolff SN, Mill WB, Lin HS, Thomas PRM, Glasgow GP, Shina DC, Herzig GP (1984) Treatment of resistant lymphoma with cyclophosphamide, total body irradiation and autologous bone marrow transplantation. N Engl J Med 310:1557-1561.
12. Herzig GP (1981) Autologous marrow transplantation in cancer therapy. Prog Hematol 12:1-23.
13. Siegel S (1956) Nonparametric statistics for the behavioral sciences. New York: McGraw-Hill, pp 96-104.

14. Kaplan EL, Meier PL (1958) Non-parametric estimation from incomplete observations. J Am Stat Assoc 53:457-481.
15. O'Reilly S, Connors J, Voss N, et al (1987) High-dose cyclophosphamide, BCNU, and etoposide (CBV) and autologous bone marrow transplantation (ABMT) in progressive Hodgkin's disease (HD). Proc ASCO 6:196.
16. Goldstone AH, Anderson CC, Linch DC (1986) Very high dose chemotherapy with autologous bone marrow transplantation (ABMT) for patients with advanced relapsed Hodgkin's disease. In Europe (ed): European Cooperative Group for Bone Marrow Transplantation, 12th Annual Meeting, Proccedings, p 120.
17. Appelbaum FR, Deisseroth AB, Graw RG, Herzig GP, Levin RS, Magrath IT, Pizzo PA, Poplack DG, Ziegler JL (1978) Prolonged complete remission following high dose chemotherapy of Burkitt's lymphoma in relapse. Cancer 41:1059-1063.
18. Appelbaum FR, Buckner CD (1986) Overview of the clinical relevance of autologous bone marrow transplantation. Clin Haematol 15:1-18.
19. Philip T, Armitage JO, Spitzer G, et al (1987) High-dose therapy and autologous bone marrow transplantation after failure of conventional chemotherapy in adults with intermediate-grade or high-grade non-Hodgkin's lymphoma. N Engl J Med 316:1493-1498.
20. Takvorian T, Canellos GP, Ritz J, et al (1987) Prolonged disease-free survival after autologous bone marrow transplantation in patients with non-Hodgkin's lymphoma with a poor prognosis. N Engl J Med 316:1499-1505.

TABLE 1. TOXICITY OF AUTOLOGOUS BONE MARROW TRANSPLANT PROTOCOLS

Protocol	Total No. of Patients	Fatal Toxicity (%)*			
		Bone Marrow	Lung	Liver	Other
CY/TBI†	96	8 (8)	11 (11)	1 (1)	5 (5)
VP/CY/TBI	54**	2 (4)	5 (9)	1 (2)	0
CBV††	42	5 (12)	2 (5)	0	1 (2)
VP/TT	6	2 (33)	0	0	0
VP/TT/CY	20	6 (30)	1 (5)	1 (5)	0

* Number of patients who died of bone marrow toxicity (infection and/or hemorrhage), lung (interstitial pneumonitis, idiopathic), liver (veno-occlusive disease), or other organ failure attributed to protocol.

** Includes patients with other hematologic malignancies for toxicity analysis

† Expanded from reference 11

†† Expanded from reference 15

TABLE 2. TOXICITY OF PHASE I VP/CY/TBI PROTOCOL*

Dose				Fatal Toxicity**		
VP-16 (mg/m^2)	CY (mg/kg)	fTBI (cGy)	Number of Patients	Bone Marrow	Lung	Liver
1800	150	1000	9	0	0	0
2250	150	1000	4	0	1	1
1800	200	1000	4	0	0	0
1800	150	1200	37	2	4	0
		Total	54	2	5	1

* See text for details

** Number of patients who died of bone marrow toxicity (infection and/or hemorrhage), lung (interstitial pneumonitis, idiopathic), or liver (veno-occlusive disease) failure.

TABLE 3. RESULTS OF AUTOLOGOUS BONE MARROW TRANSPLANTATION FOR NON-HODGKIN'S LYMPHOMAS

Protocol	No. of Patients*		Response	Alive, CCR**	
	Total	Eval	CR (%)	No.	Duration (Mo)
CY/TBI	70	58	36 (62)	12	37 (12-95)
VP/CY/TBI	32	24	16 (67)	12	9 (5-16)
VP/TT	6	4	3 (75)	3	21 (14-26)
VP/TT/CY	14	7	6 (86)	2	8,11

* See text for definition.

** Number of patients alive in continuous complete remission (CCR), unmaintained; duration in months (median, range in parentheses).

TABLE 4. RESULTS OF AUTOLOGOUS BONE MARROW TRANSPLANTATION FOR HODGKIN'S DISEASE

Protocol	No. of Patients*		Response	Alive, CCR**	
	Total	Eval	CR (%)	No.	Duration (Mo)
CY/TBI	26	24	18 (75)	9	37 (12-95)
CBV	42	35	29 (83)	23	7 (1-23)
VP/TT/CY	6	4	3 (75)	3	11 (4-12)

* See text for definition.

** Number of patients alive in continuous complete remission (CCR), unmaintained; duration in months (median, range in parentheses).

16: Long-Term Bone Marrow Culture in Autologous Transplantation: An In Vitro Biological System for Purging Leukemic Cells

L.H. Coutinho, A. Will, J. Chang, N.G. Testa, and T.M. Dexter

INTRODUCTION

Allogeneic bone marrow transplantation is now commonly used as the treatment of choice for patients with leukaemia. However, the relatively low number of patients (about 30%) with suitable HLA compatible donors and the serious complications associated with graft-versus-host disease (GVHD) are the important factors which limit the therapeutic application of this procedure. In order to widen the range of patients who could benefit from highly aggressive therapeutic regimens, autologous bone marrow transplantation is being increasingly explored as an alternative strategy.

However, a potential drawback in transplanting the patient's own marrow is the prospect of reinfusion of leukaemic clonogenic cells which could re-colonise the host. Because of this, several methods are being extensively evaluated to 'clean up' the marrow of contaminating leukaemic cells. These include ex vivo manipulation with monoclonal antibodies (1) or with pharmacological agents such as 4-hydroperoxycyclophosphamide (2).
Our efforts in this direction have emphasised the use of long-term bone marrow culture system.

RECONSTRUCTION OF THE HAEMOPOIETIC SYSTEM

The concept that all the mature blood cells take their origin from pluripotent stem cells has been supported from a variety of experimental (3) and clinical (4) studies. Furthermore clonogenic assays, using both animal and human cells, have been developed which recognise progenitor cells common to granulocytes, erythrocytes, monocytes, megakaryocytes and in some circumstances T lymphocytes (CFU-GEMM) (5-7) and for lineage committed progenitor cells of the erythrocytes (BFU-E and CFU-E), granulocytes and macrophages (CFU-GM), megakaryocytes (CFU-Mega), as well as eosinophils, basophils, T and B lymphocytes (8).

The haemopoietic progenitor cells require for their survival, growth and differentiation in colony assays the presence of exogenous growth stimulating factors which are produced by a range of different cells including those constituents of the haemopoietic system itself like activated T lymphocytes (9) monocytes (10), marrow derived stromal cells (11, 12). These assays have revealed the hierarchical structure of the haemopoietic system and also indicate that haemopoietic cell proliferation and differentiation is extrinsically regulated by mechanisms which are at least in part mediated by humoral growth factors.

When similar studies were applied to cells from patients with AML, a small subset of the leukaemic population was found to have biological characteristics analogous to those of the normal stem cell, i.e. they are self-perpetuating and are the progenitors of terminally differentiated non-proliferating blast cells (13-15). However, despite the valuable contribution of these clonogenic assays to our understanding of normal haemopoiesis and leukaemogenesis, the cultures pose problems in kinetic studies of stem cells in that differentiation is promoted at the cost of self-renewal. This is not the case in long-term bone marrow cultures (LTBMC), which allow the formation of a multi-adherent cell layer which bears structural and functional similarities to the haemopoietic microenvironment in vivo (16,17). Within this adherent cell layer, stem cell proliferation and differentiation results in long-term production of committed progenitors (mainly GM-CFC) and mature myeloid cells which are continuously released into the supernatant growth medium. In the absence of added growth factors haemopoiesis in LTBMC is sustained by regulatory mechanisms presumably mediated by close cell/cell interactions between haemopoietic and stromal cells and in situ production of growth factors by specific stromal elements (18, 19).

THE GROWTH OF LEUKAEMIC CELLS IN LTBMC

At the time of diagnosis of a leukaemia, normal haemopoiesis is suppressed by either physical replacement of stem cells or inhibition of stem cell proliferation by a leukaemia-derived humoral factor (20). Whatever mechanisms are operative in vivo, the suppressive effect of leukaemic cells on normal haemopoiesis is not exerted in the long-term bone marrow culture system. This phenomenon was first seen in cultures of marrow cells from mice with lymphoblastic leukaemia (21). In that model, culture conditions resulted in complete loss of leukaemic cells and were found to selectively favour the production of normal haemopoietic stem cells in sufficient quantity to protect lethally irradiated syngeneic mice.

Subsequently Coulombel et al. showed that in cultures from most patients with Ph' positive chronic myeloid leukaemia (22) and in some cases of AML (23) the leukaemic clone was unable to sustain its growth. Instead progenitors of normal phenotype and karyotype were continuously generated and increased in number. In continuing this line of work, we have so far studied 16 AML patients, 14 at diagnosis, 2 in relapse, and 1 at both diagnosis and relapse (KG^1 and KG^2 respectively). When marrow cells from these patients were cultured directly in a clonogenic assay aberrant leukaemic growth patterns were commonly observed except in 3 cases where only colony forming cells were detected at subnormal levels (table 1).

However, usually after 1 to 3 weeks or exceptionally after 4 weeks, apparently normal haemopoiesis was re-established in long-term cultures from over 50% of cases. As shown in table 2, in these cultures there was a total decline of leukaemic clonogenic progenitors while phenotypically normal colony forming cells (present at low levels in the initial inoculum or previously undectable) were generated and expanded to levels within the range of normal controls. In parallel, blast cells disappeared from the supernatant medium and were replaced by differentiated cells (data not shown).

That the haemopoietic progenitors and mature cells generated in LTBMC were derived from normal (rather than from leukaemic) cells is supported by cytogenetic studies of 2 AML cases where karyotype markers were present and adequate numbers of suitable metaphases were analysed (table 3). In the first case direct preparation of cells in suspension showed, on both occasions the marrow was cultured, only cells of normal karyotype. In the second patient, the abnormal karyotype (45 x y, -7 inv 2) was observed in all metaphases at the time the cells were inoculated in long-term culture. After 1 week the cells in suspension (which

Table 1

Growth Characteristics in GM-CFC Assay of Bone Marrow Cells from 16 AML Patients

Pt.	Leukaemic Growth: Absence of clones	Leukaemic Growth: Cluster formation	Normal Growth Colonies/10^5 cells*
MC		++	
PH		++	
ML	+		
SS	+		
TC		++	13
KG^1			14
MG		++	
JA		++	
AK		++	
KG^2			03
SD			07
GE	+		
BD		++	
ML		++	
PB	+		
GL		++	16
KB		++	

* Normal Values N = 13 Mean = 44 $\pm$ 2 SD 12-112

Table 2

Long-Term Bone Marrow Cultures from AML Patients: Conversion to Normal Haemopoiesis

Pt.	Leukaemic Growth 1-3	4-10 (wks)	Range of GM-CFC/Culture 1-3	4-10 (wks)
MC	-	-	142-360	360
ML	-	-	80-175	3
KG1	-	-	5-137	2
JA	-	-	5-240	0
KG2	-	-	36-504	55
SD	-	-	45-360	0
GE	+	-	5	2-29
PB	-	-	97-580	42
GL	-	-	400-2,860	30
* Normal controls			36-19320	6-970

* Range of values obtained from 13 long-term bone marrow cultures

consist mainly of differentiated non clonogenic myeloid cells) were all derived from the leukaemic clone, while the colony forming cells were cytogenetically normal. Significantly, after 2 weeks only cytogenetically normal cells were found both in the suspension and in colonies derived from the progenitor cells. This finding suggests a selective process in the long-term culture favouring the growth of residual normal stem cells. Furthermore, it should be noted that the total nucleated cell recovery in the cultures of AML patients which revert to a normal phenotype and growth pattern is similar to that of normal controls at least for 7 weeks (Fig 1). In view of the studies by Fialkow (24) which show that in the process of leukaemogenesis the acquisition of a chromosomal abnormality is a late phenomenon occurring in a pre-established clonal population, the origin of these cells may be open to discussion. However, the non-clonality of phenotypically and genotypically normal progenitor cells generated in LTBMC has been confirmed by studies of a Turner syndrome mosaic patient with chronic myeloid leukaemia (25) and more recently in cultures of a CML patient heterozygous for G-6-PD isoenzyme (26).

Table 3

Reappearance of Normal Karyotype in LTBMC from 2 AML Patients

Pt.	Karyotype	Initial Marrow	Non-adherent cells in LTBMC 1	2	3-4 (wks)
*MC	46xy de (16) (q23)	9	0	0	0
	46xy	31	15	15	9
SD	45xy, -7,inv (2)	20	20	0	0
	46xy	0	(9)	20(16)	1(16)

( ) No of metaphases obtained from individual or pooled GM colonies

* Data pooled from two samples established at different times

Figure 1

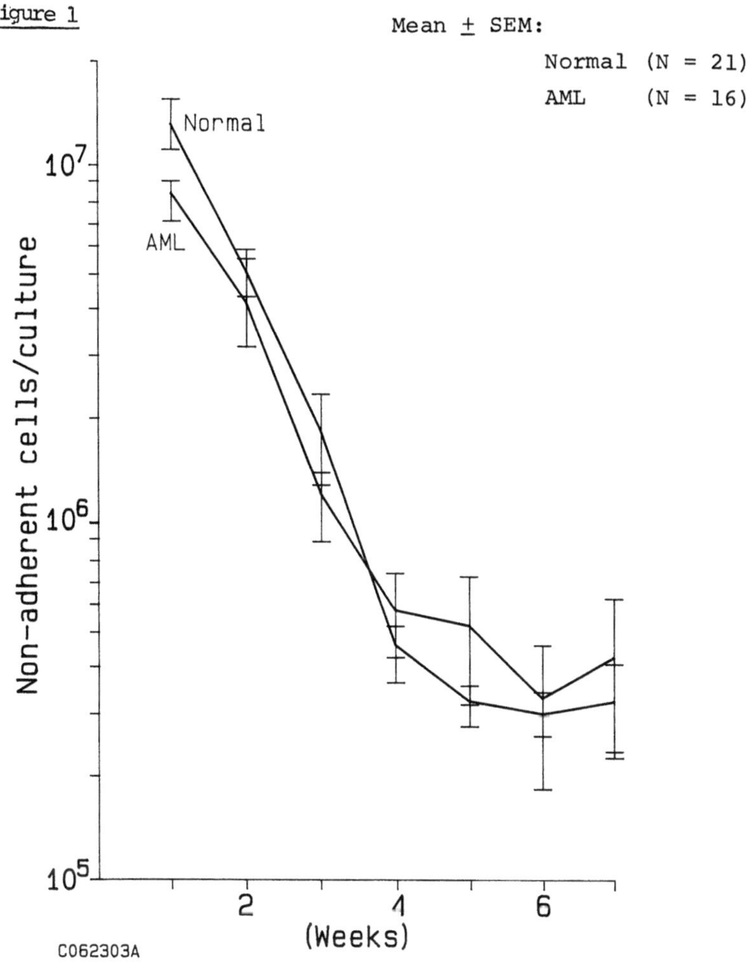

We have also examined the growth of cells in LTBMC from patients with acute lymphoblastic leukaemia. This study included 6 cases of childhood newly diagnosed ALL. All of them were C-ALL immunological type and had >80% lymphoblasts in the initial marrow sample.

Table 4 summarizes the results obtained. We divided the patients into two series (A & B) with respect to their reserve of normal haemopoietic stem cells. In 4 out of 6 patients the numbers of granulocyte-macrophage progenitors in the presentation marrow were very low or nil, which is characteristic of ALL (27) and in the other two patients GM-CFC numbers were in the lower limit of normal range. In long-term cultures of series A the expansion of normal progenitors was remarkable particularly in the first two cases of the series, and haemopoiesis was sustained throughout the culture period at levels comparable to normal controls. In cultures of series B, on the other hand, although GM-CFC production at one stage outnumbered the total input, haemopoiesis declined very quickly. This finding could suggest that the number or quality of normal stem cells was more impaired in these patients. Morphological analysis of supernatant cells from cultures of 4 patients, irrespective of the series they were allocated to, showed a total loss of lymphoblasts after 3-4 weeks with repopulation by differentiated monocytes and granulocytes.

Although this was a study of a small series of patients some valuable comments can be made. First it shows that LTBMC represent a sensitive system to determine the frequency of residual normal stem cells in leukaemic patients. Secondly unlike the situation in AML cultures where the origin of differentiated myeloid cells is uncertain, in cultures from marrow which showed initially >80% to 95% lymphoblasts differentiated granulocytypes and monocytes are unlikely to be derived from the leukaemic clone.

BONE MARROW CELLS CULTURED IN LTBMC FOR THERAPEUTIC USE

It has been clearly shown that long-term cultured bone marrow from mice is as competent as freshly isolated normal bone marrow cells in its ability to reconstitute the haemopoietic system of

Table 4

Growth of Marrow Cells from ALL Patients in LTBMC

	Pt.	Input Nucleated Cells	Input GM-CFC	Total Cumulative Production Over 6 weeks* NA Cells	GM-CFC
Series A	PG	2×10^7	0	10.7×10^6	1, 650
	LR	2×10^7	400	13.7×10^6	2,445
	KC	2×10^7	2,400	2.8×10^6	1,380
	RG	2×10^7	3,000	4.5×10^6	1,784
Series B	MA	2×10^7	200	3.9×10^6	430
	HH	2×10^7	200	8.6×10^6	460
Range of Values of normal controls (N = 16)		2×10^7	2,400-25,400	$5.4 - 66 \times 10^6$	1,097-36,083

* Taking demi-depopulation into account
NA Non-adherent

lethally irradiated animals (28). In addition mature granulocytes generated in human LTBMC were shown to be physiologically normal (29). Clearly the long-term culture system mimics haemopoiesis in vivo and the additional inability of leukaemic cells to survive in this system prompted us to investigate the possibility of using cultured bone marrow cells for autologous transplantation in leukaemic conditions.

The protocol adopted to culture bone marrow cells for this study is schematically shown in Fig 2. For a more detailed description of the methodology see report by Chang et al (30).

Figure 2

Schematic Representation of LTBMC for Autologous Transplantation

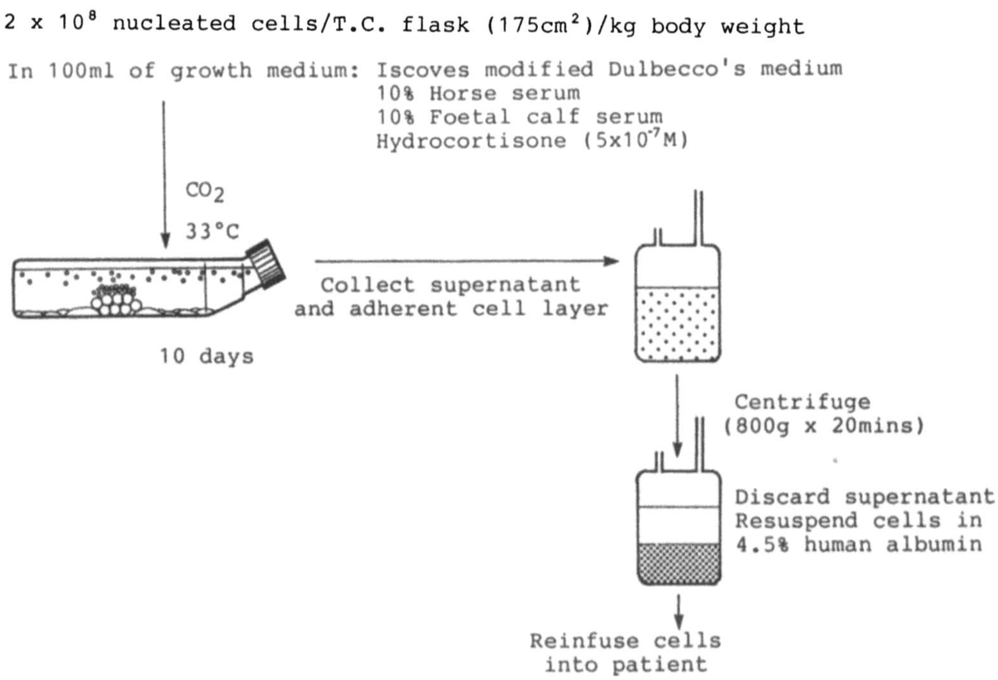

Table 5

ABMT in AML Patients Using Cells Grown in LTBMC

Pt.	Age/Sex	FAB Class	Clinical Status at ABMT	Nucleated Cells Cultured x 10^9/(% blasts)	Nucleated Cells Infused x10^9/(% blasts)	GM-CFC Number /kg b.w.
MC	14M	M_4	Relapse	8.4 (40%)	6.7 (<5%)	16,200
TC	39M	M_2	Relapse	18.0 (60%)	9.3 (12%)	10,700
FB	34F	RAEB-t	MDS	11.2 (<5%)	7.3 (<5%)	27,000
TB	18F	M_4	1st CR	14.4 (<5%)	9.3 (<5%)	98,900
JW	15F	M_2	1st CR	17.2 (<5%)	10.8 (<5%)	107,100
AF	17F	M_5	1st CR	13.0 (<5%)	9.2 (<5%)	23,400

As pre-transplantation conditioning regimen, the patients receive cyclophosphamide 1.8 g/m^2 intravenously five and four days before reinfusion and fractionated total body irradiation (200cGy twice a day) for three days. The cultured marrow is transfused after the last fraction of irradiation.

To the present date 6 AML patients, 3 in relapse and 3 in complete remission have been transplanted with autologous marrow grown in LTBMC (table 5). Sufficient volumes of marrow were cultured to ensure a cell infusion at a dose of at least 10^8 cells/kg body weight. Although the percentage recovery of total nucleated cells was in the average 65.1%,we observed a dramatic fall in the blast population of the cultured cells taken from patients in full relapse. As expected patients in remission had higher levels of normal progenitors in their processed marrow. The implication of this in the haematological outcome of the patients is not yet known.

The haematological reconstitution of patients transplanted in complete remission (table 6) was quite satisfactory and is comparable to published data from conventional autologous transplantation (31). All 3 patients are in unmaintained continuous complete remission.

The first patient transplanted in full haematological and cytogenetic relapse showed a complete haematological reconstitution with karyotypically normal cells (30). This patient presented with a chromosomal abnormality that persisted during his first remission induced by chemotherapy and which comprised the bulk of cells at the time the marrow was cultured. For this reason, we consider the apparent disappearance of the leukaemic clone following long-term culture and autologous rescue to be highly significant. Subsequent relapse occurred 9 months later but at the time cytogenetic studies revealed further abnormalities in his karyotype.

Table 6

Haematological Reconstitution Post-Transplantation

Disease Status	WCC ($x10^9$/l) 0.5 (days)	Polys ($x10^9$/l) 0.5 (weeks)	Polys >1.0 (weeks)	Plat ($x10^9$/l) 50 (weeks)	Plat >100 (weeks)	Last Transf. Plat (weeks)	Last Transf. Blood (weeks)	Survival after ABMT (weeks)	Current Status (19.6.87)
AML in Remission									
TB	22	5.5	6.5	12.5	30	6.5	6.5	109	CCR
JW	26	5	10	15	18	9	13	80	CCR
AF	28	5	7	9	24	9	9	30	CCR
AML in Relapse									
MC	37	7	8	14	37	11	11	74	+
TC	24	8	-	-	-	-	-	31	+
*FB	33	8	20	-	-	-	-	41	+

* Patients marrow had <5% blasts but was markedly myelodysplastic

\+ Deceased

The second patient transplanted in relapse never achieved a haematological remission post-transplantation. However in retrospective analysis the leukaemic cells from these two patients showed distinct biological differences in vitro in terms of persistence of leukaemia or re-growth of normal haemopoietic progenitors which conformed subsequently with their haematological outcome.

The patient who had a myelodysplastic syndrome preceding the onset of acute leukaemia, had a delayed haematological reconstitution and dysplastic features reverted in her marrow. This could suggest that her normal marrow reserve had been severely depleted and that the MDS clone persisted in long-term culture.

CONCLUSION AND PROSPECTS FOR THE FUTURE

The studies summarised here show that apparently normal haemopoietic stem cells can be expanded in LTBMC and successfully reconstitute the haemopoietic system. The procedure proved to be well tolerated and with minimal toxicity. Platelet recovery may be delayed but prolonged thrombocytopenia has also been reported in conventional autologous transplantation (31).

Obviously it is not yet possible to state the contribution that such an approach may have on the treatment of AML in first remission: this must await the result of continuing clinical studies and should be compared with standard autologous transplantation. However patients in second or greater remission or in relapse might be easier for critical evaluation. Our preliminary data indicate that some of these patients have a good normal marrow reserve which can be encouraged to grow in culture and used to rescue patients following ablative therapy. Patients with other haematological malignancies such as CML or ALL are also possible future candidates for the study.

Finally the response of leukaemic cells to recombinant growth factors known to promote differentiation and subsequently lead to clonal extinction is intriguing (32). Studies along this line are being performed to determine if the growth of normal stem cells in LTBMC can be further enhanced.

ACKNOWLEDGEMENTS

The financial support of the Cancer Research Campaign and the Leukaemia Research Fund is gratefully acknowledged.

REFERENCES

1. Ritz J, Sallan SE, Bast RC et al (1982) Autologous bone marrow transplantation in CALLA positive acute lymphoblastic leukaemia after in vitro treatment with J5 monoclonal antibody and complement. Lancet ii:60-63

2. Kaizer H, Stuart RK, Brookmeyer R et al 1985) Autologous bone marrow transplantation in acute leukaemia: a phase II study of in vitro treatment with 4-hydroperoxycyclophosphamide to purge tumor cells. Blood 65:1504-1510

3. Till JE, McCulloch EA (1961) A direct measurement of the radiation sensitivity of normal mouse bone marrow cells. Radiat Res 14:213-222

4. Fialkow PJ (1982) Cell lineages in Hematopoietic Neoplasia studied with Glucose-6-Phosphate dehydrogenase cell markers. J Cell Physiol Suppl 1:37-43

5. Fauser AA, Messner HA (1979) Identification of megakaryocytes, macrophages and eosinophils in colonies of human bone marrow containing neutrophilic granulocytes and erythroblasts. Blood 53:1023-1027

6. Messner HA, Lim B, Jamal N, Takahashi T (1983) Lymphoid cells in multilineage colonies. In Haemopoietic stem cells. Alfred Benzon Symposium, 18 Copenhagen 1982 338-345 Copenhagen: Munksgaard

7. Nakahata T, Ogawa M (1982) Identification in culture of a class of hemopoietic colony-forming units with extensive capacity to self-renew and generate multipotential colonies. Proc Nat Acad Sci (USA) 79:3843-3847

8. Metcalf D (1977) Hemopoietic colonies in vitro. In: Cloning of normal and leukemic cells. Berlin: Springer-Verlag

9. Schrader JW & Clark-Lewis I (1982) A T-cell derived factor stimulating multipotential hemopoietic stem cells: molecular weight and distinction from T-cell growth factor and T-cell derived granulocyte macrophage colony stimulating factor. J Immunol 129:30-35

10. Golde DW, Cline MJ (1972) Identification of the colony stimulating cell in human peripheral blood. J Clin Invest 51:2981-2983

11. Lanotte M, Metcalf D, Dexter TM (1982) Production of monocyte/macrophage colony stimulating factor by preadipocyte cell lines derived from murine marrow stroma. J Cell Physiol 112:123-127

12. Zipori D, Ouksin D, Tawir M, Argaman A, Toled J, Malik Z (1985) Cultured mouse marrow stromal cell lines. II Distinct subtypes differing in morphology, collagen types, myelopoietic factors and leukemic cell growth modulating activities. J Cell Physiol 122:81-90

13. Buick RN, Minden MD, McCulloch MC (1979) Self renewal in culture of proliferative blast progenitor cells in acute myeloblastic leukaemia. Blood 54:95-104

14. Moore MAS, Spitzer G, Williams N, Metcalf D, Buckley J (1974) Agar cultures studies in 127 cases of untreated acute leukaemia: The prognostic value of reclassification of leukemia according to in vitro growth characteristics. Blood 44:1-18

15. Buick RN, Till JE, McCulloch EA (1977): Colony assay for proliferative blast cells circulating in myeloblastic leukaemia. Lancet i:862-863

16. Dexter TM, Allen TD, Lajtha LG (1977) Conditions controlling the proliferation of haemopoietic stem cells in vitro. J Cell Physiol 91:335-344

17. Gartner S, Kaplan HS (1980) Long-term culture of human bone marrow cells. Proc Natl Acad Sci (USA) 77:4756-4759

18. Dexter TM, Spooncer E, Simmons P, Allen TD (1984) Long-term marrow culture: An overview of techniques and experience. In: Wright DG, Greenberger JS (eds) Long-term bone marrow culture. New York Alan R Liss, Inc

19. Gordon MY, Riley GP, Watt SM, Greaves MF (1987) Compartmentalization of a haematopoietic growth factor (GM-CSF) by glycosaminoglycans in the bone marrow microenvironment. Nature 326:483-485

20. Broxmeyer HE, Bognacki J, Dorner MH, de sousa M (1981) The identification of leukemia associated inhibiting activity (LIA) as acidic isoferritins: A regulatory role for acidic isoferritins in the production of granulocytes and macrophages. J Exp Med 153:1426-1444

21. Hays EF, Hale L (1982) Growth of normal hemopoietic cells in cultures of bone marrow from leukemic mice. Eur J Cancer Clin Oncol 18: 413-418

22. Coulombel L, Kalousek DK, Eaves CJ, Gupta CM, Eaves AC (1983) Long-term marrow culture reveals chromosomally normal haematopoietic progenitor cells in patients with philadelphia chromosome-positive chronic myelogenous leukemia. N Engl J Med 308:1493-1498

23. Coulombel L, Eaves CJ, Kalousek DK, Gupta C, Eaves AC (1985) Long-term marrow culture of cells from patients with acute myelogeneous leukemia (AML): selection in favour of normal phenotypes in some but not all cases. J Clin Invest 75:961-969

24. Fialkow PJ, Martin PJ, Najfeld V, Penfold GK, Jacobsen RJ, Hansen JA (1981) Evidence for a multi-step pathogenesis of chronic myelogenous leukemia. Blood 58:158-163

25. Dubé ID, Arlin ZA, Kalousek DK, Eaves CJ, Eaves AC (1984) Nonclonal hemopoietic progenitor cells detected in long-term marrow cultures from a Turner syndrome mosaic with chronic myeloid leukemia. Blood 64:1284-1287

26. Hogge DE, Coulombel L, Kalousek DK, Eaves CJ, Eaves AC (1987) Normal hemopoietic progenitors in a G-6PD heterozygote with CML revealed after LTBM cultures. Amer J Hematol 24:389-394

27. Moore MAS, Williams N, Metcalf D (1973) In vitro colony formation by normal and leukemic human hematopoietic cells: characterization of the colony-forming cells. J Natl Cancer Inst 50: 603-623

28. Spooncer E, Dexter TM (1983) Transplantation of long-term cultured bone marrow cells. Transplantation 35:624-627

29. Greenberg HM, Newburger PE, Parker LM, Novak T, Greenberger JS (1981) Human granulocytes generated in continuous bone marrow culture are physiologically normal. Blood 58:724-732

30. Chang J, Coutinho LH, Morgenstern G et al (1986) Reconstitution of haemopoietic system with autologous marrow taken during relapse of acute myeloblastic leukaemia and grown in long-term culture. Lancet i:294-295

31. Burnett AK, Tansey P, Watkins R et al (1984) Transplantation of unpurged autologous bone marrow in acute myeloid leukemia in first remission. Lancet ii:1068-1070

32. Souza LM, Boone TC, Gabrilove J et al (1986) Recombinant human granulocyte colony-stimulating factor: Effects on normal and leukemic myeloid cells. Science, 232:61-65

17: Allogeneic Bone Marrow Transplantation for Leukemia—Japanese Experience

T. Masaoka

ALLOGENEIC BONE MARROW TRANSPLANTATION IN LEUKEMIA: THE JAPANESE EXPERIENCE

T. Masaoka

Bone marrow transplantation (BMT) in Japan (1) began in 1975. In the first years the results were poor. The number of cases of BMT started to increase in 1980 after the formation of the Japan BMT study group of 31 hospitals supported by a grant from the Ministry of Health and Welfare of Japan. This paper reports the data obtained from the registry of the Japanese study group. Member hospitals are listed in Table 1.

Table 1. Members of the Japan BMT Study Group

Akita Univ. School of Med.	Jichi Medical College
Nihon Univ. School of Med.	Teikyo Univ. Scchool of Med.
Tokyo Univ. School of Med.	Institure of Medical Science Tokyo Univ.
Tokyo Medical and Dental Univ. School of Med.	Tokyo Womens College, of Med.
National Cancer Center	Kanagawa Children 's Medical Center
Tokai Univ. School of Med.	Shizuoka Children 's Hp.
Niigata Univ. School of Med.	Kanazawa Univ. School of Med.
Shinsyu Univ. School of Med.	Nagoya Univ. School of Med.
Branch Hp. of Nagoya Univ.	Nagoya First Red Cross Hp.
Nagoya Second Red Cross Hp.	National Nagoya Hp.
Mie Univ. School of Med.	Kyoto Univ. School of Med.
Osaka Univ. School of Med.	Kinki UNiv. School of Med.
Hyogo Medical College	Hiroshima Red Cross Hp.
Yamaguchi Univ. School of Med.	National Kyusyu Cancer Center
Matudo City Hp.	Kokura Memorial Hp.
The Cancer for Adult Diseases, Osaka	

BMT PATIENTS

As shown in Table 2, the number of BMT cases in Japan increased rapidly with the improvement of survival and exceeded 100 cases in 1985. As of 1986, 356 cases were registered, including 264 leukemia patients (74.2% of total): 112 acute lymphoblastic leukemia cases (31.5%), 106 acute non-lymphocytic leukemia cases (29.8%), and 46 hronic myelogenous leukemia cases(12.9%).

Table 2. BMT cases in Japan

	ALL	ANL	CML	MALIG LYMPH	SOLID TUMOR	AA	SCID	TOTAL
1975	1	0	0	1	0	0	0	2
76	0	1	0	0	0	0	0	1
77	1	2	1	0	0	0	0	4
78	2	0	0	1	0	1	0	4
79	4	4	0	3	0	1	0	12
80	5	6	2	3	2	1	0	19
81	5	12	3	2	5	2	0	29
82	12	11	7	5	0	6	0	41
83	22	18	6	4	2	9	0	61
84	28	27	10	2	0	13	1	81
85	32	25	17	8	3	14	3	102
TOTAL	112	106	46	29	12	47	4	356

ALL: Acute lymphoblastic leukemia
ANL: Acute non-lymphocytic leukemia
CML: Chronic myelogenous leukemia
AA: Aplastic anemia
SCID: Severe combined immune deficiency

Table 3. Causes of death after BMT

CAUSE OF DEATH	ALL	ANL	CML	MALIG LYMPH	SOLID TUMOR	AA	SCID	TOTAL
RELAPSE	21	13	8	2	2	1	0	47
GVHD	1	5	3	0	0	3	0	12
IP	18	24	9	4	2	1	1	59
SEPTICEMIA	13	6	2	3	0	4	0	28
HEMORRHAGE	3	2	0	0	1	1	0	7
RENAL FAILURE	3	1	0	0	0	0	0	4
OTHER	7	10	5	7	4	4	2	39
UNKNOWN	1	1	1	2	1	0	0	6
TOTAL	67	62	28	18	10	14	3	202

CAUSES OF FAILURE

One hundred and fifty-seven deaths (59.5%) out

of 264 leukemia patients were registered. As shown in Table 3, the main causes of death were as follows: interstitial pneumonitis (IP) (32.5%); relapse of leukemia (26.8%); septicemia (13.4%); and graft-vs-host disease (GVHD) (5.7%).

INTERSTITIAL PNEUMONITIS (IP) [2]

A step-wise reduction in the incidence of IP was found from single TBI (64%) to fractionated TBI (30%) and to the combination of fractionated TBI and selection of cytomegalovirus (CMV) antibody-negative platelet donors (13%), as shown in Table 4. These data suggest a dual mechanism for the onset of IP, i.e., lung injury by radiation and entry of virus by transfusion.

Figure 1 shows the relationship between the duration of isolation in laminar air flow (LAF) rooms and the onset of IP counted from the end of isolation. Out of 34 patients, 29 patients (85%) developed IP within 100 days (range 30-120 days) after cessation of isolation. Four patients developed IP during isolation; all of them had received both single dose TBI and platelet transfusions from random donors. In three of these patients CMV was detected. In most of the IP cases, IP developed outside the LAF room. The question of whether this is simply due to the time course of BMT or whether LAF rooms themselves have some influence on the onset of IP needs further study.

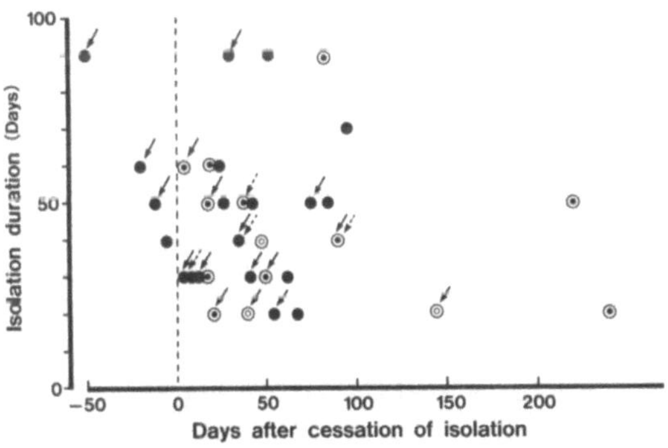

Figure 1. Onset of IP and isolation duration. / CMV pneumonia; ⁄' P. carinii pneumonia; o single TBI and CMV antibody-negative platelet donor; • single TBI and random platelet donor; **o** fractionated TBI and CMV antibody-negative platelet donor; ◉ fractionated TBI and random platelet donor. (Reprinted from <u>Bone Marrow Transplantation</u> with kind permission Ref. [2])

Table 4. TBI platelet transfusions and IP (Reprinted from <u>Bone Marrow Transplantation</u> with kind permission [Ref. 2])

TBI	Platelet transfusion	Incidence of IP	(%)
Single	Random donor	21/33	(64)
Fractioned	Random donor	10/33	(30)
Single	CMV antibody negative donor	1/8	(13)
Fractioned	CMV antibody negative donor	4/30	(13)
Total		36/104	(35)

INFECTION PREVENTION

Because the fungal infection was the most frequent complication in early stage of BMT, studies were carried out to improve infection prevention with laminar air flow rooms (LAF).

OZONE DECONTAMINATION OF LAF [3]

We have developed ozone decontamination for LAF. As shown in Table 5, ozone was very effective against fungus. Ozone has several advantages compared with other decontaminants such as formaldehyde gas or chlorhexidine spray, as shown in Table 6. Ozone decontamination is very convenient for glass and linens. The expulsion is very rapid; therefore, the days needed for decontamination are less than with formaldehyde. The most important merit of ozone decontamination is that people are acquainted with hearing about ozone concentration in air pollution information. It is very difficult to get data about chronic toxicity in humans of a decontamination drug; however, in the case of ozone, it was enough to show that the ozone concentration was below some ppm, which is often reported as oxidant concentration on the street.

Table 5. Ozone decontamination and exposure time (Reprinted with permission from Masaoka, et al, 1982 [Ref. 3])

Organism	Exposure to:	No. of colonies remaining after: 24h	48h	72h
E. coli	Ozone	4	0	0
		7	0	0
	Control	1.3×10^2	8.3×10	5.8×10
			9.5×10	2.4×10
B. subtilis	Ozone	$>10^3$	0	0
		$>10^3$	1	0
	Control	$>10^3$	$>10^3$	$>10^3$
			$>10^3$	$>10^3$
Penicillium sp.	Ozone	0	0	0
	Control	$>10^3$	$>10^3$	$>10^3$
			$>10^3$	$>10^3$

Table 6. Decontamination of clean rooms

Item \ drugs	ozone	folmaldehyde	chlorhexidine
decontamination	superficial	penetrating	fleck
resistant bacteria	-	-	+
air tight taping	+	+	-
expulsion	rapid	slow	-
inhalation	-	+	+
days	1	4	1
glass	-	-	fleck
iron	+	+	-
rubber	+	-	-
linens	dry	dry	wet

INSECTS IN LAF [4]

Insect contamination in bioclean rooms and their surroundings was surveyed every month for one year. Table 7 shows that psocoptera are the most frequently detected insects throughout the year, especially in summer.

Table 7. Insects in LAF

INSECT & ARTHROPOD	MAR-MAY	JUN-AUG	SEP-NOV	DEC-FEB	TOTAL
Diptera	2	4	4	0	10
Coleoptera	0	1	0	0	1
Psocoptera	11	26	26	3	66
Spiders	0	0	1	1	2
Mites	0	9	4	3	16

Even in a bioclean area, psocoptera were found, although the number of insects per trap was lower than in other places in the ward. Most of these insects were contaminated with fungus, as shown in Table 8. The most predominant fungus was Aspergillus, showing the importance of measures against insects for maintaining the clean condition in LAF.

Table 8. Fungus from 68 insects in LAF

ASPERGILLUS	24	27.6%
PENICILLIUM	11	12.6%
ALTERNARIA	7	8.0%
AUREOBASIDUM	1	1.1%
NIGROSPORA	6	6.9%
CLADOSPORIUM	14	16.1%
CAETOMIUM	2	2.3%
RHIZOPUS	4	4.6%
N.D.	18	20.7%

GVHD AND SURVIVAL

Figure 2 shows the survival curves of patients with acute leukemia according to their GVHD grades. Patients with GVHD grade I showed better survival than grade 0 and grade II-IV.

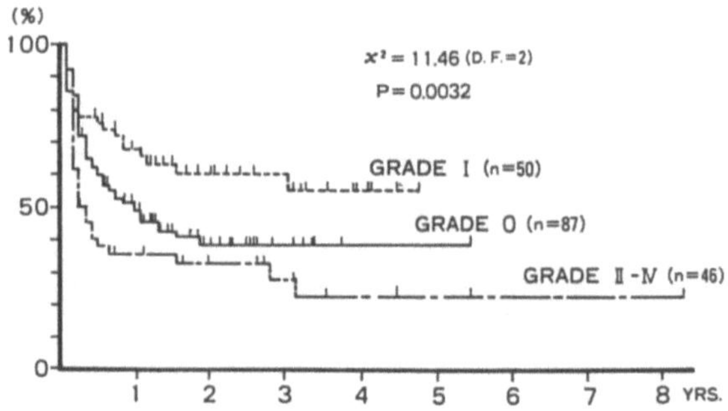

Figure 2. Survival of acute leukemia patients by GVHD grade.

As shown in Table 9, the relapse rate of acute leukemia was 38% in grade 0 group and 19% and 18% in grade I and grade II-IV group. These data may suggest the importance of graft vs. leukemia reaction (GVLR) in BMT.

Table 9. GVHD grade and relapse of leukemia

ACUTE GVHD	RELAPSE RATE (%)
0	31/83(37)
I	9/50(18)
II-IV	8/43(19)

Relapse rate was higher in the GVHD Grade 0 group than in Grade I or Grade II-IV groups.

ORAL ACYCLOVIR ADMINISTRATION AGAINST MUCOSITIS

A double-blind controlled study of oral Acyclovir from day -7 to day 35 revealed a significant reduction of viral stomatitis by Acyclovir. Virologically documented stomatitis was 0 out of 28 cases in the Acyclovir-treated group and 9 out of 29 cases in the placebo group, as shown in Table 10.

Table 10. Oral Acyclovir for herpes mucositis

Drug	Number of cases	Patients with diagnosed viral infections	
		HSV(%)	VZV(%)
ACYCLOVIR	28	0 *	0
PLACEBO	29	7(24.1%)*	2(6.9%)

HSV: Herpes simplex virus
VZV: Varicella Zoster Virus
* P <0.01

A significant difference was also obtained in the rate of oral drug intake between groups (Table 11).

Table 11.
Drug intake rate of Acyclovir

PERIOD	ACYCLOVIR	PLACEBO
Day -7 - 0	93.5%	*78.3%
Day 1 - 7	90.0%	87.1%
Day 8 - 14	82.1%	79.1%
Day 15 - 21	79.4%	72.3%
Day 22 - 28	83.4%	63.7%
Day 29 - 35	79.1%	63.7%

*P<0.01 (T-Test)

COLONY STIMULATING FACTOR

Colony-stimulating factor derived from human urine (CSF-HU) was applied to BMT. In most patients who received CSF-HU, granulocytes started to increase after 8 days, as shown in Figure 3.

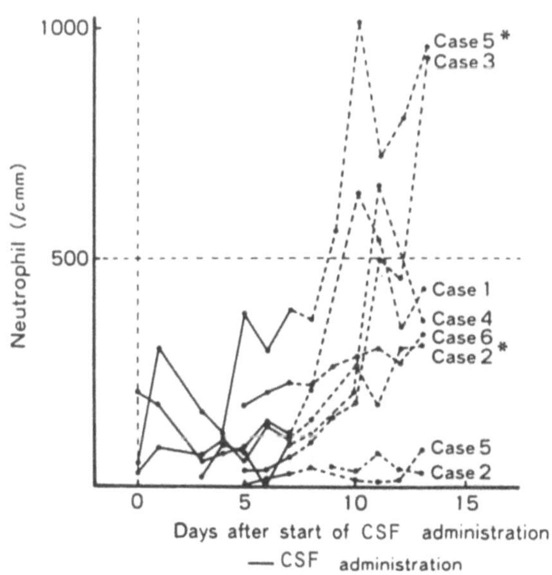

Figure 3. Neutrophil counts after start of CSF-HU administration. *=2nd administration

No side effects were observed. The days needed for the recovery of leukocytes over 1000 was 16.7 days in 30 CSF-treated patients and 25.4 days in 52 non-randomized control patients. A randomized double-blind controlled study is now being carried out.

SURVIVAL OF ACUTE LYMPHOBLASTIC LEUKEMIA (ALL)

Survival curves of patients with acute lymphoblastic leukemia are shown in Figure 4. The plateau level of survival curve was 70% in patients who received BMT during the first remission, 30% during the second or subsequent remission, and 10% during relapse.

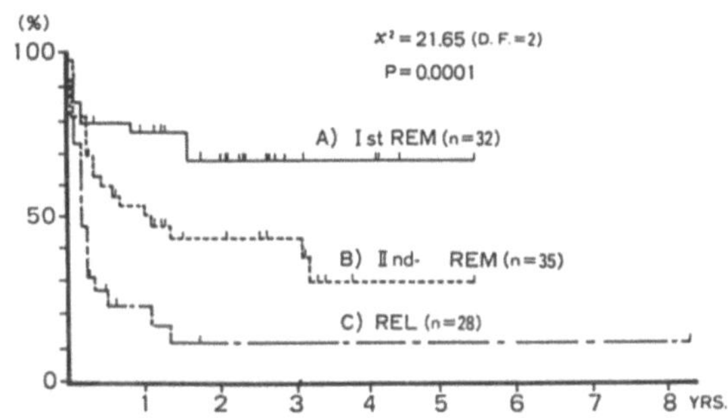

Figure 4. Survival of acute lymphoblastic leukemia patients.
REM: remission
REL: relapse

SURVIVAL OF ACUTE NON-LYMPHOCYTIC LEUKEMIA (ANL)

Long survival was obtained in 50% of BMT patients during the first remission, 30% in second or subsequent remissions, and 10% in relapse, as shown in Figure 5.

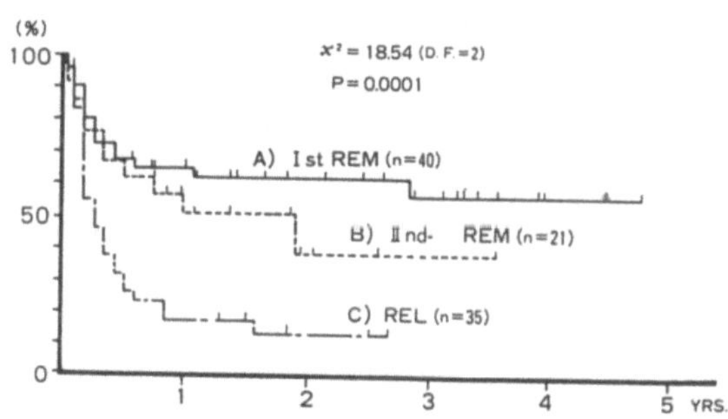

Figure 5. Survival of acute non-lymphocytic leukemia.

SURVIVAL OF CHRONIC MYELOGENOUS LEUKEMIA (CML)

Long survival was obtained in about 50% of CML patients in chronic phase and 8% in accelerated or blastic phase as shown in Figure 6.

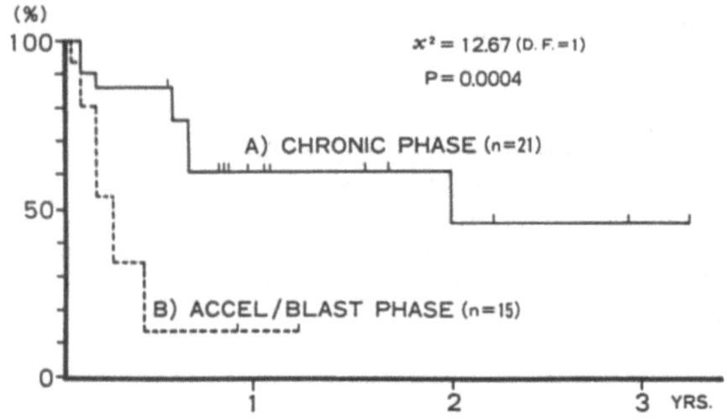

Figure 6. Survival of chronic myelogenous leukemia. ACCEL: Accelerated

INDICATION OF BMT FOR LEUKEMIA

We classify the indication of BMT into three categories, as shown in Table 12. In the first indication category we include the most favorable patients, i.e. in the first remission of acute leukemia or chronic phase of CML, age younger than 35 years, etc. However, most of the patients were introduced to us after the second indication, i.e., after the second remission of acute leukemia or accelerated or blastic phase of CML. Many BMTs have been performed for the second indication with a lower incidence of success. As the target of study, it seems also necessary to widen the indication of BMT for the less favorable patients.

Table 12. Indication for Allogeneic BMT

Factors	1st Indication	2nd	Expected
Age	35	40	45
AML	1st CR	2nd CR	relapse
ALL	1st CR	2nd CR	relapse
CML	chronic 1 year	* chronic Accelerated	blastic
Aplastic	transfusion (-)	20	20
Infection	-	-	-
Radiation	Lung (-) CNS (-)	1600 Rad	1600 Rad
HLA	complete	complete	* 1 locus mismatch
match	related	related	unrelated

IMPROVEMENT OF BMT SURVIVAL

The shortest way to improve the BMT results, however, is considered to be performing BMT in the first indication. The biggest obstacle to BMT in the early stages seems to be the fear of the failure of BMT or early death after BMT. In my center for adult diseases in Osaka, 45 BMT were done through July 1987 (Table 13). The first 20 patients belonged to the second indication, and 3 patients are alive at present. From the 21st patient on, we limited BMT only to patients in the first indication; 22 out of 25 patients are alive and disease free. Further follow up is necessary for the final results of these cases. We consider that the early death rate of the BMT in the first indication is significantly low. Thus, we feel we could have received more patients in earlier stages for BMT than before.

Table 13. BMT results of center for adult diseases, Osaka

Case No.	Period	Alive
1-20 (20 cases)	Aug. 1976- May 1984	3
21-45 (25 cases)	July 1984- June 1987	22

ITEMS OF MODIFICATION OF BMT PROCEDURES IN JAPAN

Table 14 shows the items of modification of BMT procedures in the Center for Adult Diseases, Osaka. Cyclosporin-A, fractionation of TBI, lung shielding at TBI, CMV-negative platelet transfusion, anti-CMV IgG prophylaxis, colony-stimulating factor and oral Acyclovir are the main changes during this period. By these changes we consider that BMT has become a very reliable and safe treatment for leukemia.

Table 14. Items of modification of BMT procedures

(1) Cyclosporin A..................	No. 16
(2) CSF-HU.........................	No. 18
(3) CMV (-) platelet donor..........	No. 18
(4) TBI fractionated...............	No. 19
(5) TBI lung 800 rad...............	No. 21
(6) Anti-CMV immunoglobulin.........	No. 22
(7) 1st remission & chronic phase...	No. 22

REFERENCE

1. Masaoka T (1986) Present status of bone marrow transplantation in Japan. Acta Haematol Japan 49:1491-1498
2. Teshima H et al (1986) Interstitial pneumonitis in allogeneic bone marrow transplantation: A report from the Japanese BMT study group. Bone Marrow Transplantation 1:179-183
3. Masaoka T et al (1982) Ozone decontamination of bioclean rooms. Appl Environ Microbiol 43:509-513
4. Aoki N et al (1983) The relation between isolated fungi from insect bodies and insect contamination in clinical bioclean room. J Antibact Antifung Agents 11:129-135

VI. Aplastic Anemia: R. Storb and M.M. Bortin, Chairpersons

18: Allogeneic and Syngeneic Marrow Transplantation for Aplastic Anemia: Overview of Seattle Results

Rainer Storb, Kristine Doney, E. Donnall Thomas, Claudio Anasetti, Frederick R. Appelbaum, Patrick Beatty, William Bensinger, C. Dean Buckner, Reginald Clift, Alexander Fefer, John Hansen, Roger Hill, Paul Martin, Robert McGuffin, Jean E. Sanders, Jack Singer, Patricia Stewart, Keith Sullivan, and Robert Witherspoon

INTRODUCTION

Marrow transplantation for the treatment of severe aplastic anemia has to be viewed in the context of alternate therapies for this disease. An earlier study of the International Aplastic Anemia Study Group showed that newly diagnosed patients with severe aplastic anemia treated by supportive therapy with or without androgens had a survival of only 20% at 5 years, with most patients dying within the first 6 months of diagnosis [1]. Most surviving patients had partial or complete spontaneous hematologic recoveries sufficient to live without the need for transfusions. These results were subsequently confirmed by the study group in another cohort of patients [2].

Stimulated by intriguing data from European investigators [3,4], the Seattle team began using Upjohn horse anti-human thymocyte globulin (ATG) in 1978 to treat patients with severe aplastic anemia [5]. Now, 9 years after treatment, 7 of the original 21 patients (33%) are alive; all are transfusion independent. Subsequent attempts to improve the response to ATG, and hence, survival, by additional infusion of HLA-haploidentical marrow or by added high dose corticosteroids failed to improve the results decisively [6,7]. Overall actuarial survival between 1 and 9 years for the first 123 patients 1 - 50 years old treated with ATG is close to 50% [unpublished]. A number of surviving patients have failed to respond to ATG and have remained transfusion-dependent. For comparison, the survival of 128 patients given HLAidentical marrow transplants during that same period of time is 70% [unpublished].

Because of the lack of uniform success with ATG treatment, syngeneic and allogeneic marrow transplantation have remained attractive therapeutic options. Certain in vitro tests were shown to predict the response to ATG therapy [8]. Until these early results have been confirmed, marrow transplantation seems to be the method of choice for all patients with severe aplastic anemia below 40 years of age, if a syngeneic or allogeneic marrow transplant donor is available. Once in vitro tests predictive of ATG response have become reliable, more intelligent therapeutic choices can be made for patients with aplastic anemia, and overall survival is likely to improve.

The current report presents an overview of the Seattle marrow transplant data.

SYNGENEIC GRAFTS

Nine patients with severe aplastic anemia, including 1 with an irradiation accident, were given marrow grafts from healthy monozygous twins [reviewed in 9,10]. None received immunosuppression before the first transplant. Six patients rapidly recovered normal hematopoiesis suggesting successful engraftment. All 6 are surviving between 10 and 25 years. In 3 cases, the initial marrow infusion did not result in sustained recovery. One of the 3 was next treated with ATG without effect. All 3 were subsequently given cyclophosphamide (CY), 50 mg/kg/day for four days, and a second marrow infusion. All 3 recovered their blood counts within 21 days. Two of the 3 are alive and well 4 and 8 years after grafting, respectively. The third patient, however, showed recurrence of aplastic anemia 13 months after the second marrow graft. This patient's aplastic anemia responded to subsequent treatment with ATG, and the patient is alive and well 6 years after the initial transplant. These results demonstrate that some cases of aplastic anemia reflect a qualitative or quantitative marrow stem cell defect correctable by the simple infusion of twin marrow, but other cases may be due to active suppression of hematopoiesis that can be overcome, in some cases only temporarily, by CY and twin marrow transplantation. The recurrence of aplastic anemia in one case at 13 months after preparation with CY and twin graft probably reflects the regrowth of a population of abnormal cells not completely eradicated by the preparative regimen but now responding to ATG.

ALLOGENEIC GRAFTS FROM GENOTYPICALLY HLA-IDENTICAL SIBLINGS

Rejection in Multiply-Transfused Patients Conditioned with CY. During the 1970's 93 multi-transfused patients were conditioned with CY and then given marrow infusions from HLA-identical siblings [reviewed in 11]. Graft rejection was seen in 33% of 88 evaluable patients, including 3 patients whose own marrow recovered. Mortality among rejecting patients was 80% compared with 25% among patients who did not reject their grafts. Strongly influenced by the high rate of rejection, survival in this group of 93 patients was only 46% with follow-up ranging from 6 to more than 16 years.

Experimental data in DLA-identical canine littermate marrow graft recipients suggested that rejection was due to sensitization through multiple transfusions [reviewed in 12]. Analysis of the clinical data was in agreement with the experimental findings. Among many possible factors predictive of graft rejection, the strongest association was with a unidirectional positive response in mixed leukocyte culture [13,14]. This was thought to be an expression of immunization of the patient against non-HLA antigens of the donor through transfusions. A second predictive factor was the marrow cell dose. With increasing numbers of marrow cells infused, the incidence of graft rejection decreased and vice versa. This may be related to increases in the number of stem cells or lymphoid cells infused.

Based on the clinical and experimental findings, more intensive immunosuppressive conditioning regimens were employed. The addition of procarbazine and ATG, found to be effective in experimental animals, did not decrease the rejection incidence in a prospective randomized trial in Seattle when combined with CY [15]. Similarly, the use of cyclosporine pre- or post-grafting did not overcome the problem of graft rejection [16]. A regimen similar to that used in patients with leukemia and consisting of CY combined with high dose total body irradiation (TBI) reduced the rejection rate but did not improve survival, mainly due to increased mortality from graft-versus-host disease (GVHD) and interstitial pneunomia [17].

Based on the observation that a large marrow cell dose resulted in a decreased incidence of rejection in patients and the finding of circulating hemopoietic stem cells in experimental animals, the Seattle group began using buffy coat cell infusions in addition to the marrow inoculum in early 1976 [18]. Actuarial survival between 7 and 11 years of the first 43 multiply transfused patients so treated is 67%. Graft rejection was seen in only 14% of the cases. Since then all multiply transfused patients transplanted in Seattle who are above age 18 years are conditioned with CY and given a combination of marrow and buffy coat cell infusions, while patients below age 18 are given marrow only. Buffy coat cell infusions, while having decreased the incidence of rejection, have been accompanied by an increase of de novo chronic GVHD [11]. Clearly, it would be desirable to both avoid rejection and reduce the risk of iatrogenic chronic GVHD by transplanting patients early before transfusions have to be administered.

Untransfused Patients. Studies in experimental animals and the clinical data suggested that rejection was caused by sensitization of the patient by way of blood transfusions. It seemed, therefore, desirable to carry out transplantation before transfusions had to be given. Fifty patients who had not had transfusions prior to 48 hours before the first dose of CY were given marrow transplants from HLA-identical family members following CY [11,19]. Results showed that graft failure was indeed rare. Actuarial survival is 82% with follow-up ranging from 3 to 15 years. These results further support the idea that most immunologic mechanisms causing graft failure are induced by previous blood transfusions.

Mixed Hematologic Chimerism. Ninety-six patients who were given a sex mismatched HLA-identical sibling marrow transplant following CY had sequential cytogenetic studies performed to determine both incidence and implications of post transplant mixed hematologic chimerism [20]. Fifty-six (58.3%) of the 96 were shown to be mixed chimeras with co-existing host and donor cells seen in blood or marrow 14 days or later after transplant, and 40 patients (41.7%) were complete chimeras with all cells being of donor origin. Patients with mixed chimerism had a significantly increased rate of graft rejection (31.7%) compared to only 5% in patients with complete chimerism. If patients with rejection are censored, the overall incidence of grades II - IV acute GVHD was significantly reduced in patients with mixed chimerism (23.1%) compared to an incidence of 63.2% in complete chimeras. The 5 year survival of patients with complete chimerism is 62% and 70% for mixed chimerism, excluding patients who rejected their first graft. Mixed chimerism persisted for up to 395 days post transplant, when conversion to 100% donor type cells was completed.

Second Marrow Transplants. Graft rejection has been associated with a high mortality in patients with aplastic anemia given marrow grafts from HLA-identical family members. In a study reported in the early seventies only 2 out of 29 patients undergoing graft rejection became long-term survivors [15]. A current conditioning regimen for second transplants involves CY combined with high dose ATG [21]. Of 16 recent patients undergoing second transplantation with that regimen, 12 engrafted successfully and 6 are surviving between 1 and 8 years. These data show that successful second transplants after CY and ATG are possible in most patients with aplastic anemia who have rejected their first marrow grafts; however, mortality remains high with only 40% of the patients becoming long-term survivors.

Acute and Chronic GVHD: Long-Term Survival. Aside from graft rejection, acute and chronic GVHD have had a major negative effect on survival. Through the early 1980's methotrexate has been the major drug used for GVHD prophylaxis [11]. Overall incidence of acute GVHD was 35%. The development of acute GVHD results in a dramatic decrease in overall survival, in part due to an increased risk of chronic GVHD and associated infections [22]. Actuarial survival of patients with grades 0 - I acute GVHD is approximately 82% compared to only 45% in patients with grades II - IV acute GVHD. Transplantation in a laminar airflow isolation room coupled with bacterial decontamination was associated with a decreased risk of acute GVHD and an improvement of overall survival [22], in agreement with previous data in experimental mice. Improved prevention of acute GVHD and increased survival were seen in dogs given a combination of a short course of methotrexate coupled with cyclosporine compared to dogs receiving either methotrexate or cyclosporine alone [23]. These experimental data were to some extent confirmed in a prospective randomized trial in patients with aplastic anemia [24]. This study, carried out in patients age 12 years and above, compared the combination of methotrexate and cyclosporine to methotrexate alone. The cumulative incidence of grades II - IV acute GVHD was 18% in patients receiving the combination and 55% in patients given methotrexate alone. The actuarial survival in patients given the combination was 80% compared to 55% in patients given methotrexate. We concluded that methotrexate/cyclosporine resulted in a significant decrease in the incidence and severity of acute GVHD and an improvement in survival. However, while the incidence of acute GVHD was significantly lessened by the drug combination, there was no reduction in the incidence of chronic GVHD.

Overall, the cumulative incidence of chronic GVHD is 40-50% [11]. It can be treated with prednisone, either given alone or coupled with alternating day cyclosporine. However, its management with immunosuppressive agents is still unsatisfactory. Not all patients respond to drug therapy and many suffer from potentially fatal infections related to the immunodeficiency accompanying chronic GVHD.

Nevertheless, it is gratifying to see that many patients with severe aplastic anemia are now living normal lives with successful transplants for 10 to more than 16 years without the need for any further therapy. Growth and development of children has been normal. Many patients have had normal children. There seems to be no increased incidence of secondary malignant tumors.

Special Indications For Marrow Transplantation. Most marrow transplants have been for therapy of idiopathic aplastic anemia, and in many other cases the disease has been related to chemicals or drugs. This paragraph describes transplants for patients with aplastic anemia of less frequent etiologies.

Nine Seattle patients had Fanconi anemia and were given HLA-identical sibling grafts following CY (in one case with preleukemia following CY and TBI) [25]. Five of the 9 are long-term survivors with survival ranging from 4 to more than 12-1/2 years. Fourteen patients had hepatitis associated aplastic anemia, and 11 of these are surviving between 3 and 14 years [26]. Four patients had paroxysmal nocturnal hemoglobinuria with accompanying aplastic anemia, and all are surviving between 3 and 6 1/2 years after grafting [27]. Twenty-three patients referred as aplastic anemia were found to have advanced preleukemic syndromes not related to prior therapy [28]. Three of these were prepared for transplantation with CY alone and developed leukemia within 6 months of transplantation. The remaining 20 patients were treated with CY combined with TBI. Thirteen of these 20 are alive and well 2 to more than 5 years from transplant, and 7 died from transplant associated complications. There has been no occurrence of leukemia in this group. Four additional patients grafted for preleukemia associated with severe marrow fibrosis have all died. These results suggest that for patients with life-threatening pancytopenia due to spontaneous preleukemia without severe marrow fibrosis, marrow grafting can prolong disease-free survival and may result in cure of the disease.

TRANSPLANTS FROM RELATED DONORS OTHER THAN HLA-GENOTYPICALLY IDENTICAL SIBLINGS

Twenty-four patients with severe aplastic anemia were given marrow grafts from HLA-nonidentical family members [29]. Two of these grafts were carried out after CY plus TBI, and in the remaining 22 only CY was used. All donor-recipient pairs were genotypically identical for one haplotype and phenotypically identical for a variable number of HLA-loci on the unshared haplotype. Six of the 24 patients received marrow from donors who were phenotypically matched for the second haplotype. All engrafted and are surviving. Among those 18 patients who received partially HLA-incompatible grafts, 10 had failure of engraftment and died of infections. All 7 evaluable patients achieving sustained engraftment developed grades II - IV acute GVHD. Currently, only 2 of the 18 patients who were mismatched for one or more loci on the nonshared haplotype are surviving with hematological recovery. These data show that patients with a phenotypically matched donor can benefit from a marrow transplant using only CY for conditioning. Those with partially matched donors are at high risk for graft rejection and may need additional immunosuppression such as CY and TBI to facilitate engraftment. Better GVHD prophylaxis is needed to improve survival.

CONCLUSIONS

Substantial progress has been made in marrow grafting for therapy of severe aplastic anemia since it was clinically introduced 17 years ago. Marrow recovery after transplantation is nearly always complete. The longest survivors have now been followed for more than 16 years and are leading normal lives. The problem of graft rejection has decreased, in part because of earlier transplantation, the use of leukocyte-poor transfusion products before grafting and better conditioning regimens. There have been improvements in the prevention of acute GVHD. Certain immunosuppressive regimens have been shown to favorably affect, and in a number of cases permanently arrest, the adverse course of chronic GVHD. Accordingly, survival has improved from the initial 45% to 70 - 80% depending on whether or not the patient has been transfused before transplantation. Early transplantation before transfusion is the preferred method if an HLA-identical family member is available. If transfusions are necessary, then family members should be avoided as donors. The use of leukocyte-poor red blood cell and platelet transfusions may reduce the risk of graft rejection.

Up to age 40, marrow transplantation from HLA-identical family members should be considered the therapy of choice. In patients older than 40 years, immunosuppressive therapy with ATG should be tried first.

In patients who have HLA-identical siblings, we prefer CY as the sole conditioning regimen, while in patients with HLA-nonidentical grafts CY must be combined with TBI for consistent successful engraftment. Grafts from donors other than HLA-identical siblings should only be considered after failure of immunosuppressive therapy, unless related donors are phenotypically HLA-identical. Phenotypically HLA-identical unrelated grafts are now possible but should be carried out only after unresponsiveness to ATG has been documented.

ACKNOWLEDGEMENTS

This work was supported by Grants HL 36444, CA 18221, CA 15704, and CA 18029 from the National Heart, Lung, and Blood Institute, and the National Cancer Institute, National Institutes of Health, DHHS.

REFERENCES

1. Camitta BM, Thomas ED, Nathan DG, Gale RP, Kopecky KJ, Rappeport JM, Santos G, Gordon-Smith EC, Storb R (1979) A prospective study of androgens and bone marrow transplantation for treatment of severe aplastic anemia. Blood 53:504-514

2. Camitta BM, OReilly RJ, Sensenbrenner L, Rappeport J, Champlin R, Doney K, August C, Hoffmann RG, Kirkpatrick D, Stuart R, Santos G, Parkman R, Gale RP, Storb R, Nathan D (1983) Antithoracic duct lymphocyte globulin therapy of severe aplastic anemia. Blood 62:883-888

3. Mathe G, Amiel JL, Schwarzenberg L, Choay J, Trolard P, Schneider M, Hayat M, Schlumberger JR, Jasmin Cl (1970) Bone marrow graft in man after conditioning by antilymphocytic serum. Br Med J 2:131-136

4. Speck B, Gratwohl A, Nissen C, Osterwalder B, Wursch A, Tichelli A, Lori A, Reusser P, Jeannet M, Signer E (1986) Treatment of severe aplastic anemia. Exp Hematol 14: 126-132

5. Doney KC, Weiden PL, Buckner CD, Storb R, Thomas ED (1981) Treatment of severe aplastic anemia using antithymocyte globulin with or without an infusion of HLA haploidentical marrow. Exp Hematol 9: 829-834

6. Doney KC, Dahlberg SJ, Monroe D, Storb R, Buckner CD, Thomas ED (1984) Therapy of severe aplastic anemia with anti-human thymocyte globulin and androgens: The effect of HLA haploidentical marrow infusion. Blood 63:342-348

7. Doney K, Storb R, Buckner CD, McGuffin R, Witherspoon R, Deeg HJ, Appelbaum F, Sullivan K, Thomas ED (1987) Treatment of aplastic anemia with antithymocyte globulin, high-dose corticosteroids, and androgens. Exp Hematol 15:239-242

8. Torok-Storb BJ, Doney K, Sale G, Thomas ED, Storb R (1985) Subsets of patients with aplastic anemia identified by flow microfluorometry. N Engl J Med 312:1015-1022

9. Lu D-P (1981) Syngeneic bone marrow transplantation for treatment of aplastic anaemia: Report of a case and review of the literature. Exp Hematol 9:257-263

10. Appelbaum FR, Cheever MA, Fefer A, Storb R, Thomas ED (1985) Recurrence of aplastic anemia following cyclophosphamide and syngeneic bone marrow transplantation: Evidence for two mechanisms of graft failure. Blood 65:553-556

11. Storb R, Thomas ED, Buckner CD, Appelbaum FR, Clift RA, Deeg HJ, Doney K, Hansen JA, Prentice RL, Sanders JE, Stewart P, Sullivan KM, Witherspoon RP (1984) Marrow transplantation for aplastic anemia. Semin Hematol 21:27-35

12. Storb R, Deeg HJ (1986) Failure of allogeneic canine marrow grafts after total body irradiation: Allogeneic "resistance" vs transfusion induced sensitization. Transplantation 42:571-588

13. Storb R, Prentice RL, Thomas ED (1977) Marrow transplantation for treatment of aplastic anemia: An analysis of factors associated with graft rejection. N Engl J Med 296: 61-66

14. Deeg HJ, Self S, Storb R, Doney K, Appelbaum FR, Witherspoon RP, Sullivan KM, Sheehan K, Sanders J, Mickelson E, Thomas ED (1986) Decreased incidence of marrow graft rejection in patients with severe aplastic anemia: Changing impact of risk factors. Blood 68:1363-1368

15. Storb R, Thomas ED, Weiden PL, Buckner CD, Clift RA, Fefer A, Fernando LP, Giblett ER, Goodell BW, Johnson FL, Lerner KG, Neiman PE, Sanders JE (1976) Aplastic anemia treated by allogeneic bone marrow transplantation: A report on 49 new cases from Seattle. Blood 48:817-841

16. Deeg HJ, Shulman HM, Schmidt E, Yee GC, Thomas ED, Storb R (1986) Marrow graft rejection and veno-occlusive disease of the liver in patients with aplastic anemia conditioned with cyclophosphamide and cyclosporine. Transplantation 42: 497-501

17. Storb R, Thomas ED, Appelbaum FR, Clift RA, Deeg HJ, Doney K, Hansen JA, Prentice RL, Sanders JE, Singer JW, Shulman H, Stewart PS, Sullivan KM, Dahlberg SJ, Buckner CD, Witherspoon RP (1984) Marrow transplantation for severe aplastic anemia: The Seattle experience. In: Young NS, Humphries RK, Levine A (eds), Aplastic Anemia: Stem Cell Biology and Advances in Treatment. New York: Alan R Liss, Inc.

18. Storb R, Doney KC, Thomas ED, Appelbaum F, Buckner CD, Clift RA, Deeg HJ, Goodell BW, Hackman R, Hansen JA, Sanders J, Sullivan K, Weiden PL, Witherspoon RP (1982) Marrow transplantation with or without donor buffy coat cells for 65 transfused aplastic anemia patients. Blood 59:236-246

19. Anasetti C, Doney KC, Storb R, Meyers JD, Farewell VT, Buckner CD, Appelbaum FR, Sullivan KM, Clift RA, Deeg HJ, Fefer A, Martin PJ, Singer JW, Sanders JE, Stewart PS, Witherspoon RP, Thomas ED (1986) Marrow transplantation for severe aplastic anemia: Long term outcome in 50 "untransfused" patients. Ann Intern Med 104:461-466

20. Hill RS, Petersen FB, Storb R, Appelbaum FR, Doney K, Dahlberg S, Ramberg R, Thomas ED (1986) Mixed hematologic chimerism after allogeneic marrow transplantation for severe aplastic anemia is associated with a higher risk of graft rejection and a lessened incidence of acute graft-versus-host disease. Blood 67:811-816

21. Storb R, Weiden PL, Sullivan KM, Appelbaum FR, Beatty P, Buckner CD, Clift RA, Doney KC, Hansen J, Mar-

tin PJ, Sanders JE, Stewart P, Witherspoon RP, Thomas ED (1987) Second marrow transplants in patients with aplastic anemia rejecting the first graft: Use of a conditioning regimen including cyclophosphamide and antithymocyte globulin. Blood, in press

22. Storb R, Prentice RL, Buckner CD, Clift RA, Appelbaum F, Deeg HJ, Doney K, Hansen JA, Mason M, Sanders JE, Singer J, Sullivan KM, Witherspoon RP, Thomas ED (1983) Graft-versus-host disease and survival in patients with aplastic anemia treated by marrow grafts from HLAidentical siblings: Beneficial effect of a protective environment. N Engl J Med 308:302-307

23. Deeg HJ, Storb R, Weiden PL, Raff RF, Sale GE, Atkinson K, Graham TC, Thomas ED (1982) Cyclosporin A and methotrexate in canine marrow transplantation: Engraftment, graft-versus-host disease and induction of tolerance. Transplantation 34:30-35

24. Storb R, Deeg HJ, Farewell V, Doney K, Appelbaum F, Beatty P, Bensinger W, Buckner CD, Clift R, Hansen J, Hill R, Longton G, Lum L, Martin P, McGuffin R, Sanders J, Singer J, Stewart P, Sullivan K, Witherspoon R, Thomas ED (1986) Marrow transplantation for severe aplastic anemia: Methotrexate alone compared with a combination of methotrexate and cyclosporine for prevention of acute graft-versus-host disease. Blood 68:119-125

25. Deeg HJ, Storb R, Thomas ED, Appelbaum F, Buckner CD, Clift RA, Doney K, Johnson L, Sanders JE, Stewart P, Sullivan KM, Witherspoon RP (1983) Fanconi's anemia treated by allogeneic marrow transplantation. Blood 61:954-959

26. Witherspoon RP, Storb R, Shulman HJ, Buckner CD, Deeg HJ, Clift RA, Sanders JE, Doney K, McDonald G, Sullivan KM, Appelbaum FR, Thomas ED (1984) Marrow transplantation in hepatitis-associated aplastic anemia. Am J Hematol 17:269-278

27. Szer J, Deeg HJ, Witherspoon RP, Fefer A, Buckner CD, Thomas ED, Storb R (1984) Long-term survival after marrow transplantation for paroxysmal nocturnal hemoglobinuria with aplastic anemia. Ann Intern Med 101:193-195

28. Appelbaum FR, Storb R, Ramberg RE, Shulman HM, Buckner CD, Clift RA, Deeg HJ, Fefer A, Sanders J, Self S, Singer J, Stewart P, Sullivan K, Witherspoon R, Thomas ED (1987) Treatment of preleukemic syndromes with marrow transplantation. Blood 69:92-96

29. Beatty PG, Di Bartolomeo P, Storb R, Clift RA, Buckner CD, Sullivan KM, Doney K, Appelbaum FR, Anasetti C, Witherspoon R, Sanders J, Stewart P, Martin PJ, Ciancarelli M, Hansen JA, Thomas ED (1987) Treatment of aplastic anemia with marrow grafts from related donors other than HLA genotypically matched siblings. Clinical Transplantation, in press

19: Recent Advances and Future Trends in Bone Marrow Transplantation for Severe Aplastic Anemia

E.C. Gordon-Smith

This meeting of the International Society for Experimental Hematology is an appropriate time and place to review the status of bone marrow transplantation (BMT) for the treatment of patients with severe aplastic anemia (SAA). More information is available on the effectiveness or otherwise of immuno-suppressive treatment with antilymphocyte globulin (ALG) and new methods for dealing with the problems of BMT have been introduced in the past year or so. This paper will review briefly the history of BMT for severe aplastic anemia and discuss how the indications for, and the scope of, this treatment may have changed.

BMT FOR SEVERE APLASTIC ANEMIA, 1969-1987: THE PROBLEM OF REJECTION:

The first successful allogeneic BMT for severe aplastic anemia using an HLA-identical sibling donor was carried out in Seattle in 1969 (1). The Seattle experience is reviewed in this journal and will not be quoted extensively here except to emphasise problems associated with this technique. The major problem which was encountered was that of graft rejection or failure to take which occured in about a third of the transplants (1-4). Acute graft versus host disease (aGVHD) was a less common cause of transplant related death though the proportion of evaluable patients who developed aGVHD, that is, those that did not reject the graft, was similar to that seen in patients grafted for malignant disease. These observations were thought to derive from the milder immunosuppression used for conditioning patients with aplastic anemia, namely cyclophosphamide 50ug/kg/d for four days (1) compared with the regimen used in malignant disease, cyclophosphamide 60ug/kg/d for two days with total body irradiation (10Gy) given as a single dose (5). There may be additional causes of the high rejection rate in these aplastic patients related to the immune system of the recipient. Unlike patients with leukemia, who are to some extent immunosuppressed by previous chemotherapy and their disease, patients with aplastic anemia have normal cellular and humoral immunity and are frequently immunologically stimulated by multiple transfusions of blood products before transplantation. The influence of previous transfusions on the rate of rejection was identified by the Seattle group in their study of rejection (6). In the early published series of BMT for aplastic anemia the most successful results were obtained in the multicentre, randomised trial of BMT compared with androgen therapy organised by Camitta (3) where patients were transplanted as soon after diagnosis as possible, before marked sensitisation to blood products had occured. In this series long term survival was 67% graft failure accounting for the majority of the deaths (28%).

The other major cause of death in this trial, as in other series was aGVHD (6%). This relatively low incidence of death associated with aGVHD was in part, at least, attributable to the omission of TBI from the conditioning treatment with a consequent reduction in interstitial pneumonitis (7) thought to arise from multiple factors including a GVHD, lung irradiation and cytomegalovirus. Prevention of aGVHD was attempted using methotrexate in the post graft period (1), a cytotoxic immunosuppressant which might have contributed to the incidence of graft failure.
The introduction of cyclosporin into renal transplantation and its success in preventing rejection of the kidney (8) encouraged its use in BMT, primarily to

prevent rejection in the aplastic anemia patients (9). It was hoped that additional benefit would come from a reduction also in the incidence of aGVHD (10) but this hope was not sustained though there might be some reduction in the severity of aGVHD (9).

Although cyclosporin reduced the rejection rate from the previously high levels there remained some patients who still rejected their grafts, either early following transplantation or late, following withdrawal of the drug. In the Hammersmith series out of 35 patients transplanted there were 2 early rejections and 6 late failures, the latter reversing when cyclosporin was reintroduced (9,11).

Such residual graft failure prompted other groups to give additional immunosuppression in the pregraft conditioning either as thoraco abdominal irradiation 600cGy (12) or total lymphnode irradiation TLI, as used in the treatment of Hodgkin's disease (13).

Each of these strategies reduced the rejection rate to close to zero, with survival curves which reached a plateau at 75-80%, compared with 73% for cyclosporin alone (9), for HLA-identical sibling BMT using unmanipulated donor marrow.

For patients who did suffer rejection of marrow it was sometimes possible to achieve a successful transplant from the same donor using additional immunosuppression including the use of ALG (14), though the majority failed.

Thus the clinical problem of graft failure following BMT for severe aplastic anemia using matched sibling donors seemed to be solved, leaving aGVHD as the most common cause of death with an incidence of 10-15%. This incidence of transplant related death is still higher than would be acceptable in, say a surgical procedure and much current effort is devoted to reducing aGVHD and its complications in these matched sibling donor transplants. The combined use of methotrexate and cyclosporin, reported by the Seattle group, gives some promise of improvement in these transplants (15).

The major problems which remain are the selection of patients for bone marrow transplantation in the light of improved results using ALG and what role transplantation from donors other than HLA-matched siblings may play in the management of patients who fail immunosuppressive therapy.

SELECTION OF PATIENTS - THE CRITERIA OF SEVERE APLASTIC ANEMIA

The well known criteria of severe aplastic anemia presented by Camitta and colleagues (3) were established from a multivariant analysis of patients with aplastic anemia treated by the standard therapy available at that time, namely androgens and supportive care. It had already been shown that the survival curve of such patients showed two components, a steep fall in survival in the first six months, about half the patients dying in this time, and a plateau of survival, about 20-25% of patients recovering normal marrow function (16).

The criteria of severe aplastic anemia used to define the poor risk group have stood unchallenged since their introduction but it may be appropriate to reconsider them in the light of data from ALG trials.

The criteria used for the definition of severe aplastic anemia were at least two of the following three peripheral blood values - granulocytes $< 0.5 \times 10^9/l$, platelets $< 20 \times 10^9/l$ and reticulocytes $<1\%$ (corrected for hematocrit). In addition the marrow had to be either markedly hypocellular (25% normal cellularity) or moderately hypoplastic (25%-50% of normal cellularity) with $<30\%$ of remaining cells being hematopoietic.

ANTILYMPHOCYTIC GLOBULIN FOR THE TREATMENT OF SEVERE APLASTIC ANEMIA - THE EUROPEAN EXPERIENCE

ALG was introduced for the treatment of aplastic anemia by Professor George Mathé and his colleagues in 1970 (17), but it was not until the work by Speck, Gluckman and Van Rood among others (18) that its potential became fully appreciated. The European Bone Marrow Transplant Group have collected data on 509 patients with severe aplastic anemia, 291 treated by immunosuppression, 218 by HLA-matched sibling transplants, over the period 1981-1986 (19). The patients were treated in many different centres throughout Europe. The survival curves of the two groups were identical with overlapping plateaux of 65% at 3 years. This does not indicate that the treatments are identically effective because the 35% mortality in the two groups may well affect different patients.

In an analysis of factors which may influence survival in the two groups the EBMT identified the following differences.

Age: Patients under 20 years of age with SAA survived better with HLA matched transplants than with immunosuppression, the reverse being found above 20. The differences in each group were just not statistically significant.

Neutrophil count and infection: Patients who had SAA and in whom the neutrophil count was particularly severely depressed, $<0.2 \times 10^9/l$, fared better with BMT at all ages. The difference was statistically significant. When patients with these very low counts who were infected at the time of treatment, the 39 patients treated by BMT had a greatly superior survival when compared with the 33 treated by immunosuppression (70% vs 25%, $P<0.001$). It is thus possible to identify groups of patients for whom BMT from a matched sibling donor is the first treatment of choice, but this still leaves the problem of patients who fail one or more courses of ALG (20), who do not have sibling donors.

EXPANDING THE DONOR POOL - MISMATCHED FAMILY DONORS OR MATCHED UNRELATED DONORS?

For patients with acute leukemia the use of family donors other than HLA-matched siblings the results of BMT appear to be close to those achieved with the matched sibling donors providing the family donor is phenotypically matched or is disparate at only one locus, the mismatched site being irrelevant amongst class 1 or class 11 antigens (21). This data refers to unmanipulated marrow. For patients with aplastic anemia the data base is less secure. Phenotypically matched unrelated donors, or those mismatched at one locus may provide successful grafts (22) but the evidence suggests that even one locus mismatch leads to a greater number of transplant related deaths, whether the donor is family or unrelated (23). Attempts to reduce the influence of aGVHD by T-cell depletion of the marrow lead to an unacceptable increase in graft failure unless the pregraft immuno-suppression was greatly increased (24).

However, there are some hopeful indications that such non-sibling grafts may become an acceptable form of treatment at least for patients who fail ALG treatment. These indications relate to a greater knowledge of the HLA system and its importance and to new methods of pregraft immunosuppression.

HLA-matching for non-sibling donors:

Current methods for HLA typing employ serological techniques to demonstrate identity or otherwise in BMT donors. Phenotypic identity, even within a family, does not indicate genotypic identity, as pointed out by van Rood at the EBMT meeting in 1987 (25). The question is whether this matters in the context of BMT. If this is so within a family the problem may be much greater in unrelated donor panels though fortunately the presence of positive linkage disequilibria within populations make this less of a problem than might be expected. The introduction of DNA probing techniques, particularly using restriction fragment length polymosphisms (RFLP) have made the identification of these linkeages, at least in the D region, possible for clinical use (26). A further observation is that there may be certain degrees of mismatch, particularly in the class 1 antigens, which are acceptable and others which are not based upon the degree of cross reactivity between the disparate antigens (27). The future hope is that this information may be translated into practical methods for the selection of family or unrelated donors, the RFLP providing data for the class II match, the knowledge of class 1 acceptability allowing a greater range of one antigen mismatched donors.

IMMUNOSUPPRESSION AND T-CELL DEPLETION

In this symposium Dr John Goldman has described the use of matched unrelated donors for the treatment of CGL using an immunosuppressive regimen which includes the use of in vivo anti-T cell, lytic monoclonal antibodies, TLI, TBI and busulphan. On similar principles the Hammersmith Group have devised a protocol for immunosuppression of patients with aplastic anemia for matched unrelated transplants using TLI and in vivo monoclonal antibody (Camplus-1, an 1gG2b antibody kindly supplied by Herman Waldmann and colleagues from the Department of Immunology, Addenbrooke's Hospital, Cambridge) (28). In each instance the marrow is depleted of T-cells prior to infusion. The early results for SAA are encouraging but any success may have to be paid for by an increase in long term side effects brought about by the use of radiation.

THE STATUS OF BMT FOR APLASTIC ANEMIA

The indications for bone marrow transplantation in the next few years may be summarised as follows:

(1) Patients with an HLA-matched sibling donor:

a) All patients under 50 years with SAA who have neutrophils less than $0.2 \times 10^9/l$ particularly with evidence of infection before treatment should have BMT as first line of treatment.

b) Patients under 20 years with SAA regardless of the neutrophil count have a better survival with BMT than ALG.

c) Patients between 20 and 50 years who fail to respond to ALG after four months would benefit from BMT. Likewise patients who relapse after ALG who have the appropriate donor should receive a BMT. It is not clear at this stage whether marrow and modest immunosuppression should be used, or whether increased immunosuppression with T-cell depletion is appropriate. My own preference is for the former.

2) Patients without an HLA-matched sibling donor:

For these patients a search for an acceptable family or unrelated donor, using the scheme outlined above, should be started as soon as possible after diagnosis. If a suitable donor is found BMT using increased immunosuppression and T-cell depletion should be discussed as treatment should one or two courses of ALG fail to produce remission. Again, criteria which suggest very severe disease may encourage the earlier use of such donors, and the problem of transfusion sensitisation may favour early transplant, rather than its use as a last resort.

REFERENCES

1. Storb R, Thomas ED, Buckner CD et al (1974) Allogeneic bone marrow grafting for treatment of aplastic anemia. Blood 43: 157
2. Storb R, Thomas ED, Weiden PL (1976) Aplastic anemia treated by allogeneic bone marrow transplantation. A report on 49 new cases from Seattle. Blood 48:817
3. Camitta BM, Thomas ED, Nathan DG et al (1976) Severe aplastic anemia: a prospective study of the effect of early marrow transplantation on acute mortality Blood 48: 921
4. UCLA bone marrow transplant team (1976) Bone marrow transplantation in severe aplastic anaemia Lancet ii: 921
5. Thomas ED, Buckner CD, Banaji M et al (1977) One hundred patients with acute leukemia treated by chemotherapy, total body irradiation and allogeneic bone marrow transplantation Blood 49:511
6. Storb R, Prentice RL and Thomas ED (1977) Marrow transplantation for aplastic anemia: factors associated with rejection New Engl J Med 296: 61
7. Meyers JD, Flournoy N and Thomas ED (1982) Nonbacterial pneumonia after allogeneic bone marrow transplantation A review of ten years' experience. Rev Infect Dis 4: 1119
8. Calne RY, Rolles K, White D J G et al (1979) Cyclosporin A initially as the only immunosuppresant in 34 recipients of cadaveric organs: 32 kidneys, 2 pancreases and 2 livers Lancet ii: 103
9. Hows JM, Palmer S and Gordon-Smith EC (1982) Use of cyclosporin A in allogeneic bone marrow transplantation for severe aplastic anemia Transplantation 33:382
10. Powles RL, Clink H, Spence D et al (1980) Cyclosporin A to prevent graft versus host disease in man after allogeneic bone marrow transplantation Lancet i: 327
11. Hows JM, Yin JL, Chipping PM et al (1983) Postgraft immunosuppression with cyclosporin in allogeneic bone marrow transplantation for severe aplastic anemia. Transplant Proc 15: (suppl) 2634
12. Gluckman E, Devergie A, Dutreux A et al (1978) Total body irradiation in bone marrow transplantation: Hopital St Louis results Pathol Biol (Paris) 27:349
13. Ramsay NKC, Kim TH, McGlave PB et al (1982) Successful use of total lymphoid irradiation and cyclophosphamide as a conditioning regimen for bone marrow transplantation in multiply transfused patients with severe aplastic anemia Exp Hematol 10:47
14. Storb R, Weiden DL, Sullivan KM et al (1987) Second marrow transplants in patients with aplastic anemia rejecting the first graft: use of a conditioning regimen including cyclophosphamide and antilymphocyte globulin Blood 70: 116
15. Storb R, Deeg HJ, Farewell V et al (1986) Marrow transplantation for severe aplastic anemia methotrexate alone compared with methotrexate and cyclosporin for the prevention of acute graft-versus-host disease Blood 68: 119
16. Williams DM, Lynch RE and Cartwright GE (1973) Drug induced aplastic anemia Semin Hemtol 10: 195
17. Mathé G, Amiel JL, Schwartzenberg L et al (1970) Bone marrow graft in man after conditioning with antilymphocyte globulin Brit Med J ii:131
18. Speck B, Gluckman E, Haak HC and van Rood JJ (1977) Treatment of aplastic anaemia by antilymphocyte globulin with and without allogeneic bone marrow infusion Lancet ii:1145
19. Bacigalupo A, Gordon-Smith EC, Van Lint MT et al (1987) Bone marrow transplantation (BMT) vs immunosuppression (IS) in the management of severe aplastic anaemia. Bone Marrow Transplantation 2 (suppl 1):99
20. Fairhead SM, Chipping PM and Gordon-Smith EC (1983) Treatment of aplastic anaemia with antilymphocyte globulin (ALG) Brit J Haematol 55:7
21. Beatty PG,Clift RA, Mickelson EM et al (1985) Marrow transplantation from related donors other than HLA identical siblings N Engl J Med 313: 765
22. Gordon-Smith EC, Fairhead SM, Chipping PM et al (1982) Bone marrow transplantation for severe aplastic anaemia using histocompatible unrelated volunteer donors Brit Med J ii: 835
23. Gordon-Smith EC, Hows J, Bacigalupo A et al (1987) Bone marrow transplantation for severe aplastic anaemia (SAA) from donors other than HLA-matched siblings. A report of the EBMT working party. Bone Marrow Transplantation 2 (suppl 1): 100

24. Hows JM, Yin JL, Marsh J et al (1986) Histocompatible unrelated donors compared with HLA-non-identical family donors in marrow transplantation for aplastic anemia and leukemia Blood 68: 1322
25. Van Rood JJ, (1987) Lecture to the European Bone Marrow Transplantation Group, Interlaken, Switzerland (unpublished)
26. Bradley BA, Bidwell EA, Goffin RB et al (1987) DNA probes for accurate HLA DR and DQ matching in bone marrow transplantation Bone Marrow Transplant 2 (suppl 1): 81
27. Van Rood JJ, (1987) Lecture to the Royal College of Pathologists, London (unpublished)

20: Allogeneic Bone Marow Transplantation in Leukemia

Bruno Speck, Alois Gratwohl, André Tichelli and Catherine Nissen

ALLOGENEIC BONE MARROW TRANSPLANTATION IN LEUKEMIA

Bruno Speck, Alois Gratwohl, André Tichelli and Catherine Nissen

Division of Hematology, Department of Internal Medicine, Kantonsspital, University of Basel, Basel, Switzerland

TABLE 1 PATIENT POPULATION GRAFTED BETWEEN JULY 79 AND JUNE '87 (N = 141)

DIAGNOSIS	NO.	A	D	DEAD DTX	DEAD DR
AML 1. CR	30	19	11	6	5
NOT 1. CR	19	9	10	3	7
ALL 1. CR	18	10	8	6	2
NOT 1. CR	28	8	20	7	13
CML cP	31	21	10	9	1
AP	10	5	5	4	1
MDS	2	1	1	1	-
LYMPHOMA	3	2	1	1	-
TOTAL	141	75	66	37	29

A = ALIVE DTX = DIED FROM TRANSPLANT RELATED PROBLEM
D = DEAD DR = DIED FROM RELAPSE

INTRODUCTION

Erradication of leukemia by high dose chemotherapy and total body irradiation (TBI) and the capacity of hemopoietic stem cells to repopulate the marrow form the basic concept of bone marrow transplantation (BMT) in leukemia. First attempts at allogeneic BMT were made soon after the discovery of the hemopoietic stem cell. They all failed because of rejection and Graft-versus-Host disease (GvHD) (1). The recognition of the major histocompatibility complex was the basis of the first successful BMT's in immune defiency syndromes where HLA-identical siblings served as donors (2-4). Results of BMT in leukemia, however, remained unsatisfactory because it was used almost exclusively for terminally ill patients with end-stage disease. At present it is an established therapy with predictable risks and benefits for patients with acute myelogenous (AML), acute lymphoblastic (ALL) and chronic myelogenous leukemia (CML) (5, 6). At present, experience is collected with BMT in other neoplastic disorders of the hemopoietic system.

Many aspects of the history of BMT are reflected by results obtained in our own patient population.

PATIENTS AND METHODS

The first BMT at Kantonsspital Basel was performed in January 1973. Until June 1st, 1987 a total of 209 marrow grafts were performed for malignant and non-malignant hematological disorders. The basic conditioning, Cyclophosphamide (Cy) and TBI and the basic patient care, laminar airflow-units with complete microbiological decontamination, remained identical throughout the whole period and all patients were treated and followed by essentially the same medical team. Some major changes were made in the radiation technique and in the prophylaxis against GvHD. Until June 1979 most patients were transplanted in end-stage disease, and Methotrexate was used for prophylaxis against GvHD. In the first group of patients we used high-dose combined chemotherapy immediately before starting the standard conditioning (7).

In July 1979 we changed our policy. We attempted to transplant patients earlier in their disease, acute leukemia in first complete remission and CML in chronic phase. Cyclosporin A (CsA) was now used in all patients for prophylaxis against GvHD (8, 9). Some patients continued to be referred in later stages of leukemia. Since July 1st, 1979 we have performed a total of 168 BMT, 147 for neoplastic disorders of the hemopoietic system. 141 of them had allogeneic grafts and they form the basis of this report. They are summarized in Table 1.

In all patients conditioning consisted of 2x60mg/kg Cy followed by TBI. Between October 1983 and August 1986, 24 patients at high-risk for relapse, 18 patients with advanced leukemia and 6 patients in first CR with M4 or M5 AML were given preconditioning with high-dose Ara-C and VP16 (10). Since December 1986, 6 patients at risk for relapse were given VP16 30mg/kg 2 days before Cy.

There were four different forms of giving TBI (11). From 1979 to 1985 103 patients had single dose TBI 1000 rad with a dose rate of 8 rad/min. The initial 18 ones had lung shielding to keep the lung dose at 800 rad. Since 1985 all patients are irradiated with 6 fractions of 200 rad. In 15 patients the dose rate was 20 rad/min, in the last 23 patients 3 rad/min.

TABLE 2 PATIENTS WITH T-CELL DEPLETED BONE MARROW AND IRRADIATED DONOR BUFFY COAT

UPN	AGE	SEX		ENGRAFT-MENT	MAX. GVHD	
283	35	F	MDS	+	II	A/W, NO PROBLEMS
284	27	M	AML 2.CR	+	-	A/W, NO PROBLEMS
289	35	M	CML cP	+	-	RELAPSE IN BLAST CRISIS
296	43	M	CML cP	+	-	A/W, NO PROBLEMS
299	29	M	M.HODGKIN REFRACTORY	+	IV	IP + GVHD
300	35	M	CLL	+	-	A/W, NO PROBLEMS
306	28	M	AML 1.CR	+	II	A/W, NO PROBLEMS
307	33	M	CML cP	+	-	A/W, NO PROBLEMS
312	43	M	AML 1.CR	+	II	A/W, NO PROBLEMS
315	43	M	CML cP	+	II	A/W, TOO EARLY
316	34	F	CML cP	+	-	A/W, TOO EARLY

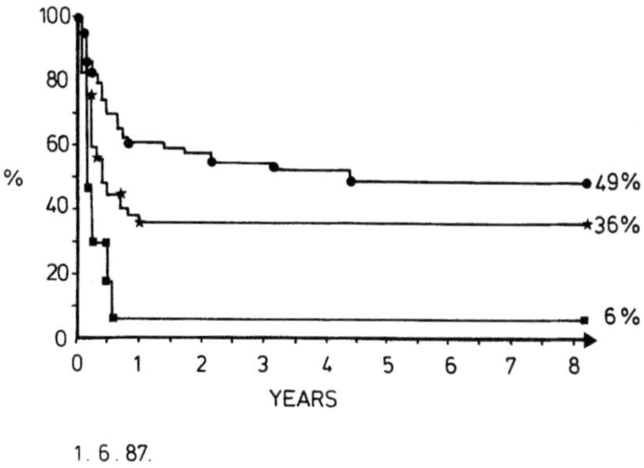

The CsA regimen for prophylaxis against GvHD remained esssentially unchanged. During the immediate pre- and post-transplant period it was given parenterally followed by a single daily oral dose for 1 year. The first 20 patients were given 20mg/kg i.m. on 7 successive days, starting on day -1. 11 patients received the same dose intravenously for 5 days. Since 1982 the CsA schedule has not been changed anymore (9): 20mg/kg as a continuous infusion on day -1, 10mg/kg as continuous for 5 days followed by 5mg/kg as continuous infusion after day +5 until the patient is able to take it orally. The oral maintenance dose is 12.5mg/kg daily for 6 months. The dose is then tapered and CsA stopped at 12 months. Doses are reduced depending on nephrotoxicity. CsA is resumed or increased if signs of GvHD appear upon withdrawl or reduction.

In 1985 we introduced T-cell depletion of the donor bone marrow for patients above the age of 25 years. A two-log depletion is performed by counterflow centrifugation (elutriation) (12). Based on our animal experiments all recipients of T-cell depleted bone marrow now receive additional irradiated buffy coat cells from the donor on days +1, +3, +5, +7 and +14 (13, 14). A total of $1x10^9$ mononuclear cells is obtained with a CS 3000 Fenwal Cell Separator, irradiated with 1500 rad and given intravenously.

All patients are nursed in sterile laminar airflow-units and in sterile environment with complete skin- and gastrointestinal decontamination. They all stay in Basel for at least 3 months after the transplant and are followed at least once per year.

Fig. 1. 8 year overall and disease-free survival. Calculation according to Kaplan and Meier (1958).

—•— Good risk patients (AML + ALL 1st CR, CML cP) N = 79
—★— Poor risk patients (AML + ALL not 1st CR, CML aP) N = 57
—■— Historical controls N = 17

RESULTS

The results are summarized in Table 1. There is no major difference between the 3 main diagnostic groups AML, ALL and CML in chronic phase. In all groups results were better when the transplant was performed in 1st CR or in CML in chronic phase (cP) compared to later stages of the disease (Fig. 1).

A total of 66 patients died, 30 of 81 good-risk patients and 36 of 60 high-risk patients. Transplant-related deaths were 21 in the good-risk and 14 in the high-risk group. Besides the stage of disease age was a major factor influencing the outcome. The proportion of transplant-related complications increases with age.

It is too early to evaluate the impact of T-cell depletion. The first 4 patients were given elutriated bone marrow without buffy coat. 2 rejected, 1 relapsed and 1 died of GvHD. On the other hand, 9 of the 11 patients given elutriated bone marrow and irradiated donor buffy coat are living and well, 8 of them without any evidence of disease, 1 with relapse (Table 2). Engraftment was complete and comparable to unseparated marrow in all patients. GvHD never exceeded grade II except in the patient transplanted for end-stage Hodgkin's disease.

DISCUSSION

Our patients reflect achievements and problems of BMT. The achievement is a clear indication for grafting and a clear definition of risk-factors. GvHD is still a major problem. We tried to solve it by T-cell depletion of the marrow by means of elutriation.

Results of BMT are better in good-risk leukemia (AML, ALL in 1st CR, CML in cP). This goes almost exclusively on the account of a lower risk of relapse. We have made great progress in the prevention of severe chronic GvHD by long-term use of CsA (8, 9). In some patients CsA is required for up to 7 years before GvHD definitely clears and tolerance is achieved. In a recent study of the European Cooperative Group for Bone Marrow Transplantation (EBMT) it was shown that among 1923 good-risk patients there is no difference in long-term disease-free survival between AML, ALL and CML (15). The same study also shows that for the same cohorts of patients long-term survival remained unchanged if transplanted before 1980, between 1980 and 84 and after 1985. It is difficult to accept that no progress has been made since 1979. This fact may reflect that there is still no ideal conditioning and no ideal prophylaxis against GvHD. Furthermore, there is a trend to transplant older patients despite the risk of transplant-related mortality by age (15, 16). Studies of the International Bone Marrow Transplant Registry (IBMTR) have shown a negative impact of T-cell depletion on leukemic relapse in acute leukemia and even more pronounced in CML (17). In our own study using elutriation for T-cell depletion, engraftment was difficult to achieve without irradiated donor buffy coat. In the last 11 patients who were treated with elutriated marrow plus irradiated donor buffy coat, engraftment was achieved as with unseparated bone marrow. Relapse rates were not unduly high. Of course, it has to be borne in mind, that the observation period in this group of patients is still relatively short and more time is required for conclusive evaluation of these data. It has been assumed, that in T-cell depleted BMT relapse is more frequent because engraftment is slower than in grafts with unseparated marrow. If this problem can be solved by enhancing engraftment with the addition of irradiated donor buffy coat, and if the presumed "healthy bone marrow effect" with its antileukemic properties can also be transferred with irradiated peripheral blood cells without risk of GvHD, this might be an enormous progress. Another potential approach to prompt engraftment of T-cell depleted bone marrow is the use of humoral hemopoietic stimulators such as GM-CSF. Such studies are currently initiated.

An important issue is the use of CsA in combination with T-cell depletion. Prentice, who reports a low incidence of relapse after T-cell depleted BMT uses no additional immunosuppression. He claims that the high incidence of relapse in other studies is due to the use of CsA (18). To date this issue is not solved yet. In the most recent surveys of EBMT and the IBMTR (15, 16), CsA did not increase the risk of relapse if unseparated marrow was grafted.

One of the greatest problems of allogeneic BMT is that it remains largely confined to young patients with an HLA-identical sibling donor. Even in this low-risk group GvHD and other transplant-related morbidity and mortality remain a great problem. The incidence of relapse has been observed to be most frequent in patients with FAB-type M5 AML, and in patients grafted within 5 months after achieving remission.

Both observations are confirmed by studies of the EBMT and the IBMTR (15, 16). Patients grafted before 5 months after reaching remission include a group of leukemias that are prone to relapse whatever treatment is applied. They eliminate themselves from this category of good-risk patients if the responsible Transplant Center postpones BMT. M5 has proved to be a type of primary resistant leukemia in most recent and several previous studies (15, 16, 19).

The impact of minimal residual disease at the time of BMT is not clear. Probably the amount of residual leukemic cells is less important than the resistance to chemo-radiotherapy used for conditioning and the allogeneic effect of BMT. This is clearly illustrated by the experience with CML-patients, where no attempt is made to reach a stage of minimal residual disease and yet relapse rates are lower than in acute leukemia (20). In ALL, high-risk remained a matter of debate as to whether the transplant should be performed in first or second remission. In a recent study of the IBMTR it was clearly shown that high-risk ALL should be transplanted in 1st CR if an HLA-identical sibling is available (21).

Other indications for BMT emerge: Myelodysplastic syndromes (MDS), multiple myeloma, lymphomas, chronic lymphocytic leukemia. From currently available information it is clear that, as in acute leukemia and CML, prognosis is better if the transplant is performed early in the course of disease.

A broader application of allogeneic BMT is to be expected from the possibility of using donors other than HLA-identical siblings. One of the possible ways is to overcome the disadvantages of T-cell depletion by replacing the "healthy bone marrow effect" by addition of irradiated donor buffy coat cells to the T-cell depleted allogeneic bone marrow. Should the "bone marrow factor" turn out to be a soluble cell product, it might even be effective as an anjuvant of antileukemic chemotherapy.

REFERENCES

1. Bortin MM (1970) A compendium of the reported human bone marrow transplants. Transplantation 9: 571-580

2. Gatti RA, Meuwissen HJ, Allen HD, Hong RA (1968) Immunologic reconstitution of sex-linked lymphopenic immunologic deficiency. Lancet II: 1366-1369

3. Bach FH, Albertini RJ, Joo P, Anderson JL, Bortin MM (1968) Bone marrow transplantation in a patient with Wiskott-Aldrich syndrome. Lancet II: 1364-1366

4. De Koning J, Dooren LJ, van Bekkum DW, van Rood JJ (1969) Transplantation of bone marrow cells and foetal thymus in an infant with lymphopenic immunologic deficiency. Lancet I: 1223-1227

5. Speck B (1984) Bone marrow transplantation. Acta haemat 72: 145-154

6. Bortin MM (1986) Increasing utilisation of bone marrow transplantation. Transplantation 42: 229-234

7. Cornu P, Speck B, Groff P, Nissen C, Sartorius J, Burri HP, Ohnacker H (1978) Allogeneic BMT for acute leukemia. Pathol Biol 26: 49-50

8. Speck B, Gratwohl A, Osterwalder B, Signer E, Nissen C, Corneo M, Jeannet M (1983) Allogeneic bone marrow transplantation: The Basel trial with cyclosporine. Transplant Proc. 15: 2617-2619

9. Gratwohl A, Speck B (1986) Bone marrow transplantation with Ciclosporin. Prog. Allergy 38: 404-431

10. Häfliger B, Gratwohl A, Tichelli A, Würsch A, Speck B. High-dose Ara-C and VP16 prior to conditioning for bone marrow transplantation in patients with high-risk leukemia. Seminars in Oncology 1987 (in press)

11. Tichelli A, Walther E, Gratwohl A, Osterwalder B, Speck B (1987) Side effects of total body irradiation before bone marrow transplantation. Basel experience July 1979 to March 1986. Strahlentherapie + Onkologie 163: 245-246

12. De Witte T, Hoogenhout J, De Pauw B, Holdrinet R, Jansen J, Wessels J, van Daal W, Hustinx T, Haanen C (1986) Depletion of donor lymphocytes by counterflow centrifugation successfully prevents acute graft versus host disease in matched allogeneic Transplantation. Blood 67: 1302-1308

13. Gratwohl A, Baldomero H, Nissen C, Speck B. Engraftment of T-cell depleted rabbit bone marrow. Acta haemat. 1987 (in press)

14. Gratwohl A, Tichelli A, Würsch, Wenger R, Nissen C, De Witte T, Speck B (1987) Irradiated donor buffy coat cells for patients with T-cell depleted bone marrow. Bone Marrow Transplantation 2 (Suppl. 1): 157

15. Gratwohl A, Hermans J, Lyklema A, Zwaan FE (1987) Bone marrow transplantation for leukaemia in Europe. Report from the Leukaemia Working Party 1987. Bone Marrow Transplantation 2 (Suppl. 1): 15-18

16. Bortin MM, Gale RP (1986) Current status of allogeneic bone marrow transplantation. A report of the International Bone Marrow Transplant Registry. In: Teresaki P (ed.) Clinical Transplants, UCLA Los Angeles, pp 17-28

17. Butturini A, Bortin MM, Seeger RC, Gale RP. Graft-vs-leukemia following bone marrow transplantation: A model of immunotherapy in man (Submitted for publication)

18. Prentice HG: Oral communication at the Annual Meeting of the EBMT, March 1-4, 1987 (unpublished)

19. Gratwohl A, Zwaan FE, Hermans J, Lyklema A (1986) Bone marrow transplantation for leukemia in Europe. Bone Marrow Transplantation 1 (Suppl. 1): 177-181

20. Speck B, Bortin MM, Champlin R, Goldman JM, Herzig RH, McGlave PB, Messner HA, Weiner RS, Rimm AA (1984) Allogeneic bone marrow transplantation for chronic myelogenous leukaemia. Lancet I: 665-668

21. Herzig RM, Barrett AJ, Gluckman E, Jacobsen SJ, Masaoka R, Ramsay NKC, Ringden O, Zwaan FE, Bortin MM, Blume KG, Horowitz MM, Marmont M, Prentice HG, Rimm AA, Speck B, Gale RP (1987) Bone marrow transplantation in high-risk acute lymphoblastic leukemia in first an second remission. Lancet I: 786-789

VII. Acute Graft-versus-Host Disease: B. Speck and D.H. Pluznik, Chairpersons

21: Bone Marrow Transplantation: The Difficulties Ahead

Mortimer M. Bortin, Mary M. Horowitz, and Alfred A. Rimm

INTRODUCTION

Between 1951, the year Lorenz et al. [1] first reported rescue of mice and guinea pigs from lethal doses of total body irradiation (TBI) by bone marrow transplantation, and 1967, at least 200 allogeneic bone marrow transplants in humans were attempted; none was successful as measured by long-term disease-free survival [2]. Between 1968, when the first successful allogeneic bone marrow transplants were performed [3-5], and the mid-1970's, there was progressive improvement in results [6]. Much of the improvement was based on information gained from studies in animal models, selection of patients in earlier phases of disease, improved measures to prevent and treat infection, improved supportive care and, perhaps most important, expanded understanding of the fundamentals of immunogenetics and transplantation biology.

Scientists involved in allogeneic bone marrow transplantation are well aware of the major causes of treatment failure (Table 1). Many seem to believe that these problems, while persisting, have had a decreasing incidence since the mid-1970's, but have they? The incidence, case fatality and mortality rates associated with these complications during the past decade are presented in this paper. In addition, the incidences for the period 1978-1982 are compared with those for 1983-1987.

Table 1. Main causes of treatment failure following allogeneic bone marrow transplantation.

A. Acute graft-versus-host disease
B. Interstitial pneumonitis
C. Posttransplant infection
D. Recurrence of underlying disease

MATERIALS AND METHODS

Data submitted to the International Bone Marrow Transplant Registry by 145 transplant teams worldwide reporting on 5,945 patients were analyzed using univariate statistical methods. Included in the analyses were 993 consecutive patients with acute lymphoblastic leukemia (ALL), 1080 with acute myelogenous leukemia (AML), 798 with chronic myelogenous leukemia (CML) and 657 with severe aplastic anemia (SAA). All 3,528 of these patients received bone marrow from HLA-identical siblings between 1978 and 1987. Data for 2,417 patients with other diseases, donors other than HLA-identical siblings and whose transplants were performed prior to 1978 were excluded from analysis. Due to the highly significant association between disease status at the time of transplantation and relapse, leukemia patients were grouped by disease status for analyses of recurrent or persistent leukemia. Chi square analyses were used to test differences between incidences; P values < 0.01 were considered to be statistically significant. The reader should bear in mind that the results are based on pooled data from 145 teams. Individual teams may have had higher or lower rates.

RESULTS

Magnitude of the Problem

Data presented in Table 2 show the impact of each of the major complications of allogeneic bone marrow transplantation on outcome for the 10-year period 1978-1987.

Although the incidence of moderate to severe acute graft-versus-host disease (AGVHD) varies widely in selected subsets (e.g., high when no prophylaxis against AGVHD is used and low in patients receiving grafts depleted of T-cells), the overall incidence was 42% (Table 2). Thirty-four percent of the patients who developed moderate to severe AGVHD died with it as a primary or contributing cause. The mortality rate due to AGVHD was 14% among 3,301 patients at risk.

The overall incidence of interstitial pneumonitis (IPn) in this series was 24% with a mortality rate of 18% (Table 2). As indicated

Table 2. Overall incidence, case fatality rate and mortality rate (± 95% confidence interval) for the major causes of treatment failure following HLA-identical bone marrow transplantation for leukemia and severe aplastic anemia between 1978 and 1987.

Cause of Treatment Failure	N	Incidence(%)	Case Fatality Rate (%) [a]	Mortality Rate (%) [b]
A. Acute GVHD	3301 [c]	42(± 2)	34(± 2)	14(± 1)
B. Interstitial Pneumonitis	3484	24(± 1)	75(± 1)	18(± 1)
C. Posttransplant Infection	3484	69(± 2)	35(± 2)	24(± 1)
D. Recurrent Disease				
Severe Aplastic Anemia	625 [d]	11(± 2)	54(± 4)	6(± 2)
ALL 1st Remission	285	14(± 4)	64(± 6)	9(± 3)
ALL 2nd Remission	377	28(± 5)	79(± 4)	22(± 4)
ALL More Advanced	331	37(± 5)	89(± 3)	33(± 5)
AML 1st Remission	663	11(± 2)	86(± 3)	10(± 2)
AML 2nd Remission	161	22(± 7)	94(± 4)	20(± 6)
AML More Advanced	256	37(± 6)	86(± 4)	32(± 8)
CML Chronic Phase	471	8(± 2)	13(± 3)	1(± 1)
CML Accelerated Phase	256	21(± 5)	72(± 6)	16(± 5)
CML Blastic Phase	71	31(±11)	73(±11)	23(±10)

Footnotes on next page.

[a] Percent of patients developing the complication who died with it as a primary or contributory cause of death.

[b] Percent of transplanted patients who died with the complication as a primary or contributory cause of death.

[c] Number of patients at risk, i.e., patients surviving at least 21 days with engraftment.

[d] Number of patients at risk, i.e., patients surviving at least 21 days.

by the case fatality rate of 75%, IPn is usually fatal when it occurs.

Infections are common both early after bone marrow transplantation when immune defenses are not yet restored, and later on, often in association with the impaired immune competence that accompanies acute or chronic GVHD. Of the 3,484 patients in the study, 69% developed infections posttransplant of sufficient consequence to be reported, with a case-fatality rate of 35%. Infection is a common primary cause of death or terminal event, with a mortality rate of 24%.

There were 625 patients with SAA who survived at least 21 days and thus could be evaluated for evidence of engraftment; 557 of these had stable engraftment of donor marrow. Among the 68 patients whose graft failed or was rejected, the case fatality rate was 54% with a mortality rate of 6%. Once a graft has failed the likelihood of death was higher than 50%. The case fatality rate was less than 100%, however, because some patients achieved stable engraftment after a subsequent transplant, others had improvement in the disease with partial engraftment or mixed chimerism and others had autologous recovery of hematopoiesis.

Among patients with leukemia, the incidence of relapse and the mortality rate due to recurrent or persistent leukemia was lowest among patients with ALL or AML transplanted in first remission and among patients transplanted in the chronic phase of CML. The case fatality rate reflects the likelihood of death due to relapse among those who relapse and, with the exception of CML in the chronic phase, it was uniformly high. It was less than 100%, however, because some patients achieved remission after a second transplant or after treatment with chemotherapy, while others with recurrent disease were still alive at the time of their last follow-up report. With continued follow-up the incidence, case fatality and mortality rates due to relapse are expected to increase.

TEN-YEAR PROGRESS REPORT

There has been a highly significant ($P<0.0006$ - $P<0.0001$) decline in the incidence of AGVHD, IPn and posttransplant infections in the past five years in comparison with the previous five years (Figure 1).

The incidence of graft failure or rejection in severe aplastic anemia has decreased from 12% between 1978-1982 to 10% in the past five years; the difference is not statistically significant (Figure 2).

A comparison of the frequency of relapse following bone marrow transplantation for ALL in first remission, AML in first remission and CML in chronic phase between 1978 to 1982 and 1983 to 1987 is presented in Figure 3. It should be noted that essentially all patients receiving transplants for ALL in first remission were considered to be at high risk of relapse if treated with chemotherapy. The data show a consistent decrease in the incidence of relapse over time but in no instance is the decrease statistically significant.

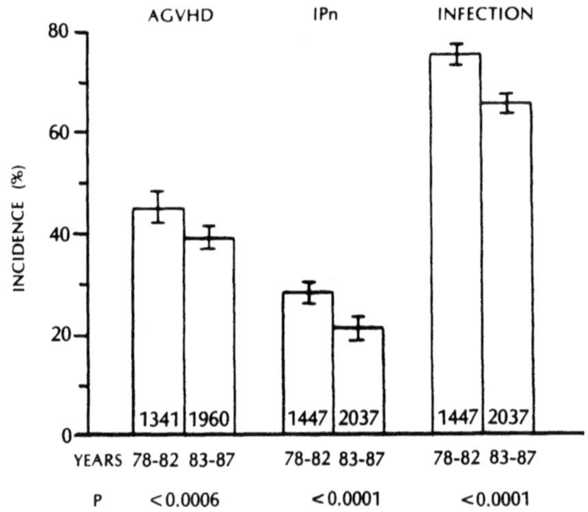

Figure 1. Incidence of acute graft-versus-host disease (in patients at risk), interstitial pneumonitis and posttransplant infections during the periods 1978 to 1982 and 1983 to 1987. Numbers within bars represent number of patients in the group. Vertical brackets are 95% confidence intervals.

Among patients transplanted for ALL and AML in second remission and CML in accelerated phase a consistent trend again was observed showing a decrease in the incidence of recurrent leukemia over the ten-year period 1978 to 1987 (Figure 4). Although the decreased incidence among patients transplanted in the accelerated phase of CML in the past five years is considerable (18% vs 29% in the previous five years), the difference is not statistically significant ($P<0.07$).

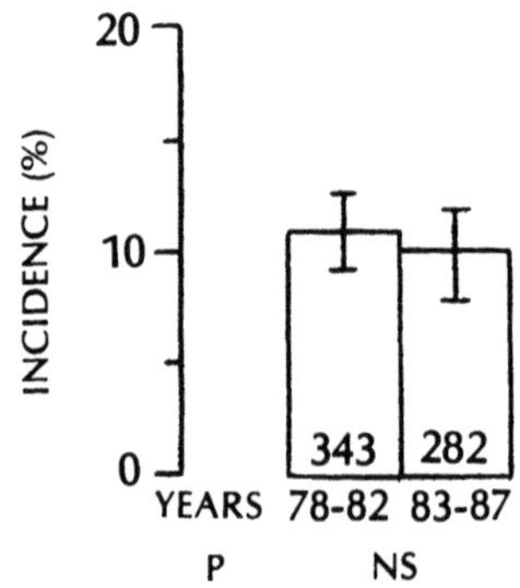

Figure 2. Incidence of graft failure/rejection during the periods 1978 to 1982 and 1983-1987. Numbers within bars represent number of patients at risk. Vertical brackets are 95% confidence intervals.

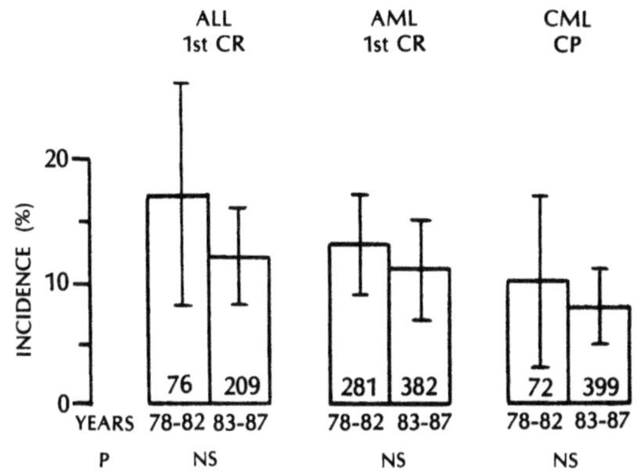

Figure 3. Incidence of relapse 1978-1982 and 1983-1987 following bone marrow transplantation for leukemia early in the course of the disease. Numbers within bars represent number of patients in the group. Vertical brackets are 95% confidence intervals.

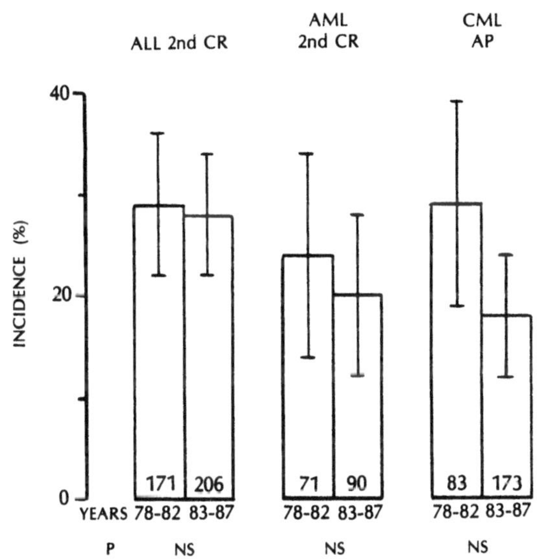

Figure 4. Incidence of relapse 1978-1982 and 1983-1987 following bone marrow transplantation for acute leukemia in second remission and CML in the accelerated phase. Numbers within bars represent number of patients in the group. Vertical brackets are 95% confidence intervals.

No improvement in the incidence of recurrent or persistent leukemia occurred during the period of study among patients whose disease was advanced at the time of bone marrow transplantation (Figure 5). During the past five years there has been a significant increase in the incidence of recurrent or persistent leukemia among patients with CML transplanted in the blastic (acute) phase ($P<0.006$); this finding should be interpreted with caution, however, because only 71 patients were available for study.

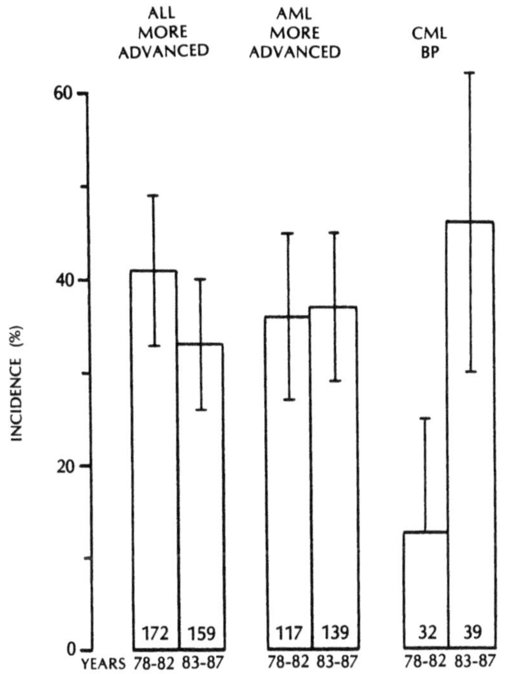

Figure 5. Incidence of recurrent or persistent leukemia 1978-1982 and 1983-1987 following bone marrow transplantation for patients with advanced disease. Numbers within bars represent number of patients in the group. Vertical brackets are 95% confidence intervals.

DISCUSSION

Preliminary analyses of data reported to the IBMTR confirm that AGVHD, IPn, infection and recurrent disease are the major problems encountered following allogeneic bone marrow transplantation. The incidence and adverse influence of these complications on survival are documented in Table 2. As shown in Figures 1-5, there has been both progress and lack of progress against these complications over the past decade. For example, in comparison with transplants performed between 1978 and 1982, there has been a recent and (statistically) highly significant decrease in the incidence of AGVHD, IPn and infection. Although these decreases are certainly a move in the right direction, by clinical standards the pace has been slow and the degree of improvement, modest.

The decreased incidence of AGVHD can be accounted for largely by a concomitant increase in the use of bone marrow treated ex vivo to decrease or eliminate donor T-lymphocytes. Numerous reports document that this approach is highly effective at reducing the risk and severity of AGVHD [7-11]. T-lymphocyte depletion is, however, a two edged sword because, as presently applied, it also is associated with an increased risk of recurrent leukemia and of graft failure/rejection in most series [12-17]. These decreased and increased risks tend to counterbalance one another and, as a consequence, there is no clear evidence that use of T-depleted marrow improves the probability of disease-free survival [13]. Challenge for the future: What can be done to further decrease the risk of AGVHD without introducing problems of comparable magnitude?

The IBMTR is currently investigating the reasons to account for the declining incidence of IPn, from 28% to 21%. The most likely explanations include an increased use of blood products from CMV seronegative donors and prophylactic use of CMV immune globulin [18,19], an increased use of T-depleted marrow with its attendant decrease in the incidence of AGVHD which predisposes to IPn [20,21], and increased use of cyclosporine as prophylaxis against AGVHD rather than methotrexate, the latter being associated with an increased risk of IPn [22,23]. Challenge for the future: What additional measures should be used to reduce the incidence and lethality of IPn?

The decreased incidence in posttransplant infections from 75% between 1978 and 1982 to 65% in the past five years is due in large measure to better patient selection, improved infectious disease surveillance, and prophylactic use of improved antimicrobial and antiviral agents as well as CMV immune globulin. Challenge for the future: Are there other steps that can be taken to cause a further reduction in the risk of life-threatening infections posttransplant?

Progress in the past decade against recurrent disease has been less impressive. Although the trends are mostly favorable, there have been no statistically significant reductions overall in the incidence of graft failure or rejection in SAA or in persistent disease or relapse in leukemia. Challenge for the future: What can be done to decrease the risk of recurrent disease?

Among other difficulties that lie ahead is the problem that most patients who might benefit from a bone marrow transplant lack an HLA-identical sibling. Early indications are that the risk and severity of several major complications of bone marrow transplantation are magnified when either related or unrelated, partially or fully matched donors are substituted for HLA-identical siblings. Challenge for the future: Can methods be found to circumvent the problems of histoincompatibility in bone marrow transplantation?

The questions posed above are truly difficult and no one knows the answer to any of them. The field of bone marrow transplantation, with its intellectual challenges and its promise to cure the incurable, has attracted and continues to attract brilliant scientists. With all that talent, the slowness of progress is eloquent evidence of the complexity and fundamental nature of the difficulties that lie ahead. Analyses are in progress at the IBMTR to identify approaches that have failed and those that have succeeded in efforts to reduce the risk of the causes of treatment failure. It is hoped that the results of these studies will help provide leads for future directions of research in bone marrow transplantation.

ACKNOWLEDGEMENTS

Support for this study was provided by grant CA 40053 from the National Cancer Institute, DHHS, contracts N01-AI-62530 from the National Institute of Allergy and Infectious Diseases, DHHS, B16-084-US from the Commission of European Communities and grants from the A.J. Bitker Memorial Foundation, Frank G. Brotz Family Foundation, Lester Glen Family Foundation, Hilda T. Harris, William Randolph Hearst Foundation, Heller Foundation, William L. Law Foundation, Ambrose Monell Foundation, Elsa U. Pardee Foundation, Procter and Gamble Co., RGK Foundation, Sandoz Research Institute, Joan and Jack Stein and the Swiss Cancer League.

This 51st report from the International Bone Marrow Transplant Registry was prepared for the Advisory Committee: R.P. Gale, Los Angeles (Chairman); F.H. Bach, Minneapolis; A.J. Barrett, London; D.W. van Bekkum, Rijswijk; J.C. Biggs, Sydney; K.G. Blume, Los Angeles; M.M. Bortin, Milwaukee; K.A. Dicke, Houston; E. Gluckman, Paris; J.M. Goldman, London; R.A. Good, St. Petersburg; R. Hong, Madison; R.H. Herzig, Cleveland; J.H. Kersey, Minneapolis; H.J. Kolb, Munich; A. M. Marmont, Genoa; T. Masaoka, Osaka; H.A. Messner, Toronto; R.J. O'Reilly, New York; R.L. Powles, London; A.A. Rimm, Milwaukee; O. Ringden, Huddinge; J.J. van Rood, C. Rozman, Barcelona; B. Speck, Basel; R.S. Weiner, Gainesville; and F.E. Zwaan, Leiden.

We thank Ms. D'Etta Koser and Ms. Sharon Gurgul for help with data analysis and Ms. Karen Witkowski for typing the manuscript.

The bone marrow transplant teams at the institutions listed below contributed the patient data used in this study.

Argentina: British Hospital of Buenos Aires, Buenos Aires. Australia: Institute of Medicine, Adelaide; Royal Prince Alfred Hospital, Camperdown; St. Vincent's Hospital, Darlinghurst; Royal Children's Hospital, Parkville; Royal Melbourne Hospital, Parkville; Royal Perth Hospital, Perth; Alfred Hospital, Prahran; Prince of Wales Children's Hospital, Randwick; Westmead Centre, Westmead; Queen Elizabeth Hospital, Woodville. Austria: Med. Univ.-Klinik, Vienna; Belgium: Cliniques Univ. Saint-Luc, Bruxelles; University of Leuven, Leuven. Brazil: Instituto Nacional de Cancer, Rio de Janeiro; Hospital de Clinicas, Curitiba. Canada: Tom Baker Cancer Centre, Calgary; McMaster University, Hamilton; Montreal Children's Hospital, Montreal; Princess Margaret Hospital, Toronto. China: Beijing Medical University, Beijing; Lanzhou General Hospital, Lanzhou. Denmark: Rigshospitalet, Copenhagen. England: Queen Elizabeth Medical Center, Birmingham; University Hospital of Wales,

Cardiff; St. James's University Hospital, Leeds; Charing Cross & Westminster Med. School, London; Institute of Child Health, London; The London Clinic, London; Royal Free Hospital, London; Royal Marsden Hospital, London; Royal Postgraduate Medical School, London; Westminster Children's Hospital, London; Royal Victoria Infirmary, Newcastle. Finland: University of Helsinki, Helsinki; Turku University, Turku. France: Angers University, Angers; Centre Regional de Transfusion Sanguine, Besancon; Hôpital des Sablons, Grenoble; Hôpital Debrousse, Lyon; Hôpital Eduoard Herriot, Lyon; Institut J. Paoli I. Calmettes, Marseille; Hôpital des Enfants Malades, Paris; Hôpital des Enfants Pediatrie, Paris; Hôpital Saint-Antoine, Paris; Hôpital Saint-Louis, Paris; Groupe Hôspitalier du Hau Leveque, Pessac; Hôpital Jean Bernard, Poiters; Hôpital Nord, St. Etienne; Hôpital Purpan, Toulouse; Groupe Hôpital Paul-Brousse, Villejuif. East Germany: Karl Marx Universitat, Leipzig. West Germany: Universitatsklinikum Charlottenburg, Berlin; Christian-Albrechts-Universitat, Kiel; der Universitats Kinderklinik, Munich; Universitat Muenchen, Munich; Med Universitatsklinik, Tubingen; Universitat Ulm, Ulm/Donau. Holland: Academisch Ziekenhuis, Leiden; University Hospital, Leiden; University of Nijmegen, Nijmegen; Rotterdam Radio-Therapeutic Institute, Rotterdam. Hungary: National Institute of Haematology, Budapest; Semmelweis University, Budapest. India: Tata Memorial Hospital, Bombay. Ireland: St. James's Hospital, Dublin. Israel: Hadassah University Hospital, Jerusalem. Italy: S. Orsola University Hospital, Bologna; Ospedale San Martino, Genoa; University of Milan, Milan; Ospedale Civile, Pesaro; Universita Chieti, Pescara; University degli Studi La Sapienza, Rome; University of Rome, Rome. Japan: Tokai University School of Medicine, Kanagawa; Kanazawa University School of Medicine, Kanazawa-shi; Nagoya Second Red Cross Hospital, Nagoya; Center For Adult Diseases, Osaka; Jichi Medical School, Tochigi-ken; University of Tokyo, Tokyo. Korea: St. Mary's Hospital, Seoul. New Zealand: Christchurch Hospital, Christchurch. Norway: Rikshospitalet, Oslo. Poland: Postgraduate Medical Center, Warsaw. Saudi Arabia: King Faisal Specialist Hospital, Riyadh. Scotland: Royal Infirmary of Edinburgh, Edinburgh; Glasgow Royal Infirmary, Glasgow. South Africa: University of Cape Town Medical School, Cape Town. Spain: Hospital Infantil Vall d'Hebron, Barcelona; University of Barcelona, Barcelona; Hospital "Reina Sofia", Cordoba; Clinica Puerta de Hierro, Madrid; Hospital de la Princesa, Madrid; Hospital "M. De Valdecilla", Santander; Hospital "La Fe", Valencia. Sweden: Huddinge Hospital, Huddinge; University of Lund, Lund; Kantonsspital, Basel; Kantonsspital, Zurich; Kinderspital, Zurich. Taiwan: National Taiwan University Hospital, Taipei; Taoyuan General Hospital, Taoyuan. United States: Emory University, Atlanta; Alta Bates Hospital, Berkeley; NIAID, Bethesda; Roswell Park Memorial Institute, Buffalo; Rush-Presbyterian-St. Lukes, Chicago; University of Chicago Hospital, Chicago; Children's Hospital, Cincinnati; University of Cincinnati Medical Center, Cincinnati; Case Western Reserve University, Cleveland; Cleveland Clinic, Cleveland; University of Colorado Health Science Center, Denver; City of Hope, Duarte; Duke University Medical Center, Durham; University of Florida, Gainesville; Baylor College of Medicine, Houston; Children's Hospital, Houston; M.D. Anderson Hospital, Houston; University of Kansas, Kansas City; Wilford Hall Medical Center, Lackland AFB; University of Kentucky, Lexington; Arkansas Children's Hospital, Little Rock; University of California/Medicine, Los Angeles; University of California/Pediatrics, Los Angeles; University of Wisconsin/Medicine, Madison; University of Wisconsin/Pediatrics, Madison; Marshfield Clinic, Marshfield; Loyola University, Maywood; Medical College of Wisconsin, Milwaukee; University of Minnesota, Minneapolis; Memorial Sloan-Kettering, New York City; The Mount Sinai Hospital, New York City; Children's Hospital Medical Center, Oakland; University of Oklahoma, Oklahoma City; Bishop Clarkson Memorial Hospital, Omaha; University of Nebraska, Omaha; Children's Hospital, Philadelphia; Hahnemann University, Philadelphia; Oregon Health Sciences University, Portland; Latter Day Saints Hospital, Salt Lake City; Pacific Medical Center, San Francisco; University of California, San Francisco; All Children's Hospital, St. Petersburg. Yugoslavia: Klinika za Unutrasnje bolesti KBC-Rebro, Zagreb.

REFERENCES

1. Lorenz E, Uphoff D, Reid TR, et al. (1951) Modification of irradiation injury in mice and guinea pigs by bone marrow injections. J Natl Cancer Inst 12:197-201.

2. Bortin MM (1970) A compendium of reported human bone marrow transplants. Transplantation 9:571-587.

3. Bach FH, Albertini RJ, Joo P, et al. (1968) Bone marrow transplantation in a patient with Wiskott-Aldrich syndrome. Lancet 2:1364-66.

4. Gatti RA, Allen HD, Meuwissen HJ, et al. (1968) Immunological reconstitution of sex-linked lymphopenic immunological deficiency. Lancet 2:1366-69.

5. deKoning J, Dooren LJ, van Bekkum DW, et al. (1969) Transplantation of bone-marrow cells and fetal thymus in an infant with lymphopenic immunological deficiency. Lancet 1:1223-27.

6. Thomas ED Storb R, Clift RA, et al. (1975) Bone marrow transplantation. N Engl J Med 282:832-43, 895-902.

7. Reisner Y, Kapoor N, Kirkpatrick D, et al. (1981) Transplantation for acute leukemia with HLA-A and B nonidentical parental marrow cells fractionated with soybean agglutinin and sheep red blood cells. Lancet 2:327.

8. Prentice HG, Blacklock HA, Janossy G, et al. (1984) Depletion of T lymphocytes in donor marrow prevents significant graft verus host disease in matched allogeneic leukemia marrow transplant recipients. Lancet 1:472.

9. Waldmann H, Or R, Hale G, et al. (1984) Elimination of graft versus host disease by in vitro depletion of alloreactive lymphocytes using a monoclonal rat anti-human lymphocyte antibody (CAMPATH-1). Lancet 2:483.

10. Lowenberg B, Wagemaker G, van Bekkum DW, et al. (1986) Graft-versus-host disease following transplantation of 'one log' versus 'two log' T-lymphocyte-depleted bone marrow from HLA-identical donors. Bone Marrow Transplantation 1:133-40.

11. Hale G, Waldmann H (1986) Depletion of T-cells with Campath-1 and human complement. Analysis of GvHD and graft failure in a multi-centre study. Bone Marrow Transplantation 1(Suppl 1):93.

12. De Witte T, Janssen J, Drenthe-Schonk A, et al. (1986) A high incidence of autologous repopulation after allogeneic bone marrow transplantation using lymphocyte depleted donor marrow. Exp Hematol 14:448, (Abstract).

13. Gale RP (1987) T cells, bone marrow transplantation, and immunotherapy: use of monoclonal antibodies. In: Immune interventions in disease. Fahey JL (moderator). Ann Intern Med 106:257-74.

14. Apperley JF, Jones L, Hale G, et al (1986) Bone marrow transplantation for chronic myeloid leukaemia: T-cell depletion reduces the risk of graft-versus-host disease but may increase the risk of leukaemic relapse. Bone Marrow Transplantation 1:53-66.

15. Pollard CM, Powles RL, Millar JL, et al (1986) Leukaemic relapse following Campath 1 treated bone marrow transplantation for leukaemia. Lancet 2:1343-44.

16. Trigg ME, Billing R, Sondel PM, et al (1985) Clinical trial depleting T lymphocytes from donor marrow for matched and mismatched allogeneic bone marrow transplants. Cancer Treat Rep 69:377-86.

17. Goldman JM, Gale RP, Bortin MM, et al (1987) Bone marrow transplantation for CML in chronic phase: Increased risk of relapse associated with T-cell depletion. Submitted.

22: Predictive Models of Graft versus Host Disease

G.B. Vogelsang, A.D. Hess, M. Silanskis, K. Friedman, E. Farmer, and G.W. Santos

Graft-versus-host disease (GVHD) remains a major cause of mortality and morbidity following allogeneic bone marrow transplant (BMT) despite major histocompatibility complex (MHC) identity of both the donor and recipient. One of the difficulties in studying GVHD in this setting has been the lack of an in vitro model capable of detecting reactivity to minor histocompatibility antigens. Furthermore, many factors may contribute to GVHD in the intact animal including toxicity from the preparative regimen, infection, and the effects of the immunosuppressive therapy given.

We have previously reported on our initial experience with a skin explant model in GVHD (1,2) Briefly, the model utilizes sensitized lymphocytes co-cultured with recipient skin and changes of GVHD are seen histologically in positive explants. We have also adapted this model to use in animal systems. We wish to report on our experiences using this model to probe the immunobiology of graft-versus-host disease.

MATERIALS AND METHODS

Informed Consent. All protocols were reviewed and approved by the Johns Hopkins University Institutional Review Board.

Patient Selection. Seventy patients undergoing BMT for acute lymphocytic leukemias, acute myelogenous leukemia, chronic myelogenous leukemia, lymphoma, or aplastic anemia and their normal genotypic HLA-identical donors were included in the study. In general, patients with acute lymphocytic leukemia, chronic myelogenous leu-kemia and lymphoma received cyclophosphamide 50 mg/kg for 4 days followed by total body irradiation 300 rads per day for 4 days. Patients with acute myelogenous leukemia received busulfan 4 mg/kg for 4 days and cyclophosphamide 50 mg/kg for 4 days. Patients with aplastic anemia received cyclophosphamide plus total body irradiation or plus cyclosporine depending on the date of the transplant. Nineteen patients received cyclophosphamide plus methylprednisolone, 9 received cyclosporine plus methylprednisolone and the remainder received cyclosporine as GVHD prophylaxis. The patients ranged in age from 7 to 50 years, reflective of the patients receiving BMT except for the exclusion of patients and donors under 7 years of age.

Lymphocyte Isolation. Human peripheral blood lymphocytes were obtained from patients and donors by Ficoll-hypaque (Pharmacia Piscataway, NJ) density centrifugation. The mononuclear cells at the interface were removed, washed 3 times and then resuspended at a concentration of 2 x 10^6 cells per ml in complete media which contained RPMI 1640, 20% heat inactivated, pooled normal serum supplemented with 1% l-glutamine, penicillin (100 units/ml), and streptomycin (100 ug/ml).

Mixed Lymphocyte Cultures. Bulk mixed lymphocyte cultures were established using 6 x 106 responding cells co-cultured with the same number of irradiated (1500 rads) stimulating cells with 6 mls of complete media in 30 ml culture flasks (Tissue culture flasks, Corning glass works, Corning, NY) at 37o. Cells were incubated for 7 days.

Skin Explants. Bulk lymphocyte cultures were harvested at 7 days. The cells were harvested, washed, and resuspended in fresh complete media. The cells were then placed in round bottom microtiter plates (LINBRO

Chemical Co., New Haven, Conn.) at a con-centration of .8 x 10 cells. A 4 mm punch biopsy was obtained in a sterile manner from the donor and recipient. One half ml sections of skin from the donor or recipient were placed in co-culture with the cells. After 3 days, the explants were removed and placed in 10% buffered formalin. After sectioning and staining with hematoxylin and eosin, the histopathology was evaluated by a dermatopathologist in a blinded fashion. GVHD was rated in a standard fashion: grade O-normal skin, grade 1 vacuolization of the basil layer, grade 2 dyskeratosis, grade 3-subepidermal cleft formation, grade 4 complete epidermal separation. Only grade 2 or greater histologic GVHD was considered positive. All explants were done in duplicate. All experiments were performed in two to three positive donor-recipient pairs.

Separation of Lymphocyte Population of a Fluorescein Activated Cell Sorter (FACS). The cells were pelleted by centrifugation at 500 g for 20 minutes and then incubated for 1 hour at 4o in the presence of 150 ng anti Leu-1, anti Leu-2, anti Leu-3, and anti Leu-5 monoclonal antibodies (Becton Dickenson, Mountain Grove, CA). Control samples were incubated with PBS. The cells were then subjected to analysis and sorting.

Drugs. Cyclosporine (generous gift of Sandoz Ltd., Basel) was dissolved in 95% ethanol and diluted to the specified concentration in PBS with .05% Tween 80. Recombinant Interleukin-2 (RIL2-Cetus Coup., Emeryville, CA) was diluted in sterile water to the specified concentration. Gamma Interferon (Biogen Corp., Cambridge, MA) was also diluted in sterile water.

RESULTS

Predictive Model. To date 70 HLA identical patient donor pairs have been tested using the skin explant model. Of 35 patients predicted by this model to develop GVHD 32 have developed at least grade II histologic GVHD and a skin rash involving 25-50% of their body. Of the 35 patients with negative explants, 30 have had no GVHD.

T Cell Enrichment. Explants were performed with cells sorted for pan T, helper, and suppressor cytotoxic subsets at the time of initiation of bulk cultures and at the time of co-culture with skin. As shown in Table 1, when cells were sorted prior to initiation of bulk cultures there was little effect of enriching for each of these cell population. However, when the cells were sorted after sensitization, more severe changes of GVHD were seen in the cytotoxic suppressor cell subsets. GVHD however, was found in skin co-cultured with the helper subset, although much less severe.

Gamma Interferon. Gamma interferon at a concentration of 50 units/ml was added both to the bulk MLC and to the explant, as shown in Table 2. Addition of gamma interferon to the cells during sensitization had no effect on eventual grade of GVHD. Addition of gamma interferon to the actual explant resulted in more severe GVHD.

IL-2. Addition of RIL-2 at a concentration of 50 units/ml to the bulk MLR but not to the sensitized cells at the time of skin addition resulted in more severe GVHD, as shown in Table 2. There was no effect of the R-IL2 on autologous controls.

Cyclosporine. Cyclosporine at 5 X 10-6 M/ml was added to cultures again at the initiation of bulk MLC and at the time the addition of the sensitized cells to the skin, as shown in Table 2. Addition to cyclosporine to the bulk MLC resulted in ablation or marked reduction of the severity of GVHD seen. Addition of cyclosporine once sensitization had occurred was ineffective in changing the degree of GVHD seen in explants.

DISCUSSION

The present study provides both an update on the skin explant model for predicting GVHD and information on the use of the model as a probe to study GVHD. Our initial report of the skin explant model for predicting GVHD in patients undergoing genotypic HLA identical marrow transplant included 32 patients (2). At that time of the 18 recipient donors that were positive 16 patients were found to have histologic grade 2 or higher graft-versus-host disease of the skin on biopsy and only 3 of the 14 negative pairs developed GVHD. Now, 70 HLA matched recipient donor pairs have been studied perspectively. Explants were set up pretransplant and all received post transplant GVHD prophylaxis. Patients were followed post transplant without knowledge of explant results. Of the 35 patients with positive explants, 32 have developed at least grade 2 histologic GVHD and a rash involving greater than 25% of their bodies. Of the 35 patients with negative explants 30 have had no GVHD. Of those patients with negative explants who developed GVHD, 3 had very mild cutaneous only GVHD and 2 had systemic GVHD of late onset. Thus the model has continued to highly predictive. Currently we are beginning a protocol to use the explant to decide post-transplant GVHD prophylaxis. Patients with negative explants will receive no therapy to see if indeed these patients will not develop GVHD. Should less than 15% of the patients so identified develop GVHD, this technique will be used to select only high risk patients for GVHD prophylaxis studies.

There have been logistic problems with using the explant model for the study of the immunobiology of GVHD. Since half of the explants are negative, evaluation of manipulation performed in the explants were limited to positive explant. Thus, half of the experiments performed were uninterpretable because the unmanipulated explant was negative. To maximize each human HLA matched explant, the model was adapted to an animal system so that initial experiments could be conducted in the animal model and verified in the human system: Thus, all experiments were first performed in a rat major mismatched combination, a rat minor mismatch combination, and finally in the human HLA identical situation. There have been no disagreements between the rat and human data.

Explants performed using major mismatch combinations in the rat and human always showed more intense changes of GVHD. Matched human explants and minor antigen rat mismatched explants showed less intense reaction of GVHD and were mild to moderate grade 2.

When lymphocytes were sorted into pan T, helper T, and suppressor/ cytotoxic T cell subsets prior to initiation of bulk cultures, all subsets of T cells cause GVHD and of approximately equal intensity. However, when the cells were sorted after sensitization, more severe GVHD was seen and the explant cultured with the cytotoxic/suppressor subset. This difference and intensity may be because the separation process allowed the 10-20% contaminating lymphocytes to regrow so the purity of the cell population at the end of sensitization was decreased. This could be checked by restaining the cells prior to coculture with the end organ. An alternative hypothesis is that many cell populations are necessary for sensitization of the cells needed to generate a cytotoxic effector. Once this effector cell is generated, these other cell populations become relatively less important. Enriching for the effector cells results in more significant GVHD reaction. This hypothesis is currently being tested by adding blocking antibodies at various time points to the culture.

Different immune modulators were added to the explants. Both IL-2 and gamma interferon increased the degree of GVHD seen and cyclosporine was capable of ablating this reaction without effecting the autologous controls for any of the three agents. However, the timing of the addition of these agents was very important. Both IL-2 and cyclosporine had to be added the initiation of bulk cultures to enhance GVHD. Thus, both of these agents seem to be affecting the generation of the effector cell. These results in the case of cyclosporine have been demonstrated in other systems where it can be shown that once a effector cell has been generated, increasing doses of cyclosporine are necessary to down regulate the cell (3). This model may then also be useful in looking at cyclosporine sensitivity by adding different concentrations in the cultures. Gamma interferon was only effective when added directly to the cells and tissue. This suggests that the gamma interferon was either working on the target organ or the sensitized effector cell. It has been suggested that Gamma interferon increases Ia expression in skin thus strongly supporting the notion that the target is being effected in this particular case. Other evaluation of this hypothesis can be tested by addition again of blocking antibodies. Current experiments in the lab are directed at growing out epidermal cells to also examine what is the target of GVHD.

Thus, this model of GVHD has both been proven to be accurate and predictive for GVHD as shown by the continued success in the 70 patients tested and to be a useful tool to study the immunobiology of GVHD. The two other models reported in the literature for predicting GVHD lack this adaptability to a workable model situation. Delmonte et al. (4) described a complex system which probably detected minor histocompatibility antigen differences. The test is based on generating inhibitory activity against the growth of colony-forming units in culture by initially culturing radioresistant non-T cells derived from the marrow of HLA-identical pairs. Among 20 patients, this model correctly predicted the presence of absence of GVHD in 18. This model has a great deal of research interest (i.e. mechanism of action of this effect), but the technical difficulty of the assay, the length of the assay, and the need for donor and recipient marrow make this test impractical. Bageet et al. (5) used epidermal cell lymphocyte reaction between donor lymphocytes and host epidermal cells isolated from suction blisters to predict GVHD. In 30 patient-donor pairs, 21 pairs showed reactivity in the epidermal cell-lymphocyte cultures. In the patients developing GVHD, the ratio of the mixed-epidermal-lymphocyte cell reactions counts per minute to the mixed lymphocyte reaction was greater (mean 4.12 + 2.84) than in patients without GVHD (mean 1.27 + 1.16). These models, although very intriguing, do not incorporate the end organ and are based on statistical associations for predicting GVHD. Thus, we believe the skin explant model shows the most promise of the three for continued work and development for understanding graft-versus-host disease.

REFERENCES

1. Berkman A, Farmer E, Tutschka P, Hess A, and Santos G. (1982) Skin explant culture as a model for cutaneous graft-versus-host disease. Exp Hematol 10:33-40.

2. Vogelsang GB, Hess AD, Berkman A, Tutschka PJ, Farmer E, Converse P, and Santos, GW. (1985) An in vitro predictive test for graft-versus-host disease in patients with genotypic HLA-identical bone marrow transplants. N Engl J Med 313:645-650.

3. Hess AD, Colombani PM, Esa AH (1986) Cyclosporine and the immune response: Basic aspects. CRC Critical Reviews in Immunology 6:123-149.

4. Delmonte L, O'Reilly RJ, Kirkpatrick D, Kapoor N (1982) In vitro model for detection of alloreactivity between HLA-matched donor-host pairs. Transplantation 34:100-103.

5. Bagot M, Cordonnier C, Tilkin AF, Heslan M, Vernan TP, Dubertret L, Levy JP (1986) A possible predictive test for graft-versus-host disease in bone marrow graft recipients: The mixed epidermal cell-lymphocyte reaction. Transplantation 41:316-319.

Table 1: Effect of different T cell populations on GVHD in the skin explant model

Effector cell subset	Grade GVHD Sorted prior to Sensitization	Grade GVHD Sorted after Sensitization
Unsorted	2	2
Pan T cell	2	3
Helper T cell	2	2
Suppressor T cell	2	4

Table 2: Effect of different immunomodulator on grade of GVHD seen in explant

Mediator	Grade GVHD Added to MLC*	Grade GVHD Added to co-culture
gamma interferon	2	3
RIL2	4	2
CsA	0	2

* MLC represents mixed lymphocyte culture.

23: Prevention of Severe GVHD Employing Cyclosporine in HLA-Matched Marrow Transplant for Leukemia

Peter J. Tutschka and Edward A. Copelan

INTRODUCTION

The success of clinical allogeneic bone marrow transplantation (BMT) is often compromised by the development of acute graft-versus-host disease (GVHD), considered by many to be the central problem of allogeneic marrow grafting. In an attempt to prevent this serious complication, two approaches are presently being used. One involves the elimination of immunocompetent lymphocytes from the donor marrow inoculum by purging with various physico-chemical or immunological methods, the other utilizes post transplant immunosuppression in an attempt to tolerize the graft against the host. Although to some extent effective, both approaches are associated with considerable problems. Ex vivo depletion of T-lymphocytes from the donor marrow inoculum has been associated with a high degree of non-engraftment. Furthermore, successful purging is thought to possibly result in decreased immunocompetence of the resulting graft either due to a delayed recovery of the immune system or due to the lack of adoptively transferred immunity. Lastly, in several studies an almost prohibitively high rate of relapse of the underlying hematologic malignancy has been reported (1).

Post transplant immunosuppression with cytotoxic agents such as cyclophosphamide (CY) or methotrexate (MTX), although effective, is associated with a relatively high incidence of acute and chronic GVHD and, furthermore, might be responsible for the relatively long delay in bone marrow recovery after marrow transplantation. The introduction of cyclosporine A (CsA), an immunosuppressive but not cytotoxic drug, seemed to overcome that problem, and several uncontrolled studies indicated a possible advantage over conventional GVHD prophylaxis with cytotoxic agents (2,3,4). This observation, however, could not be verified in controlled trials where CsA did not appear to be more effective than MTX (5,6).

In a previous trial we investigated the combination of CsA and methylprednisolone (MP) for GVHD prevention, a regimen that was compared in a randomized double-blind study to a combination of CY and MP (7). Although this combination regimen appeared to be more effective than CsA alone, when compared to historical controls and also appeared to be more effective than a combination of CY and MP, incidence and severity of GVHD were still relatively high. Therefore, we developed a modified regimen that again combined CsA and MP. We report here the results of a pilot study of 50 consecutive adult patients transplanted for leukemia who were treated with CsA and MP as prophylaxis of GVHD.

METHODS

Protocols

All protocols were reviewed and approved by The Ohio State University Institutional Review Board. Informed consent was obtained from each patient or, in the case of minors, from their parent or guardian.

Patient Population

A total of 50 adult patients were consecutively entered into the study. All patients transplanted carried the diagnosis of acute lymphocytic, acute non-lymphocytic or chronic myelogenous leukemia regardless of the remission status. All patients were ambulatory, had an HLA identical sibling donor and were more than 15 and $\leq$ than 50 years of age with a median age of 28 years. All data are analyzed as of February 14, 1987. The patients were transplanted between February 13, 1984 and August 14, 1986. The patients were divided into two groups. A standard risk group consisted of patients with acute leukemia in the first or second remission or chronic myelogenous leukemia in the chronic phase. Twenty patients, 11 with acute non-lymphocytic leukemia in remission, 2 with acute lymphocytic leukemia in remission and 7 with chronic myelogenous leukemia in chronic phase were in this group. The high risk group consisted of 30 patients with refractory acute leukemia, acute leukemia in relapse or chronic myelogenous leukemia in accelerated or blastic phase. In this high risk group were 12 patients with acute non-lymphocytic leukemia, 4 with acute lymphocytic leukemia and 14 patients with chronic myelogenous leukemia in accelerated (n=9) or blastic phase (n=5) of the disease. Thirty-four patients were sex matched with their recipients and 16 patients were sex mismatched. All patients were identical for the A, B, C, D/Dr loci with the allogeneic sibling donors. Where possible genotypical analysis of the entire family was performed. In 7 patients there were major blood group mismatches with their donors.

Bone Marrow Donors

All donors were required to give informed consent prior to the procedure which was carried out under general anesthesia. All donors tolerated the marrow aspiration well. A mean number of $5.7 \times 10^8 \pm 0.25$ ($\pm$ 1 SE) nucleated cells per kilogram body weight of the recipient was infused into the patients.

Preparative Regimen

All patients were given methotrexate intrathecally (10 mg/m_2 of body surface) 10 days prior to marrow transplantation. All patients regardless of their diagnosis received a combination of busulfan (BU) and CY. BU was given orally at a dose of 1 mg/kg of ideal body weight 4 times daily for 4 consecutive days to a total dose of 16 mg/kg. CY was given at a daily dose of 60 mg/kg of ideal body weight and was administered intravenously over a one hour period for 2 consecutive days. Bone marrow was infused 2 days after the final dose of CY.

Supportive Care

All patients were placed in ultraclean rooms on the day of hospitalization and treated in strict isolation. "Sterile diet" with very low bacterial content was begun on day -4 together with oral clotrimazole and oral trimethoprim-sulfamethoxazole. The patients were given intravenously a commerically available immunoglobulin preparation at a dose of 500 mg/kg every 2 weeks for 4 months after transplantation. Furthermore, the same immunoglobulin preparation was given orally at a dose of 50 mg/kg daily during the first 4 weeks after transplantation. During the first 30 days after transplantation, a median of 5 units of packed red blood cells and 5 single donor platelet concentrates were transfused.

Post Transplant Immunosuppression

All patients received a combination of CsA and MP to prevent GVHD. CsA therapy was initiated one day prior to transplantation and was administered as a continuous infusion of 5 mg/kg daily for 4 days. After that time, the dose of CsA was reduced to 3 mg/kg given intravenously over 6 hours daily until day 14. This dose reduction was done to decrease the possibility of nephrotoxicity during the time of aplasia when nephrotoxic antibiotics such as aminoglycosides might become necessary. From day 14 through day 35, during the time when the possibility of developing acute GVHD was highest, the dose of CsA was increased to 3.75 mg/kg given intravenously over 6 hours. Thereafter, CsA was slowly tapered until day 180, after which time CsA was discontinued. MP was started on day 7 at a dose of 0.5 mg/kg per day given in 2 daily doses of 0.25 mg/kg. On day 14, during the time of risk for acute GVHD the dose was increased to 1 mg/kg per day given until day 28. From there on until day 72 the MP was slowly tapered. Table 1 displays the details of this immunosuppressive regimen. Dose reductions of CsA were made when the serum creatinine reached 2.2 mg/dl. At this point CsA was reduced to the next lower level (from 5 to 3.75, from 3.75 to 3, from 3 to 2 mg/kg, respectively). If the creatinine exceeded 4 mg/dl, the CsA was held until the creatinine level returned to less than 4 mg/dl.

Table 1
Schema of Post-Transplant Immunosuppression

Day after Transplant	CsA Dose	MP Dose
0	5 mg/kg iv	0.25 mg/kg bid iv
4	3 mg/kg iv	
7		0.25 mg/kg bid iv
15	3.75 mg/kg iv	0.50 mg/kg bid iv
29		0.40 mg/kg bid iv
36	5 mg/kg bid po	
43		0.25 mg/kg bid iv
57		0.10 mg/kg bid iv
64		0.10 mg/kg bid iv qod
72		DC drug
84	4 mg/kg bid po	
98	3 mg/kg bid po	
120-180	2 mg/kg bid po	

Evaluation Criteria

Engraftment was documented indirectly by peripheral blood counts and periodic marrow examinations. Where available engraftment was measured directly by cytogenetic markers, red cell enzymes and red cell antigens. Engraftment was assumed when peripheral white count exceeded 1.0×10^9 per liter together with a platelet count of $>40 \times 10^9$ per liter and a reticulocyte count of >1%.

Graft-versus-Host Disease

Incidence and severity of GVHD were recorded using criteria previously described in the literature (8). Chronic GVHD was assessed using descriptive criteria reported in the literature (9). Patients were considered to have developed chronic GVHD if they had either the typical features of the disease and/or were given adrenal steroids after day 100. To judge the severity of GVHD we used the following grades. Grade 1 disease consisted of mild symptoms that resolved within 2 months, grade 2 disease consisted of mild symptoms that required 2 to 6 months for resolution without sequelae, and grade 3 disease consisted of marked symptoms that required more than 6 months of therapy.

Remission Status

Patients were considered to be in complete remission after transplantation for acute leukemia if they showed a completely normal bone marrow and peripheral blood status together with the absence of lymphohematopoietic cells of recipient origin by cytogenetic analysis. Patients were considered to be in complete remission after transplantation for chronic myelogenous leukemia if they showed a completely normal bone marrow and peripheral blood picture together with the absence of lymphohematopoietic cells of recipient origin by cytogenetic analysis. Patients who showed the presence of the Philadelphia chromosome prior to transplantation required the complete and persistent disappearance of this cytogenetic abnormality. Relapse was defined as reappearance of the Philadelphia chromosome or reappearance of an abnormal, leukemic picture in the bone marrow.

Interstitial Pneumonia

Interstitial pneumonia was diagnosed by characteristic bilateral infiltrates on chest x-ray with a concominant fall in arterial PO_2 and histologic verification where clinically possible.

Toxic Side Effects of CsA

Renal failure was defined as elevated creatinine serum levels greater than 2.5 mg/dl sustained over more than 7 days. Hyperkalemia was defined as showing a serum potassium of $\geq$ 5.4 m Eq/l on three occasions. Hypertension was defined as high blood pressure that required antihypertensive medications for $\geq$ 7 consecutive days.

Statistical Analysis

Estimates of survival probabilities and the probability of being in remission were computed by using the product-limit estimates of Kaplan and Meier (10).

RESULTS

Of the 50 patients entered into the study, 2 could not be evaluated for engraftment. One patient died on day +2 from cardiac failure, the other patient showed a recovery marrow on day +14 but never reached a white blood count that exceeded 1.0×10^9/liter or a platelet count of 14×10^9/liter prior to his death. The remaining 48 patients all showed complete and sustained engraftment with only donor cells being found at $\geq$ 100 days post transplantation by cytogenetic analysis. The patients reached a white blood count above 1.0×10^9/liter at a median of 15 days (range 11 through 36) and a self-sustaining platelet count of 40×10^9/liter at 19 days (range 11 through 38) after transplantation.

Infectious complications during the first 30 days after transplantation

Eleven high risk and 8 standard risk patients (38%) did not develop a temperature of >100.5°F in the first 30 days and required no therapeutic antibiotics. Only 1 patient was given amphotericin B for a suspected fungal infection. One patient was documented to have bacteremia with pseudomonas aeruginosa, probably derived from a cutaneous pseudomonas abscess that antedated the transplant procedure. Two patients developed stomatitis herpes simplex virus and 3 patients developed candida esophagitis documented from endoscopy. All of these infectious complications responded promptly to the institution of appropriate antibiotics. The median day of discharge of all patients from the inpatient bone marrow transplant unit was 22 days (range 18 through 71).

Interstitial pneumonia

Interstitial pneumonia occurred in 6 patients, 4 of whom died with the disease. In 2 patients the histology of interstitial pneumonia could not be established. In 2 patients cytomegalovirus could be identified and in 1 patient each the pneumonia was associated with legionella and pneumocystis carnii.

Graft-versus-host disease (GVHD)

Acute GVHD of grade I manifested as a skin rash of less than 25% body surface distribution, was seen in 11 patients. Four patients showed clinically significant GVHD, 1 displaying grade II disease, 2 showing grade III disease and 1 showing grade IV disease. All 3 patients with severe GVHD grades III and IV died in part from the GVHD. Forty-five patients survived for more than 100 days after transplantation. Therefore, the incidence of clinically significant GVHD of grades II through IV has only been 8.8%.

Chronic GVHD of grade I was seen in 5 patients, of grade II was seen in 15 patients and chronic GHVD of grade III was seen in 5 patients. Chronic GVHD resolved with no sequela in all but 2 patients, but was associated with death in 2 patients with grade III disease. Of the 45 patients surviving more than 100 days, 19 or 42% have shown clinically significant chronic GVHD of grade II or greater any time during their transplant.

MAJOR SIDE EFFECTS OF THE GVHD PREVENTION REGIMEN

Renal failure

Renal function abnormalities, in particular elevations of the serum creatinine level, were frequently observed. Serum creatinine levels $\geq$ 2 were observed in 25 patients, levels of $\geq$ 3 in 8 patients and $\geq$ 4 mg/dl in 4 patients. Renal failure, defined by elevated creatinine serum levels $\geq$ 2.5 sustained over more than 7 days was seen in 6 patients. Four of these patients had persistent renal failure until the time of their death, while 2 of the 6 patients recovered. The 4 patients that died in renal failure had additional major organ system complications such as interstitial pneumonia and severe graft-versus-host disease.

Hyperkalemia

Hyperkalemia defined as a serum potassium concentration of ≥ 5.4 mEq/liter on three occasions was seen in 16 patients. In none of these patients did hyperkalemia result in clinical problems, but often required the application of ion exchange resins. With the decrease of Cyclosporine as prescribed by the protocol, the hyperkalemia resolved in all instances.

Hypertension

Hypertension defined as requiring anti-hypertensive therapy for more than 7 consecutive days was seen in 20 patients. This hypertension was clearly dependent on the dose of Cyclosporine and with the reduction of the dose of Cyclosporine over time, as prescribed by the protocol, hypertension disappeared and anti-hypertensive therapy could be discontinued.

Survival and remission status

Of the 50 patients transplanted, 35 remain alive in unmaintained clinical remission. Thus, the actuarial three year survival rate of this patient population is 65%. Of the 20 patients transplanted in the standard risk group, 19 are alive and only 1 patient has died from an aspergillus infection associated with chronic GVHD. The patient, however, was in complete remission at the time of death. Of the 30 patients transplanted in the high risk group, 16 are alive at present in unmaintained clinical remission. The actuarial remission rate of patients transplanted in the standard risk group is 100% at 3 years. Actuarial remission rate for patients transplanted in the high risk group is 65.5% ± 11.1 (S.E.). Actuarial disease-free survival for patients transplanted in the standard risk group is 88.9% ± 10.5 (S.E.). Probability of disease-free survival for patients transplanted in the high risk group at 3 years is 50.6% ± 9.6 (S.E.).

DISCUSSION

Although not a controlled trial, this pilot study of 50 patients indicates several important points. To effectively prevent GVHD it is not necessary to purge donor marrow inocula *ex vivo* prior to transplantation. Post grafting immunosuppression, in the present trial with a combination of two non-myelotoxic immunosuppressive agents, resulted in an incidence of <10% of clinically significant (grade 2 or greater) acute GVHD, even in an adult patient population with a relatively high median age where 44% of patients were more than 30 years old.

We attribute this result of our new regimen that has been designed to better accommodate the post grafting phases of marrow transplantation. In this regimen a high initial dose of CsA is reduced drastically during the phase of aplasia to mimimize toxic side effects especially to the kidney, when potentially nephrotoxic broad spectrum antibiotics have to be used. Once engraftment has occurred and nephrotoxic antibiotics have been discontinued, the dose of CsA is increased to better counteract the high probability of acute GVHD present at that stage of marrow transplantation.

By combining CsA and MP we not only intended to increase the immunosuppressive power of the regimen but we intended to provide graft-versus-host protection even during the phase when CsA dose was low and thus possibly inadequate to prevent GVHD.

The toxicities observed were indeed quite manageable clinically. In this study CsA levels were not used to make dose changes. Instead serum creatinine levels were followed exclusively as guidelines. This proved sufficient to prevent major renal toxicity. Although renal function abnormalities were seen frequently, permanent renal damage attributable to CsA was not encountered. Similarly, the other two major side effects seen in this patient population, hyperkalemia and hypertension, could be easily managed clinically and fortunately disappeared over time with the protocol prescribed dose reductions of CsA.

Despite the low incidence of GVHD the relapse rate from the underlying hematologic malignancy was very low. To date none of the patients transplanted in the standard risk group has relapsed, the actuarial relapse of patients transplanted in the high risk group with far advanced disease being a comfortingly low 35%. This indicates either that the regimen did not affect the cellular components responsible for the graft-versus-leukemia effect, or that the preparative regimen used, namely a combination of BU and CY, had an exceedingly high antileukemic efficacy.

In this study we have not only observed a low incidence of GVHD and a gratifyingly high overall disease free survival but also a low complication rate, especially as far as infections are concerned. We attribute this low infection rate to several components in the overall transplant support system that were applied, such as avoidance of total body irradiation, implementation of gnotobiotic principles, use of cytomegalovirus negative blood component therapy and aggressive use of immunoglobulin therapy. Since at least in preclinical animal models infections can trigger graft-versus-host reactions, it is possible that the low infection rate seen here contributed in a significant way to the reduction and incidence and severity of GVHD. Studies are underway in our transplant center to identify the possible contribution that these various support measures might make in reducing graft-versus-host reactions.

REFERENCES

1. O'Reilly RJ (1987) Current developments in marrow transplantation. Transpl Proc XIX:92-102
2. Powles RL, Clink HM, Spence D, Morgenstern G, Watson JG, Selby PJ, Woods M, Barrett A, Jameson B, Sloane J, Lawler SD, Kay HEM,

Lawson D, McElwain TJ, Alexander P (1980) Cyclosporine A to prevent graft-versus-host disease in man after allogeneic bone marrow transplantation. Lancet 1:327-329
3. Gluckman E, Devergie A, Archimbaud E, Poirier O, Lokiec F (1983) Clinical results of Cyclosporine A prophylactic treatment of graft-versus-host disease. Exp Hematol 11:41
4. Tutschka PJ, Beschorner WE, Hess AD, Santos GW (1983) Cyclosporin-A to prevent graft-versus-host disease: A pilot study in 22 patients receiving allogeneic marrow transplants. Blood 61:318-325
5. Deeg HJ, Storb R, Thomas ED, Flournoy N, Kennedy MS, Banaji M, Appelbaum FR, Bensinger WI, Buckner CD, Clift RA, Doney K, Fefer A, McGuffin R, Sanders JE, Singer J, Stewart P, Sullivan KM, Witherspoon RP (1985) Cyclosporine as prophylaxis for graft-versus-host disease: A randomized study in patients undergoing marrow transplantation for acute nonlymphoblastic leukemia. Blood 65:1325-1334
6. Storb R, Deeg HJ, Thomas ED, Appelbaum FR, Buckner CD, Cheever MA, Clift RA, Doney KC, Flournoy N, Kennedy MS, Loughran TP, McGuffin RW, Sale GE, Sanders JE, Singer JW, Stewart PS, Sullivan KM, Witherspoon RP (1985) Marrow transplantation for chronic myelocytic leukemia: A controlled tiral of Cyclosporine versus methotrexate for prophylaxis of graft-versus-host disease. Blood 66:698-702
7. Santos GW, Tutschka PJ, Bookmeyer R, Saral R, Beschorner WE, Bias WB, Braine HG, Burns, Farmer ER, Hess AD, Kaizer H, Mellitis D, Sensenbrenner LL, Stuart R, Yeager AM (1987) Cyclosporine plus methylprednisolone versus cyclophosphamide plus methylprednisolone as prophylaxis for graft-versus-host disease: A randomized double-blind study in patients undergoing allogeneic marrow transplantation. Clin Transpl 1:21-28
8. Glucksberg H, Storb R, Fefer A, Buckner CD, Neiman PE, Clift RA, Lerner KG, Thomas ED (1974) Clinical manifestations of graft-versus-host disease in human recipients of marrow from HLA-matched sibling donors. Transplantation 18:295
9. Sullivan KM, Shulman HM, Storb R, Weiden PL, Witherspoon RP, McDonald GD, Schubert MM, Atkinson K, Thomas ED (1981) Chronic graft-versus-host disease in 52 patients: Adverse natural course and successful treatment with combination immunosuppression. Blood 57:267-276
10. Kaplan EL, Meier P (1958) Nonparametric estimation from incomplete observations. J Am Stat Assoc 53:457

VIII. Chronic Graft-versus-Host Disease: P.J. Tutschka and R. Parkman, Chairpersons

24: Chronic Graft-versus-Host Disease: Pathogenesis, Diagnosis, Treatment, and Prognostic Factors

Keith Sullivan, Robert Witherspoon, Rainer Storb, Frederick R. Appelbaum, Patrick Beatty, William Bensinger, Carolyn Bigelow, C. Dean Buckner, Martin Cheever, Reginald A. Clift, Kristine Doney, Alexander Fefer, Philip Greenberg, John Hansen, Paul Martin, Dana Matthews, George McDonald, Joel Meyers, Finn Bo Petersen, Jean Sanders, Howard Shulman, Jack Singer, Patricia Stewart, and E. Donnall Thomas

INTRODUCTION

Chronic graft-versus-host disease (GVHD) and associated infections are major determinants of late morbidity and mortality in 25-50% of long-term survivors of allogeneic marrow transplantation [1]. With improving supportive care during transplant, broadening criteria for donor selection and expanding indications and numbers of centers for transplant, an increasing number of long-term survivors are reported [2-4]. For primary care hematologists and oncologists, recognizing and treating late complications is of increasing importance. The following reviews the pathogenesis, diagnosis, treatment and prognosis of chronic GVHD.

DEFINITION AND INCIDENCE

Chronic GVHD is a clinicopathologic syndrome with autoimmune-like features developing 100-400 days after allogeneic marrow transplantation [5]. Although most patients with chronic GVHD have had preceding acute GVHD, 20-30% will have a <u>de novo</u> onset without prior acute GVHD. In others, chronic GVHD has a <u>progressive</u> onset as a direct extension of acute GVHD or follows a <u>quiescent</u> period after acute GVHD resolution. Acute GVHD is considered an alloimmune T-cell mediated disorder, while the immunopathogenesis of chronic GVHD resembles an autoimmune disorder [6].

Clinical chronic GHVD developed in 52 of 175 (30%) marrow recipients who survived >150 days after allogeneic transplant [7]. Analysis of crude incidence data suggested a greater frequency in patients receiving transplants for aplastic anemia (42%) than for leukemia (21%) [7]. Cumulative hazard rate analyses, correcting for competing hazards such as death from relapse, show that there is no difference in incidence for patients receiving transplants for aplastic anemia, acute nonlymphocytic leukemia, or acute lymphocytic leukemia [8].

Increasing patient age and degree of prior acute GVHD increase the risk for chronic GVHD [7-9]. The administration of viable donor buffy coat cells also increases the risk [9,10]. One report suggests a higher risk for chronic GVHD in recipients of marrow from older donors [10]. Data have been presented for [11] and against [12] an association of preceding cytomegalovirus (CMV) infection and subsequent development of chronic GVHD.

The relationship of age and acute GVHD to the development of chronic GVHD may be influenced by other factors. When published clinical trials are reviewed, it appears that although the incidence of acute GVHD can be substantially increased when posttransplant immunosuppression is withheld [13] or significantly decreased when posttransplant methotrexate and cyclosporine (CSP) are given [14], the incidence of chronic GVHD appears unaltered by these manipulations of acute GVHD and correlates predominantly with patient age [8].

IMMUNOPATHOGENESIS

Age may influence GVHD kinetics by means of thymic function. It has been postulated that stable graft-host tolerance requires a functioning thymus. Acute GVHD has been shown to damage thymic epithelium [15]. Absence of thymic function might prevent development of antigen-specific suppressor T cells thought to mediate tolerance and thus lead to the development of chronic GVHD [16]. Such a relationship is supported by demographic, pathology and laboratory studies showing thymic atrophy and low serum thymic hormone levels in children with chronic GVHD [5,7,17].

Although acute GVHD has been shown to be mediated by donor-derived cytotoxic T lymphocytes with specificity for recipient restricted histocompatibility antigens, the immunopathogenesis of chronic GVHD and its associated "disordered immunity" is less clear [18]. Several studies have shown differences in cellular effector mechanisms in acute and chronic GVHD [19]. Results from preclinical and human studies suggest that chronic GVHD derives from the chimera's generation of alloantigen nonspecific suppressor cells and inability to generate antigen-specific suppressor T cells [16,18,20].

Clonal analyses of T lymphocytes in a murine model of chronic GVHD have recently demonstrated additional effector mechanisms. Noncytotoxic T lymphocytes with autologous Ia specificity have been identified in mice developing chronic GVHD [21, 22]. These autoreactive helper clones appear to release lymphokines which stimulate collagen synthesis leading to scleroderma and fibrosis. Further description of the role of these autoreactive cells is presented by Parkman and colleagues in another section of this volume.

PATHOLOGY

The skin is the most thoroughly studied target organ in chronic GVHD [23]. In the generalized form there is an initial inflammatory phase with eosinophilic body formation and lichenoid reaction at the basal layer. In the late phase the epidermis becomes atrophic and fibrosis is observed throughout the dermis and adnexal structures. A variant or localized form of chronic GVHD shows only modest inflammation with little or no lichenoid reaction or eosinophilic body formation. The deeper reticular dermis exhibits nodular fibrosis. Liver histology resembles lobular hepatitis, chronic persistent or chronic active hepatitis [5,24]. Late hepatic changes include reduction or absence of small bile ducts and marked cholestasis. Chronic GVHD has been likened to primary biliary cirrhosis [25].

Oral biopsies and ocular tissues show lymphoplasmacytic infiltrates and fibrous destruction of the lacrimal and salivary glands similar to Sjogren's syndrome [26]. Pulmonary lesions include fibrous obliteration of the lumen of the bronchioles similar to late findings in human heart/lung transplants or naturally occurring autoimmune disease [27].

Although chronic GVHD resembles autoimmune diseases such as progressive systemic sclerosis (PSS), lichen planus, Sjogren's syndrome, rheumatoid arthritis, lupus erythematosus, and eosinophilic fasciitis, there appear to be several differences. Investigators in Paris report a predominance of sclerosis in the upper dermis in chronic GVHD as opposed to deeper dermis and hypodermis involvement in PSS [28]. Renal and neurologic involvement is rare in chronic GVHD [5] and esophageal manifestations do not include characteristic muscle or neuronal abnormalities seen in PSS [24].

CLINICAL MANIFESTATIONS

Dermal involvement is the most frequent clinical feature of chronic GVHD [8]. Erythema, dyspigmentation, poikiloderma, and lichenoid lesions may be observed. Without therapy, the skin becomes progressively indurated and sclerotic, leading to joint contractures and disability. Liver function abnormalities are predominantly cholestatic but hepato-cellular dysfunction may make it difficult to distinguish chronic GVHD from viral hepatitis. Isolated hepatic abnormalities without other target organ involvement has not been observed in chronic GVHD.

Oral lesions include erythema, atrophy and lichen planus-like findings [29]. Ocular abnormalities include keratoconjunctivitis sicca, conjunctivitis and uveitis [30]. Desquamative esophagitis [31], polyserositis [5], vaginal stenosis [32], and myasthenia gravis [33] are less common manifestations.

Over the last several years, the spectrum of chronic GVHD appears to have been altered as an increasing proportion of patients are treated with immunosuppressive therapy. The frequency of disabling joint contractures has fallen from 40-50% to 5-10% and the generation of autoantibodies appears lessened as patients are more intensively treated [34]. Pulmonary complications including obliterative bronchiolitis are more recently recognized features in 10-15% of patients with chronic GVHD [35-37].

DIAGNOSIS AND GRADING

Table 1 summarizes criteria for the diagnosis of chronic GVHD [5]. Patients with limited disease represent only 10% of the total and are important to identify because they have a favorable course without therapy. In contrast, patients with extensive (i.e., multi-organ) disease have an unfavorable natural history.

The clinician relies upon biopsy material to establish the diagnosis and assess the response to treatment. A full-thickness 3 mm punch biopsy of the skin is obtained from involved areas. Biopsy of the sun-exposed forearm area can show diagnostic changes even in the absence of dermal lesions. Oral mucosal biopsies are also obtained [26]. A battery of screening tests are obtained before day 100 to help detect early disease [8]. The diagnosis of clinical chronic GVHD is made if the patient has multi-organ clinical manifestations and positive skin and oral biopsies. Sub

Table 1. Clinicopathologic Classification of Chronic GVHD [5]

Limited chronic GVHD

Either or both:

1. Localized skin involvement
2. Hepatic dysfunction due to chronic GVHD

Extensive chronic GVHD

Either:

1. Generalized skin involvement or
2. Localized skin involvement and/or hepatic dysfunction due to chronic GVHD

Plus:

3. a. Liver histology showing chronic aggressive hepatitis, bridging necrosis or cirrhosis, or
   b. Involvement of eye: Schirmer's test with less than 5 mm wetting, or
   c. Involvement of minor salivary glands or oral mucosa demonstrated on labial biopsy specimen, or
   d. Involvement of any other target organ

---

clinical chronic GVHD is defined in patients who have characteristic pathology findings on both the blind oral and skin biopsies in the absence of clinical signs or symptoms of chronic GVHD.

The severity of individual organ involvement correlates poorly with overall survival. The cumulative effect of the multi-tissue abnormalities does correlate with the functional performance of the patient. For this reason, we have graded the severity of chronic GVHD by its impact on the patient's daily functional activity as measured by the Karnofsky Performance Score.

IMMUNODEFICIENCY AND INFECTION

Multiple B and T cell abnormalities have been reported in patients developing chronic GVHD [38-40]. Severe immunodeficiency appears to persist for as long as the disease remains active. Humoral recovery, reconstitution of cellular immunity, opsonization and granulocyte chemotaxis are all impaired. Generation of nonspecific suppressor T lymphocytes further increases the risk of infection [41]. Damage to the skin and intestinal tract from chronic GVHD may serve as additioal risk factors for infection.

The most important clinical aspect of chronic GVHD is immune suppression and associated infection. The relative risk of late non-varicella zoster infection is 2.2-fold increased in patients developing chronic GVHD compared to long-term survivors without chronic GVHD [41]. Sinusitis, bronchitis, otitis media, bacterial pneumonia, bacteremia, and interstitial pneumonia may be observed after day 100 [41]. Encapsulated organisms such as *S. pneumoniae* and *H. influenzae* are common while fungal infections are relatively infrequent despite prolonged use of corticosteroids. Meyers and colleagues review posttransplant infections in another section of this volume.

PREVENTION

Attempts at augmenting thymic function with thymopentin administration or functioning thymic transplants have not been successful in preventing chronic GVHD [42,43]. Prevention of infection during chronic GVHD has focused on methods of accelerating immune reconstitution, antibiotic or intravenous immune globulin prophylaxis and immunosupressive treatment to control GVHD-induced immune dysregulation. Administration of thymosin has not hastened the tempo of immune recovery [44]. Adoptive transfer of specific immune responsiveness may be of benefit in the future [45]. The mainstay of infection prophylaxis has been the administration of daily trimethoprim sulfamethoxazole (TMP-SMX). With this prophylaxis, the incidence of interstitial pneumonia in patients with chronic GVHD has been reduced from 28% to 8% [46]. Moreover, it appears that pneumococcal bacteremia and pneumonia are reduced in patients receiving daily antibiotic prophylaxis.

Although serum IgG is usually quantitatively normal after transplant, several observations indicate that the immunoglobulin produced may be functionally deficient [39,40,47,48]. *In vitro* synthesis and *in vivo* response to specific antigen challenge are impaired. Moreover, conversion from IgM to IgG in the secondary response is blunted. These qualitative IgG defects combined with quantitative serum and secretory IgA deficiencies could contribute to the recurrent sinopulmonary infection and late obstructive lung disease observed in patients with chronic GVHD [34,41]. Administration of polyspecific immunoglobulin preparations during the first 100 days after transplant has been shown in controlled trials to lower the incidence of interstitial pneumonia and CMV infection [49]. Septicemia following engraftment appears reduced in immune globulin recipients [50]. Long-term prophylaxis with immunoglobulin may be of benefit in patients developing chronic GVHD and is currently being evaluated in controlled trials. Prevention and treatment of infections after marrow transplant is reviewed by Winston and colleagues in another section of this volume.

Another approach at preventing late infection focuses on the treatment and control of chronic GVHD-associated immune dysregulation. Prior studies have shown that without immunosuppressive treatment, infections and mortality were common in patients with clinical extensive chronic

GVHD [7]. Titration of the amount of immunosuppression needed to control GVHD without inducing additional risk for infection is a delicate and vital aspect of therapy.

TREATMENT

Without treatment, approximately 20% of patients with clinical extensive chronic GVHD survive with Karnofsky scores ≥70% [7]. Immunosuppressive therapy with antithymocyte globulin and/or corticosteroids given late in the course of the disease provides little apparent benefit. In a pilot study of cytotoxic agents combined with corticosteroids, 16 of 21 patients survived free of disability [7]. However, comparing results of azathioprine and prednisone therapy to prior experience with prednisone alone was complicated by the fact that patients given the combination were treated in more recent years when earlier diagnosis and better supportive care and follow-up were employed.

Between 1980 and 1983 we conducted a double-blind, controlled clinical trial comparing prednisone and placebo to prednisone and azathioprine (1.5 mg/kg-/day) given as early treatment of extensive chronic GVHD [51]. Patients with thrombocytopenia were placed into therapy with corticosteroids. All three groups of patients received similar doses of prednisone (1 mg/kg/QOD) and prophylactic TMP-SMX (1 DS PO BID). Nonrelapse mortality and infections were increased in patients randomized to azathioprine compared to patients randomized to placebo [34]. Early treatment with prednisone alone appeared superior to prednisone plus azathioprine in normal risk chronic GVHD. However, patients with thrombocytopenia had increased infections and only approximately 25% survived despite steroid therapy [34,51].

In late 1982 we started a pilot study of additional therapy in patients with high-risk chronic GVHD who either failed prior treatment or who were previously untreated but had persisting thrombocytopenia [52,53]. Oral cyclosporine (6 mg/kg/q 12 hours/QOD) was combined in an alternating-day regimen with prednisone (1 mg/kg/QOD). Toxicity appeared acceptable and long-term survival has increased to over 50% in these high-risk patients.

Small numbers of patients with chronic GVHD have been treated with thymosin, transfer factor, penicillamine, hydroxychloroquine or electron beam irradiation without success [7,54]. Four patients with progressive extensive chronic GVHD were treated by the Ulm group with cyclosporine and three survive 9 months after transplant [55]. Recently investigators from Baltimore reported success with thalidomide treatment in a rat model of chronic GVHD [56]. Clinical studies of this therapy are currently in progress.

PROGNOSTIC FACTORS

Patients with a limited form of clinical chronic GVHD have a favorable outcome without treatment while those with clinical extensive disease have an unfavorable natural course. Among patients with extensive chronic GVHD, mortality is highest in those with a progressive type onset, intermediate in those with a quiescent onset and lowest in those with a de novo onset of chronic GVHD [7,34].

Thrombocytopenia is a major but poorly understood adverse prognostic factor in patients with clinical extensive chronic GVHD [34,51,57]. Although some patients may have an autoimmune-like origin of thrombocytopenia [58], most have hypocellular marrow aspirates. Viral-induced or cell-mediated suppression of megakaryocytopoiesis could account for this persisting thrombocytopenia.

Increasing patient age appears to result in increased mortality from chronic GVHD [7,34]. Patients failing the initial treatment also have a poor prognosis [34].

Patients with subclinical chronic GVHD have less transplant-related complications than patients with clinical disease. However, even with early immunosuppressive therapy, survival is not improved in patients with subclinical disease due to an increased risk of leukemia relapse when compared to patients with clinical chronic GVHD [34].

GRAFT-VERSUS-LEUKEMIA EFFECT

Previous analyses have shown that patients developing acute or chronic GVHD have a higher probability of remaining free of leukemia than patients not developing GVHD [59]. Patients with the de novo onset of chronic GVHD have the highest probability of long-term disease-free survival [59]. A recent update of patients with acute leukemia given unmodified allogeneic marrow grafts in Seattle between 1970 and 1986 has been reported [60]. Among 450 patients surviving in remission 150 days after HLA-identical transplant, recurrent leukemia was highest in patients developing neither acute nor chronic GVHD and lowest in patients developing both acute and chronic GVHD (52% versus 28%, p=0.0001).

Effector mechanisms mediating this apparent graft-versus-leukemia effect in animals have been described [61]. Causality is a central issue for it is not known whether the apparent graft-versus-leukemia effect in man is a primary immunologic event in association with GVHD or whether the lack of GVHD is simply a marker of persistent donor-host chimerism (and leukemia). Of concern is the fact that as new technologies are employed to deplete the bone marrow graft of viable T lymphocytes to prevent GVHD, an increased rate of relapse of leukemia may be observed [62].

CONCLUSIONS

The success of marrow transplantation has occasioned a new set of challenges. Good risk candidates are transplanted in hundreds of centers worldwide and an increasing proportion of patients are cured of their malignant disorders. Attention has now shifted to the quality of life of these long-term survivors and events after they leave the transplant center.

Early diagnosis of chronic GVHD is critical so that treatment can be started before clinical deterioration. Early therapy with prednisone has been successful in patients with normal risk chronic GVHD and disabling complications are now infrequent. However, late infections continue to be common events and better methods to accelerate immune reconstitution and prevent infection are needed. A new alternating-day regimen of prednisone and cyclosporine appears to improve survival in patients with high-risk chronic GVHD. Other controlled clinical trials are now in progress in different prognostic factor groups. Improved understanding of the pathogenesis, diagnosis, treatment and prognostic factors of this disorder has reduced the late morbidity of allogeneic marrow transplantation.

ACKNOWLEDGEMENTS

This work was supported in part by grants CA 18221, CA 15704, CA 18029 from the National Cancer Institute and HL 36444 from the National Heart, Lung, and Blood Institute, National Institutes of Health, DHHS.

REFERENCES

1. Sullivan KM, Deeg HJ, Sanders JE, Shulman HM, Witherspoon RP, Doney K, Appelbaum FR, Schubert MM, Stewart P, Springmeyer S, McDonald GB, Storb R, Thomas ED (1984) Late complications after marrow transplantation. Semin Hematol 21:53-63

2. Thomas ED (1983) Marrow transplantation for malignant diseases (Karnofsky Memorial Lecture). J Clin Oncol 1:517-531

3. Beatty PG, Clift RA, Mickelson EM, Nisperos B, Flournoy N, Martin PJ, Sanders JE, Storb R, Thomas ED, Hansen JA (1985) Marrow transplantation from related donors other than HLA-identical siblings. N Engl J Med 313:765-771

4. Bortin MM, Rimm AA (1986) Increasing utilization of bone marrow transplantation. Transplantation 42:229-234

5. Shulman HM, Sullivan KM, Weiden PL, McDonald GB, Striker GE, Sale GE, Hackman R, Tsoi M-S, Storb R, Thomas ED (1980) Chronic graft-versus-host syndrome in man: A long-term clinicopathological study of 20 Seattle patients. Am J Med 69:204-217

6. Sullivan KM (1986) Acute and chronic graft-versus-host disease in man. Int J Cell Cloning 4(Suppl 1):42-93

7. Sullivan KM, Shulman HM, Storb R, Weiden PL, Witherspoon RP, McDonald GB, Schubert MM, Atkinson K, Thomas ED (1981) Chronic graft-versus-host disease in 52 patients: Adverse natural course and successful treatment with combination immunosuppression. Blood 57:267-276

8. Sullivan KM, Witherspoon R, Deeg HJ, Doney K, Appelbaum F, Sanders J, Lum L, Loughran T, Hill R, Anasetti C, Shields A, Nims J, Shulman H, Storb R, Thomas ED (1987) Chronic graft-versus-host disease in man. In: Gale RP, Champlin R, eds. Progress in bone marrow transplantation. New York: AR Liss, 473-487

9. Storb R, Prentice RL, Sullivan KM, Shulman HM, Deeg HJ, Doney KC, Buckner CD, Clift RA, Witherspoon RP, Appelbaum FA, Sanders JE, Stewart PS, Thomas ED (1983) Predictive factors in chronic graft-versus-host disease in patients with aplastic anemia treated by marrow transplantation from HLA-identical siblings. Ann Intern Med 98:461-466

10. Ringden O, Paulin T, Lonnqvist B, Nilsson B (1985) An analysis of factors predisposing to chronic graft-versus-host disease. Exp Hematol 13:1062-1067

11. Lonnqvist B, Ringden O, Wahren B, Gahrton G, Lundgren G (1984) Cytomegalovirus infection associated with and preceding chronic graft-versus-host disease. Transplantation 38: 465-468

12. Meyers JD, Flournoy N, Thomas ED (1986) Risk factors for cytomegalovirus infection after human marrow transplantation. J Infect Dis 153: 478-488

13. Sullivan KM, Deeg HJ, Sanders J, Klosterman A, Amos D, Shulman H, Sale G, Martin P, Witherspoon R, Appelbaum FR, Doney K, Stewart P, Meyers J, McDonald GB, Weiden P, Fefer A, Buckner CD, Storb R, Thomas ED (1986) Hyperacute GVHD in patients not given immunosuppression after allogeneic marrow transplantation. Blood 67: 1172-1175

14. Storb R, Deeg HJ, Whitehead J,

Appelbaum F, Beatty P, Bensinger W, Buckner CD, Clift R, Doney K, Farewell V, Hansen J, Hill R, Lum L, Martin P, McGuffin R, Sanders J, Stewart P, Sullivan K, Witherspoon R, Yee G, Thomas ED (1986) Methotrexate and cyclosporine compared with cyclosporine alone for prophylaxis of acute graft versus host disease after marrow transplantation for leukemia. N Engl J Med 314:729-735

15. Seddik M, Seemayer TA, Lapp WS (1980) T cell functional defect associated with thymic epithelial cell injury induced by a graft-versus-host reaction. Transplantation 29:61-66

16. Tsoi M-S (1982) Immunologic mechanisms of graft-versus-host disease in man. Transplantation 33:459-464

17. Atkinson K, Incefy GS, Storb R, Sullivan KM, Iwata T, Dardenne M, Ochs HD, Good RA, Thomas ED (1982) Low serum thymic hormone levels in patients with chronic graft-versus-host disease. Blood 59:1073-1077

18. Tutschka PJ (1987) Mechanisms of chronic GVHD. In: Gale RP, Champlin R, eds. Progress in bone marrow transplantation. New York: AR Liss, 457-472

19. Gleichmann E, Pals ST, Rolink AG, Radaszkiewicz T, Gleichmann H (1984) Graft-versus-host reactions: Clues to the etiopathology of a spectrum of immunological diseases. Immunol Today 5:324-332

20. Beschorner WE, Tutschka PJ, Santos GW (1983) Chronic graft-versus-host disease in the rat radiation chimera. III. Immunology and immunopathology in rapidly induced models. Transplantation 35:224-230

21. Parkman R (1986) Clonal analysis of murine graft-versus-host disease. I. Phenotypic and functional analysis of T lymphocyte clones. J Immunol 136:3543-3548

22. Parkman R, DeClerck Y, Champagne J, Walker S (1987) Chronic graft-versus-host disease is an autoimmune disease. In: Gale RP, Champlin R, eds. Progress in bone marrow transplantation. New York: AR Liss, 497-504

23. Shulman HM, Sale GE, Lerner KG, Barker EA, Weiden PL, Sullivan K, Gallucci B, Thomas ED, Storb R (1978) Chronic cutaneous graft-versus-host disease in man. Am J Pathol 91:545-570

24. McDonald GB, Shulman HM, Sullivan KM, Spencer GD (1986) Intestinal and hepatic complications of human bone marrow transplantation. Gastroenterology 90:460-477, 770-784

25. Epstein O, Thomas HC, Sherlock S (1980) Primary biliary cirrhosis is a dry gland syndrome with features of chronic graft-versus-host disease. Lancet 1:1166-1168

26. Sale GE, Shulman HM, Schubert MM, Sullivan KM, Kopecky KJ, Hackman RC, Morton TH, Storb R, Thomas ED (1981) Oral and ophthalmic pathology of graft versus host disease in man: Predictive value of the lip biopsy. Hum Pathol 12:1022-1030

27. Burke CM, Theodore J, Dawkins KD, Yousem SA, Blank N, Billingham ME, Van Kessel A, Jamieson SW, Oyer PE, Baldwin JC, Stinson EB, Shumway NE, Robin ED (1984) Post-transplant obliterative bronchiolitis and other late lung sequelae in human heart-lung transplantation. Chest 86:824-829

28. Gluckman E, Janin-Mercier A (1987) Is chronic graft-versus-host disease similar to autoimmune diseases. In: Gale RP, Champlin R, eds. Progress in bone marrow transplantation. New York: AR Liss, 489-495

29. Schubert MM, Sullivan KM, Morton TH, Izutsu KT, Peterson DE, Flournoy N, Truelove EL, Sale GE, Buckner CD, Storb R, Thomas ED (1984) Oral manifestations of chronic graft-versus-host disease. Arch Intern Med 144:1591-1595

30. Jack MK, Jack GM, Sale GE, Shulman HM, Sullivan KM (1983) Ocular manifestations of graft-v-host disease. Arch Ophthalmol 101:1080-1084

31. McDonald GB, Sullivan KM, Schuffler MD, Shulman HM, Thomas ED (1981) Esophageal abnormalities in chronic graft-versus-host disease in humans. Gastroenterology 80:914-921

32. Corson SL, Sullivan K, Batzer F, August C, Storb R, Thomas ED (1982) Gynecologic manifestations of chronic graft-versus-host disease. Obstet Gynecol 60:488-492

33. Bolger GB, Sullivan KM, Spence AM, Appelbaum FR, Johnston R, Sanders JE, Deeg HJ, Witherspoon RP, Doney KC, Nims J, Thomas ED, Storb R (1986) Myasthenia gravis after allogeneic bone marrow transplantation: Relationship to chronic graft-versus-host disease. Neurology 36:1087-1091

34. Sullivan KM, Witherspoon RP, Storb R, Weiden P, Flournoy N, Dahlberg S,

Deeg HJ, Sanders JE, Doney KC, Appelbaum FR, McGuffin R, McDonald G, Meyers J, Schubert MM, Gauvreau J, Shulman HM, Sale GE, Anasetti C, Loughran T, Strom S, Nims J, Thomas ED. Prednisone and azathioprine compared to prednisone and placebo for treatment of chronic graft-versus-host disease: Prognostic influence of prolonged thrombocytopenia after allogeneic marrow transplantation. (submitted for publication)

35. Ralph DD, Springmeyer SC, Sullivan KM, Hackman RC, Storb R, Thomas ED (1984) Rapidly progressive air-flow obstruction in marrow transplant recipients: Possible association between obliterative bronchiolitis and chronic graft-versushost disease. Am Rev Respir Dis 129:641-644

36. Witherspoon RP, Buckner CD, Sullivan KM, Fisher L, Clark J, Storb R, Thomas ED. Causes of late failure in patients transplanted for acute leukemia. Bone Marrow Transplantation, (in press)

37. Clark JG, Schwartz DA, Flournoy N, Sullivan KM, Crawford SW, Thomas ED. Risk factors for development of airflow obstruction in marrow transplant recipients. Ann Intern Med, (in press)

38. Lapp WS, Ghayur T, Mendes M, Seddik M, Seemayer TA (1985) The functional and histological basis for graft-versus-host-induced immunosuppression. Immunol Rev 88:107-133

39. Witherspoon RP (1986) Suppression and recovery of immunologic function after bone marrow transplantation. J Natl Cancer Inst 76:1321-1324

40. Lum LG (1987) A review: The kinetics of immune reconstitution after human marrow transplantation. Blood 69:369-380

41. Atkinson K, Farewell V, Storb R, Tsoi M-S, Sullivan KM, Witherspoon RP, Fefer A, Clift R, Goodell B, Thomas ED (1982) Analysis of late infections after human bone marrow transplantation: Role of genotypic nonidentity between marrow donor and recipient and of nonspecific suppressor cells in patients with chronic graft-versus-host disease. Blood 60:714-720

42. Atkinson K, Storb R, Ochs HD, Goehle S, Sullivan KM, Witherspoon RP, Lum LG, Tsoi M-S, Sanders JE, Parr M, Stewart P, Thomas ED (1982) Thymus transplantation after allogeneic bone marrow graft to prevent chronic graft-versus-host disease in humans. Transplantation 33:168-173

43. Witherspoon RP, Navari R, Storb R, Sullivan KM, Doney K, Beatty P, Lum LG, Thomas ED (1987) Treatment of marrow graft recipients with thymopentin. Bone Marrow Transplantation 1:365-371

44. Witherspoon RP, Hersman J, Storb R, Ochs H, Goldstein AL, McClure J, Noel D, Weiden PL, Thomas ED (1983) Thymosin fraction 5 does not accelerate reconstitution of immunologic reactivity after human marrow grafting. Br J Haematol 55: 595-608

45. Lum LG, Seigneuret MC, Shiobara S, Noges J, Munn N, Shough N, Jin N-R, Beatty P, Martin P, Sullivan K, Storb R, Thomas ED. Adoptively transferred immunity persists in human marrow graft recipients. In: Truitt RL, Gale RP, Bortin MM, eds. Cellular immunotherapy of cancer. New York: AR Liss, (in press)

46. Sullivan KM, Meyers JD, Flournoy N, Storb R, Thomas ED (1986) Early and late interstitial pneumonia following human bone marrow transplantation. Int J Cell Cloning 4(Suppl 1):107-121

47. Witherspoon RP, Storb R, Ochs HD, Flournoy N, Kopecky KJ, Sullivan KM, Deeg HJ, Sosa R, Noel DR, Atkinson K, Thomas ED (1981) Recovery of antibody production in human allogeneic marrow graft recipients: Influence of time post transplantation, the presence or absence of chronic graft-versus-host disease, and antithymocyte globulin treatment. Blood 58:360-368

48. Korsmeyer SJ, Elfenbein GJ, Goldman CK, Marshall SL, Waldmann TA (1982) B cell, helper T cell and suppressor T cell abnormalities contribute to disordered immunoglobulin synthesis in patients following bone marrow transplantation. Transplantation 33:184-190

49. Sullivan KM. Immunoglobulin therapy in bone marrow transplantation. Am J Med, (in press)

50. Petersen FB, Bowden RA, Thornquist M, Meyers JD, Buckner CD, Counts GW, Nelson N, Newton BA, Sullivan KM, McIver J, Thomas ED. The effect of prophylactic intravenous immune globulin on the incidence of septicemia in marrow transplant recipients. Bone Marrow Transplantation, (in press)

51. Sullivan KM, Storb R, Flournoy N, Weiden P, Shulman H, Deeg HJ, Witherspoon R, Thomas ED (1982) Preliminary

analysis of a randomized trial of immunosuppressive therapy of chronic graft-versus-host disease (GVHD). Blood 60 (Supp 1):173a, (abstr)

52. Sullivan KM, Deeg HJ, Storb R, Nims J, Witherspoon R, Doney K, Appelbaum F, Thomas ED (1986) Alternating-day cyclosporine and prednisone improve survival in patients with high-risk chronic graft-versus-host disease. Exp Hematol 14:529, (abstr)

53. Sullivan KM, Witherspoon RP, Storb R, Deeg HJ, Dahlberg S, Sanders JE, Appelbaum FR, Doney KC, Weiden P, Anasetti C, Loughran T, Hill R, Shields TP, Shulman H, Nims J, Strom S, Thomas ED. Alternating day cyclosporine and prednisone for treatment of high-risk chronic graft-versus-host disease. (submitted for publication)

54. Summerfield GP, Bellingham AJ, Bunch C, Woodrow JC (1983) Successful treatment of chronic cutaneous graft-versus-host disease (GVHD) with penicillamine. Clin Lab Haemat 5:313-318

55. Bunjes D, Heit W, Arnold R, Schmeiser T, Heimpel H (1986) Cyclosporine as an alternative to cyclophosphamide in the treatment of chronic graft-versus-host disease. Transplantation 41:170-172

56. Vogelsang GB, Taylor S, Gordon G, Hess AD (1986) Thalidomide, a potent agent for the treatment of graft-versus-host disease. Transplant Proc 18:904-906

57. First LR, Smith BR, Lipton J, Nathan DG, Parkman R, Rappaport JM (1985) Isolated thrombocytopenia after allogeneic bone marrow transplant and chronic thrombocytopenic syndromes. Blood 65:368-374

58. Anasetti C, Sullivan K, Deeg J, Slichter S (1986) Graft-versus-host disease (GVHD) is associated with autoimmune-like thrombocytopenia. J Cell Biochem Suppl 10D:222, (abstr)

59. Weiden PL, Sullivan KM, Flournoy N, Storb R, Thomas ED, the Seattle Marrow Transplant Team (1981) Anti-leukemic effect of chronic graft-versus-host disease: Contribution to improved survival after allogeneic marrow transplantation. N Engl J Med 304:1529-1533

60. Sullivan KM, Fefer A, Witherspoon R, Storb R, Buckner CD, Weiden P, Schoch G, Thomas ED. Graft-versus-leukemia in man: Relationship of acute and chronic graft-versus-host disease to relapse of acute leukemia following allogeneic bone marrow transplantation. In: Truitt RL, Gale RP, Bortin MM, eds. Cellular immunotherapy of cancer. New York: AR Liss, (in press)

61. Greenberg PD, Cheever MA, Fefer A (1981) Eradication of disseminated murine leukemia by chemo-immunotherapy with cyclophosphamide and adoptively transferred immune syngeneic Lyt 1^+2^- T lymphocytes. J Exp Med 154:952-963

62. Mitsuyasu RT, Champlin RE, Gale RP, Ho WG, Lenarsky C, Winston D, Selch M, Elashoff R, Giorgi JV, Wells J, Terasaki P, Billing R, Feig S (1986) Treatment of donor bone marrow with monoclonal anti-T-cell antibody and complement for the prevention of graft-versus-host disease: A prospective, randomized, double-blind trial. Ann Intern Med 105:20-26

25: The Role of Autoreactive T Lymphocytes in Graft-versus-Host Disease (GVHD)

Robertson Parkman, Josette Champagne, Maxwell Cooper, Veronica Draper, Yves DeClerck, and Sharyn Walker

Chronic graft versus host disease (GVHD) has many clinical and histopathological features that are similar to human autoimmune diseases including pulmonary fibrosis, sclerodermatous skin changes, esophageal dysmotility, and an increased frequency of autoantibodies.[1-3] It has been difficult, however, to study chronic GHVD in animal models because most models of GVHD lead to the early death of the animals or the surviving animals do not have the histopathological features seen in human chronic GVHD.[4,5]

We have established a murine model of histocompatible GVHD due to antigenic differences at minor histocompatibility loci (non-H-2). The donor, LP, and recipient, C57Bl/6 (B6), strains are H-2 identical, MLC non-reactive and Mls identical.[6] With the transplantation of escalating numbers of donor T lymphocytes, animals developed no GVHD, both acute and chronic GVHD or only fatal acute GVHD.[7] Thus, the model has many similarities to histocomaptible human bone marrow transplantation and produces a significant number of animals with sclerodermatous skin changes, allopecia and fibrosis, changes that are clinically similar to human chronic GVHD. Thus, the LP-B6 model is both immunologically and pathologically similar, if not identical, to human chronic GVHD.

To study the effector mechanisms involved in acute and chronic GVHD, T lymphocyte clones were generated from the spleens of B6 recipients of LP spleen cells. Clones were established from animals with acute GVHD 14-17 days following transplantation and from animals with clinically detectable chronic GVHD 50 days following transplantation.[8] The recipient spleen cells were initially expanded with irradiated recipient (B6) spleen cells and then cloned by limiting dilution with irradiated B6 spleen cells and exogenous IL 2. The resultant clones were phenotyped and tested for their blastogenic specificity and dependency on exogenous IL 2 for their in vitro blastogenesis. The effect of their secreted cytokines on fibroblast proliferation and collagen synthesis was determined.

All clones derived from animals with chronic GVHD had a phenotype of Thy 1.2^+, Lyt 1.2^+, Lyt 2.2^-, and $L3T4^+$. In vitro assays of blastogenesis demonstrated that the chronic GVHD clones were stimulated equally by LP and B6 spleen cells. Further analysis with congenic mice defined the shared stimulating antigen as Ia^{-b}, the Ia shared by LP and B6; thus, all the clonagenic T lymphocytes in the spleens of mice with chronic GVHD were autoreactive, i.e., they responded to antigens expressed on the donor LP cells.[Table 1]

In parallel, the clones derived from the spleens of mice with acute GVHD were studied. Two thirds of the clones displayed a Thy 1.2^+, Lyt 1.2^+, Lyt 2.2^+ and $L3T4^-$ phenotype and B6 specific blastogenesis in vitro.[8] All clones were dependent upon exogenous IL 2 for in vitro blastogenesis. The majority of the clones were cytotoxic and were phenotypically and functionally identical to clones derived from LP animals immunized with B6 spleen cells; thus, the B6 specific, acute GVHD clones were classic immune cytotoxic T lymphocytes (CTL). The other 1/3 of clones derived from acute GVHD mice had a Lyt 2^-, $L3T4^+$ phenotype, were non-cytotoxic and required no exogenous IL 2 for in vitro blastogenesis. The specificity of the $L3T4^+$ clones derived from acute GVHD mice was Ia^{-b} in in vitro blastogenesis assays; thus, the autoreactive clones derived from animals with acute GVHD were similar, if not identical, to the clones derived from animals with chronic GVHD and suggested that the cellular events that culminate in clinical chronic GVHD are initiated during acute GVHD.

To determine the cytokine, that supported the autocrine in vitro blastogenesis of the autoreactive T lymphocyte clones derived from animals with chronic GVHD, antibodies to IL 2 and IL 4 were added to the in vitro cultures with irradiated B6 spleen cells as stimulator cells. The addition of IL 4 produced a greater than 80% inhibition of blastogenesis where the addition of anti-IL 2 produced no such inhibition demonstrating that the autoreactive cells were producing IL 4 and that IL 4 was cytokine responsible for their autocrine growth support.(R. Parkman, Unpublished observations) Supernatants of chronic GVHD clones were also tested for the production of gamma interferon, and two out of ten clones studied produced significant levels of gamma interferon (270 and 990 International units/ml).

Because increased collagen deposition is the major histopathological finding in chronic GVHD, the supernatants of the chronic GVHD clones were tested for their capacity to stimulate total collagen production, collagen production per fibroblast and fibroblast proliferation. Four of nine chronic GVHD clones stimulated total collagen production by increasing the amount of collagen produced per fibroblast.[9] The stimulatory supernatants had no effect on fibroblast proliferation. In contrast, when the supernatants of clones derived from animals with acute GVHD were tested, supernatants from B6 specific, Lyt 2.2^+ clones stimulated fibroblast proliferation but had no effect on collagen production per fibroblast. Thus, during acute GVHD there is the release of cytokines capable of stimulating fibroblast proliferation while during chronic GVHD there is the production of cytokines capable of stimulating collagen production on a per fibroblast basis. It is, therefore, possible that the increased collagen deposition seen in chronic GVHD is a consequence of both fibroblast proliferation and increased collagen synthesis. The synergy between acute and chronic GVHD cytokines would explain in part the observation that the incidence of chronic GVHD is greater in individuals who have suffered from acute GVHD.

Interleukin 4(IL 4) was originally called B cell stimulatory factor 1 (BSF-1).[10-12] However, it is now clear that, in addition to its effects on B cells (stimulation of IgE synthesis and Ia expression on resting B cells), IL 4 has effects on T lymphocytes. IL 4 is capable of stimulating resting T lymphocytes when they are co-stimulated with PMA. IL 4 is an autocrine growth factor for some autoreactive helper T lymphocytes derived from animals with GHVD. Preliminary experiments have indicated that IL 4 is uniquely capable of stimulating fibroblast collagen production on a per fibroblast basis as compared to other cytokines (IL 1, IL 2, IL 3, and gamma interferon) tested. The other cytokines may stimulate fibroblast proliferation but have no stimulatory effect on fibroblast collagen production. Thus, IL 4 may be a central cytokine in the production of chronic GVHD and other autoimmune diseases since it is capable of the autocrine stimulation of autoreactive helper T lymphocytes and of stimulating fibroblast collagen synthesis. In addition, IL 4 may stimulate autoreactive B lymphocytes (Lyt 1^+ B cells in mice or Leu 1^+ B cells in humans) to produce autoantibodies.[13,14]

The clonal analysis of animals with chronic GVHD has revealed that the only clonagenic T lymphocytes in the spleens of animals with chronic GVHD are autoreactive T lymphocytes, the majority of which are capable of the in vitro production of IL 4, which is sufficient for their in vitro blastogenesis. The IL 4 produced by these cells may be capable of stimulating increased fibroblast collagen production, autoantibody production and Ia expression. Thus, the autoreactive cells are capable of supporting their own growth, stimulating the expression of their stimulating antigen and releasing cytokines that increase collagen production. This murine model of autocrine stimulation may be applicable to human chronic GVHD and other fibrotic diseases characterized by increased collagen deposition.

References

1. Sullivan KM, Parkman R (1983) The pathophysiology and treatment of graft-versus-host disease. In: Clinics in Haematology, D.G. Nathan (ed.), W.B. Saunders Company Ltd. (pubs.), Chapter 8.
2. Shulman HM, Sale GE, Lerner KG (1978) Chronic cutaneous graft-versus-host disease in man. Am J Path 91:545-570.
3. Graze PR, Gale RP (1979) Chronic graft-versus-host disease: A syndrome of disordered immunity. Am J. Med 66:611-620.
4. Korngold R, Sprent J (1978) Lethal graft-versus-host disease after bone marrow transplantation across minor histocompatibility barriers in mice. Prevention by removing mature T cells from marrow. J Exp Med 148: 1687-1698.
5. Korngold R, Sprent J (1983) Lethal graft-versus-host disease across minor histocompatibility barriers in mice. Clin Haematol 12:681-693.
6. Hamilton BL, Brevan MJ, Parkman R (1981) Anti-recipient cytotoxic T lymphocyte precursors are present in the spleen of mice with acute graft-versus-host disease due to minor histocompatibility antigens. J. Immunol 126:621-625.
7. Hamilton BL, Parkman R (1983) Acute and chronic graft-versus-host disease induced by minor histocomaptibility antigens in mice. Transpalntation 36:150-155.
8. Parkman R (1986) Clonal analysis of murine graft-versus-host disease. I. Phenotypic and functional analysis of T lymphocyte clones. J Immunol 136:3543-3548.
9. DeClerck Y, Drpaer V, Parkman R (1986) Clonal analysis of murine graft-versus-host disease. II. Leukokines that stimulate fibroblast proliferation and collagen synthesis in graft-versus-host disease. J Immunol 136:3549-3552.
10. Howard M, Farrar J, Hilfiker M (1982) Identification of a T cell-derived B cell growth factor distinct from interleukin 2. J Exp Med 155:914-923.
11. Roehm NW, Liebson J, Zlotnick A, et al (1984) Interleukin-induced increase in Ia expression by normal mouse B cells. J Exp Med 160: 679-694.
12. Coffman RL, Carty J (1986) A T cell activity that enhances polyclonal IgE production and its inhibition by interferon-gamma. J Immunol 136:949-954.
13. Herzenberg LA, Stall AM, Lalor PA, et al (1986) The Ly-1 B cell lineage. Immunol Rev 93:81-102.
14. Gadol N, Ault KA (1986) Phenotypic and functional characterization of human Leu 1 (CD5) B cells. Immunol Rev 93:21-31.

TABLE 1
CHARACTERISTICS OF T LYMPHOCYTE CLONES DERIVED FROM MICE WITH GVHD

GVHD	PHENOTYPE	SPECIFICITY	IL 2 INDEPENDENCE	FIBROBLAST COLLAGEN PRODUCTION
Chronic	Lyt 2^-, $L3T4^+$ (100%)	Ia^{-b}	3/6	4/9
Acute	Lyt 2^+, $L3T4^+$ (70%)	B6 minor antigens	0/15	2/8
	Lyt 2^-, $L3T4^+$ (30%)	Ia^{-b}	5/6	2/3

26: Predictive Factors for Chronic Graft-versus-Host Disease and Leukemic Relapse After Allogeneic Bone Marrow Transplantation

N. Jacobsen, J.H. Badsberg, B. Lönnqvist, O. Ringdén, L. Volin, T. Ruutu, J. Rajantie, M.A. Siimes, J. Nikoskelainen, A. Toivanen, H.K. Andersen, N. Keiding, and G. Gahrton for the Nordic Bone Marrow Transplantation Group

ABSTRACT

A retrospective multicenter study was carried out in 190 patients who were treated with cyclophosphamide, total body irradiation and allogeneic bone marrow transplantation due to ALL (N=86), AML (N=72), malignant lymphoma (N=6), myelofibrosis (N=2) or CML (N=24). Chronic GvHD occurred in 44 patients. Using Cox multivariate regression analysis with time dependent covariates, donor age >20 years, female donor >20 years to male recipient and preceding acute GvHD were found to predispose for chronic GvHD. When donor age was excluded from the model, cytomegalovirus (CMV) seropositive bone marrow donor was found to be a risk factor for chronic GvHD. However, the donor age effect on chronic GvHD could only in part be explained by an increased ratio of CMV seropositive donors with age.

Posttransplant relapse risk factors were analysed using multivariate analysis in 163 patients with acute leukaemia or malignant lymphoma. Relapse occurred in 36 cases. Disease stage further advanced than 1.remission, transplantation during relapse and donor age >20 years were found to increase the risk of relapse, whereas a protective effect was observed when donor was CMV-seropositive or when using female donor to male recipient.

This study calls for further analyses of donor factors that may determine the risk of complications and relapse after allogeneic bone marrow transplantation.

INTRODUCTION

Chronic Graft-versus-Host Disease (GvHD) is a donor T-lymphocyte mediated systemic inflammatory reaction that may cause severe morbidity and increased mortality after allogeneic bone marrow transplantation (1,2). Several factors have been shown to predispose patients to chronic GvHD: Occurrence of preceding moderate-severe (grade II-IV) acute GvHD, increasing patient age, and posttransplant infusion of unirradiated buff-coat cells obtained from the bone marrow donor (3). More recently, Lönnqvist et al. reported that cytomegalovirus (CMV) infection was associated with and preceded chronic GvHD (4). Furthermore, using univariate analysis, donor CMV seropositivity was found to be a risk factor for chronic GvHD (5).

Patients with acute leukaemia who develop GvHD have a reduced risk of posttransplant relapse suggesting an antileukaemic activity associated with GvHD (6). Furthermore, using univariate analysis, patients with posttransplant CMV infection (7) and AML patients with CMV seropositive donors (8) have been reported to be at decreased risk of relapse.

We here present the results of a retrospective multicenter study using Cox regression analysis of risk factors for chronic GvHD and posttransplant relapse.

METHODS

A consecutive series of 190 allograft recipients was analysed retrospectively in a multicenter study. The median interval from transplantation to either last follow up, leukaemic relapse or death was 281 days (range 12-1960 days). 158 patients had acute leukaemia (AML, N=72, ALL, N=86). Six patients had malignant lymphoma which in all cases had involved the bone marrow. The 164 patients with acute leukaemia or lymphoma were transplanted during induction failure (N=6), 1.remission (N=69), 2.-4. remission (N=72) or 1.-3. relapse (N=16). In one additional case, it was unclear whether the patient had induction failure or was in 1.relapse. 24 patients had CML in chronic or accelerated phase and two patients had myelofibrosis.

All patients received intraveneous chemotherapy, usually cyclophosphamide, 120 mg/kg, followed by total body irradiation (9). Bone marrow cells were obtained from HLA identical, MLC nonreactive siblings (166 cases) or haploidentical family donors (24 cases). No T-cell depletion was employed. Posttransplant methotrexate (N=66), cyclosporine (N=114) or a combination of methotrexate and cyclosporine (N=10) was given as prophylaxis against acute GvHD. Acute and chronic GvHD were diagnosed and graded according to generally accepted criteria (1,9). In the present analysis no distinction was made between limited and extensive chronic GvHD. Donor and recipient sera were studied in each center prior to transplantation with ELISA technique for IgG antibodies to CMV. Criteria for diagnosis of posttransplant CMV infection was based on serologic examinations and/or virus isolation in culture as described previously (10).

STATISTICAL METHODS

The basic response variable was time until occurence of the relevant event (chronic GvHD and relapse respectively). Death, last follow up or (in the analysis of chronic GvHD) relapse was counted as censoring. Multivariate regression analysis was performed according to Cox including pretransplant characteristics as fixed covariates and posttransplant CMV infection as well as acute GvHD as time-dependent covariates. Minimal models were obtained using a modified stepwise procedure, in two cases deliberately excluding a significant covariate (e.g. donor age) in order to identify alternative models of possible biologic or prognostic importance. The Cox regression model expresses the effect of each covariate on the intensity (event/time unit) as a multiplicative intensity factor $e^{\beta 1}$. The intensity factors are quoted below together with corresponding P values which pertain to a test concerning exclusion of the relevant covariates given all other retained (11).

RESULTS AND DISCUSSION

Correlations were observed between donor and patient ages. Furthermore, the proportion of CMV seropositive individuals increased with the age.

Chronic GvHD occurred in 44 of 190 patients and was diagnosed between 70 and 400 days (median 135 days) after transplantation. The overall probability at 500 days was 34%. Using multivariate Cox regression analysis risk factors for chronic GvHD could be described by the following model:

	Factor	
Donor >20 yrs	2.6	P=0.01
Female >20 yrs to male	2.9	P=0.003
Preceding acute GvHD (gr.II-IV)	1.9	P=0.04

In this model the following factors did not influence the probability of chronic GvHD: Patient age, underlying disease, stage of disease, patient CMV immune status, posttransplant CMV infection, HLA mismatch, male-to-female transplantation and type of GvHD prophylaxis.

Thus, the study showed that donor age had a marked influence on the incidence of chronic GvHD but failed to confirm an effect of patient age. This observation is in contrast to results obtained by others (3) and suggests that the cellular composition of the graft may be much more important than environmental recipient factors.

Female donor to male recipient has been found to predispose for acute GvHD, but has not previously been described as a risk factor for chronic GvHD (12,13). This factor was associated with an increased chronic GvHD incidence even in models including acute GvHD, indicating that even when the female-to-male effect on the incidence of acute GvHD was taken into account, a separate strong effect on the risk of chronic GvHD was observed. This effect may be due to an immunologic reaction against the Hy antigen of male recipients (14). Female donor to male recipient was a risk factor only when the donor was more than 20 years old. One possible explanation is that presensitation against Hy antigen through pregnancies with male fetus had taken place in a larger proportion of these donors.

Since donor age was correlated to seropositive CMV immune status, which was a significant risk factor for chronic GvHD in univariate analysis (5), we tested the hypothesis that the CMV immune status of the donor was the determinant that predisposed recipients from older donors for chronic GvHD. In a second model excluding the donor age, CMV seropositive donor was found to be associated with a marked increase in the chronic GvHD incidence:

	Factor	
Donor CMV seropositive	2.7	P=0.002
Female-to-male	2.5	P=0.003
Preceding acute GvHD (gr.II-IV)	2.2	P=0.01

Possible explanations for this association have been discussed previously (5). Briefly, this association could be due to cross-reactions between viral and (minor) transplantation antigens or to non-specific immune stimulation or failure to establish tolerance as a result of a donor cell mediated anti-CMV immune reaction. In this context it is of interest that an increased number of CD8+ HNK1+ T cells has been found in bone marrow obtained from CMV seropositive donors (15). CMV-seropositive donor is a risk factor for posttransplant CMV-infection in seronegative patients (16). This raised the question whether post-transplant CMV infection per se induced chronic GvHD, as indicated by a previous study by the Swedish group (4). However, with the statistical methods used in the present analysis, CMV infection could not be shown to be a risk factor for chronic GvHD.

Likelihood ratio tests indicated that the first model offered a better description of chronic GvHD risk factors than the second model.An interpretation of this is that other donor age-related factors than CMV seropositivity,such as presensitation against other antigens, played an additional role for the development of chronic GvHD.

As an extension of the present analysis, we have studied risk factors for post-transplant leukaemic relapse in 163 recipients with acute leukaemia or malignant lymphoma, in whom the stage of disease at the time of transplantation could be accurately determined.Thirtysix of 163 patients with acute leukaemia or malignant lymphoma had posttransplant relapse, which occurred between 15 and 1005 (median 197) days after transplantation.

The following factors were found by multivariate analysis to influence the risk of posttransplant relapse:

	Factor	
BMT later than 1.remission	8.9	P<0.001
BMT during relapse	5.0	P=0.006
Donor >20 yrs	3.7	P=0.005
Donor CMV seropositive	0.18	P=0.002
Chronic GvHD	0.07	P=0.001

In this model the following factors had no influence on the risk of relapse: Patient age, underlying disease, patient CMV immune status, posttransplant CMV infection, HLA mismatch, female donor to male recipient, other sex combinations, acute GvHD and type of GvHD prophylaxis.

Thus, the most important predictive factors for posttransplant relapse were transplantation at a disease stage later than 1.remission and during relapse (17-20). Furthermore, the analysis supported the notion that the occurrence of chronic GvHD was associated with a decreased posttransplant relapse probability (6). Morover, a marked reduction of the risk of posttransplant relapse was observed in recipients with CMV seropositive donors, even in a model that included chronic GvHD and donor age. As with respect to chronic GvHD, the effect of immune donors was apparently not mediated through increased occurrence of CMV infection, since posttransplant infection was not a risk factor. Finally, donor age per se had an adverse effect by increasing the relapse risk after transplantation.

In a model excluding chronic GvHD, female donor (irrespectively of age) to male recipient was found to be an additional protective factor against posttransplant relapse (factor 0.28, P<0.008).

CONCLUSION

This study has demonstrated

1. Donor age and female donor to male recipient are important predisposing factors for chronic GvHD.
2. Donor CMV immune status may in part be the factor that determines recipients with older donors for chronic GvHD.
3. Donor CMV immunity significantly reduces the risk of posttransplant relapse even in a Cox model including chronicGvHD.
4. Female donor to male recipient is a proxy for chronic GvHD that predicts continuous posttransplant remission.
5. Donor age >20 years predisposes for relapse.

ACKNOWLEDGEMENTS

Supported by Danish Medical Research Council (12-6591), The Danish Cancer Society (87-286), The Swedish medical Research Council, The Swedish Cancer Society and by Sigrid Juselius Foundation, Finland.

REFERENCES

1. Shulman HM, Sullivan KM, Weiden PL et al (1980) Chronic graft-versus-host syndrome in man. A long-term clinico-pathologic study of 20 Seattle patients. Am J Med 69:204-217
2. Sullivan KM, Shulman HM, Storb R et al (1981) Chronic graft-versus-host disease in 52 patients:Adverse natural course and successful treatment with combination immunosuppression. Blood 57:267-276
3. Storb R, Prentice RL, Sullivan KM et al (1983) Predictive factors in chronic graft-versus-host disease in patients with aplastic anaemia treated by marrow transplantation from HLA-identical siblings. Ann Intern Med 98:461-466
4. Lönnqvist B, Ringdén O, Wahren B, Gahrton G et al (1984) Cytomegalovirus infection associated with and preceding chronic graft-versus-host disease. Transplantation 38:465-468

5. Jacobsen N, Andersen HK, Skinhøj P et al (1986) Correlation between donor cytomegalovirus immunity and chronic graft-versus-host disease after allogeneic bone marrow transplantation. Scand J Haematol 36:499-506
6. Weiden PL, Sullivan KM, Flournoy N et al (1981) Antileukemic effect of chronic graft-versus-host disease. Contribution to improved survival after allogeneic marrow transplantation. N Engl J Med 304:1529-1533
7. Lönnqvist B, Ringdén O, Ljungman P et al (1986) Reduced risk of recurrent leukaemia in bone marrow transplant recipients after cytomegalovirus infection. Brit J Haematol 63:671-679
8. Jacobsen N, Keiding N, Ryder L et al (1987) Graft-versus-leukaemia activity associated with cytomegalovirus antibody positive bone marrow donors in acute myeloid leukaemia (letter) Lancet 1:456-457
9. Thomas ED, Storb R, Clift RA et al (1975) Bone marrow transplantation. N Engl J Med 292:832-843, 895-902
10. Jacobsen N, Lönnqvist B Ringdén O et al (1987) Graft-versus-leukaemia activity associated with cytomegalovirus seropositive bone marrow donors but separated from graft-versus-host disease in allograft recipients with AML. Eur J Haematol 38:350-355
11. Kalbfleisch JD, Prentice RL (1980) The statistical analysis of failure time data. New York: Wiley
12. Atkinson K, Farrell C, Chapman G et al (1986) Female marrow donors increase the risk of acute graft-versus-host disease: Effect of donor age and parity and analysis of cell subpopulations in the donor marrow inoculum. Brit J Haematol 63:231-239
13. Gale RP (1986) Acute graft-vs-host disease in humans: Prognostic factors. Exp Haematol 14:430
14. Goulmy E, Blokland E, Bradley BA et al (1977) Y-antigen killing by T-cells of women is restricted by HLA. Nature 266:544-545
15. Gratama JW, Fibbe WE, Naipal AMIH et al (1986) Cytomegalovirus immunity and T lymphocytes in bone marrow donors and acute graft-versus-host disease. Bone Marrow Transplantation 1:141-146
16. Meyers JD, Flournoy N, Thomas ED (1986) Risk factors for cytomegalovirus infection after human marrow transplantation. J Infect Dis 153: 478-488
17. Zwaan FE, Hermans J, Barrett AJ et al (1984) Bone marrow transplantation for acute nonlymphoblastic leukaemia: A survey of the European group for bone marrow transplantation (EGBMT). Brit J Haematol 56:645-653
18. Zwaan FE, Hermans J, Barrett AJ et al (1984) Bone marrow transplantation for acute lymphoblastic leukaemia: A survey of the European group for bone marrow transplantation (EGBMT). Brit J Haematol 58:33-42
19. Gale RP, Kay HEM, rimm AA et al (1982) Bone marrow transplantation for acute leukaemia in first remission. Lancet 2:1006-1009
20. Gale RP, Kersey JH, Bortin MM et al (1983) Bone marrow transplantation for acute lymphoblastic leukaemia. Lancet 2:663-667

IX. Infections After Bone Marrow Transplants: W.H. Burns and V. Rizzoli, Chairpersons

27: Viral Infection Following Bone Marrow Transplantation

William H. Burns and John R. Wingard

Virus infections, along with graft-versus-host disease (GVHD), are a major impediment to the success of allogeneic bone marrow transplantation (BMT). The list of viruses often infecting these patients is long. The herpesviruses infect patients following transplant in a manner temporally related to the time of transplant (1) and form the basis of this report.

HERPES SIMPLEX VIRUS

Reactivated herpes simplex virus (HSV) infections previously occurred in 70% of seropositive BMT patients with occasional mortality. These infections have been essentially eliminated during the initial inpatient stay by the use of intravenous (2) or oral (3) acyclovir (ACV) prophylaxis, usually beginning several days prior to transplant and given in our unit until hospital discharge. We have no evidence that this approach results in emergence of resistant HSV. On the contrary, we have argued that the suppression of HSV before reactivation, at a time of minimal numbers of replicating viral genomes, will result in selection of resistant virus less frequently than initiating therapy after infection is established (4). We have treated several hundred BMT patients with close to 100% efficacy and had no emergent resistant virus during prophylaxis. We have isolated six resistant HSV isolates from BMT patients after the transplant when they were being treated for established HSV infections (4,5). These infections were generally mild and none were fatal. In one case, four months after resolution of the resistant HSV infection, the patient reactivated his original sensitive virus. All resistant isolates had mutations in the thymidine kinase (TK) structural gene or sequences that control its expression and detailed enzymatic studies of the thymidine kinases of three of these isolates indicated that mutations can result in alterations in either the amount of TK produced or in changes in the affinity for thymidine or antiviral analogues (6). Interestingly, studies in collaboration with G. Hayward comparing endonuclease restriction cleavage patterns have shown that the resistant HSV isolates from 3 of the 6 patients probably represent different virus from the original sensitive isolates (7).

In conclusion, HSV infections are no longer a clinical problem for BMT patients in the early transplant period if ACV prophylaxis is provided. Later HSV infections have not resulted in emergence of resistant virus and usually resolve with or without ACV treatment as the patients are more immunocompetent at that time than in the first few weeks following BMT. Resistant virus has been isolated after ACV treatment of established infections but such infections usually have been mild. In some cases the resistant isolates represent a different virus from the original isolate and subsequent reactivation may occur with the original sensitive virus.

CYTOMEGALOVIRUS

Historically, cytomegalovirus (CMV) has been the most important pathogen following BMT, causing a usually fatal interstitial pneumonitis (IP) and accounting for the deaths of approximately 15% of all allogeneic transplant patients. Although much has been learned about the epidemiology and predisposing factors of CMV IP in this patient population, many aspects of its pathogenesis are still unclear. Certain clinical observations, such as the timing of the syndrome post transplant, the predilection of the virus for the lungs, the predisposing influence of the allogeneic state and acute GVHD and the importance of the mode of virus acquisition, must be addressed in any comprehensive description of the pathogenesis of the syndrome. In addition, factors to explain recent changes in the epidemiology of the syndrome should be sought to provide a logical basis to further control of occurrence of the syndrome.

The experience of the Seattle group with CMV IP has been reported with the most recent published analysis of 952 allogeneic recipients through 1982 (8). The incidence of CMV IP was 15% overall and 17% in the leukemia patients. In their multivariate analysis, they identified predisposing factors included the diagnosis of leukemia, increasing age, the use of cytotoxic agents other than cyclophosphamide in the leukemia conditioning regimen, acute GVHD, and seropositivity before transplant. We recently analyzed our experience with 386 allogeneic patients through October, 1985. Our overall incidence of CMV IP was 12% and our multivariate analysis also indicated that a diagnosis of leukemia, age, acute GVHD, CMV excretion, and seropositivity were important predictors for the syndrome. As had been reported by the International Bone Marrow Transplant Registry (9), we also found that the use of cyclosporine A rather than other agents for GVHD prophylaxis decreased the risk for CMV IP.

However, two surprising new observations emerged. First, we have had a marked decrease in the incidence of CMV IP (but not idiopathic IP) from 1983 to the present. In fact, as of June, 1987, we have experienced only 1 case of CMV IP in 186 allogeneic recipients in the past 3 years. Possible explanations for this decline include more effective prevention of severe acute GVHD, the use of high dose ACV (500 mg/m2 every 8 hours intravenously) prophylactically for CMV seropositive recipients, and the use of seronegative blood products for seronegative recipients having seronegative BM donors. However, the high dose ACV prophylaxis was begun in April, 1984 and the incidence of CMV IP in seropositive patients had already begun to decrease before that time. The policy of furnishing seronegative blood products was instituted in November, 1983, and obviously applies only to seronegative recipients. Currently, we favor the decrease in severe GVHD as probably the most important factor for the dramatic decrease in CMV IP.

The second surprising observation was our finding that only 1 of 115 seronegative allogeneic recipients developed CMV IP. Sixty-eight (59%) of these patients did not receive screened blood products. Although the recent Seattle report had clearly demonstrated the advantage of the seronegative state prior to BMT (13% incidence of CMV IP versus 21% for seropositive recipients), we were struck by our incidence of 2% in seronegative recipients receiving unscreened blood products (and 0% in those receiving screened blood products). It is difficult to know why our results are so different. One possibility is that the ELISA assay we use is more sensitive than the complement fixation assay used earlier in Seattle and that false seronegative patients are included in their seronegative group. Their finding that 56% of their patients were seronegative compared to 26% of our allogeneic patients prior to 1983 suggests that the serological assays do have different sensitivities, or there is always the possibility that the two centers are dealing with very different patient populations in re CMV status. In any case, our data clearly indicate that patients reactivating the virus endogenously are at much higher risk of developing CMV IP than are those acquiring the virus exogenously (from blood products), and this finding must be included in pathogenetic considerations.

Although epidemological observations and the recognition of risk factors have provided valuable insights concerning CMV IP in BMT patients, many aspects of its pathogenesis are poorly understood. The allogeneic setting and acute GVHD are important risk factors. CMV IP occurs historically in about 15% of allogeneic patients but only rarely in syngeneic patients and in only 2% (3 of 143) of our autologous BMT patients and 4% of 70 autologous patients reported by Seattle (10). Previous suggestions that allogeneic stimulation might increase virus activation are not supported by our finding that CMV excretion was the same (about 30% of patients) regardless of GVHD status and excretion rates were similar in autologous and syngeneic BMT patients. It is clear that virological factors alone do not explain the syndrome and GVHD is probably having its influence through mechanisms other than virus activation.

Immunological factors are of obvious importance. The capacity to mount a lymphocyte-mediated cytotoxic response, particularly an HLA-restricted T cell response, is an important determinant of survival from CMV infections (11,12). Patients developing acute GVHD are thought to have abnormal or inappropriately regulated immune responses and also receive additional prophylaxis and therapeutic immunosuppression. The form of immunosuppression varies at different transplant centers and we and others (9) have found the use of cyclosporine prophylaxis lowers the risk of CMV IP. Whether this is due to better GVHD control or other factors is not clear. It is difficult to relate these findings to the pathogenesis of CMV IP in a specific mechanistic way since few experimental studies in animal models have addressed these issues. Immunosuppression per se is not the only immunological factor involved since the syndrome does not develop in the period of greatest immunosuppression but as the immune system reconstitutes. Other immunological factors could include thymic injury from GVHD and the possibility that target cells for virus replication may be more virogenic in this environment, as is the case for mouse hepatitis virus replication in macrophages taken from a thymic-deficient environment (13). The role of physical damage to the lung by the conditioning regimen is also unclear.

In the past we have hypothesized that the clinical syndrome of CMV IP results from the timing and extent of virus replication in the lung and the timing and strength of the lymphocyte-mediated responses (14). A strong cell-mediated response at a time when virus replication in the lung is limited would result in a small immunopathological effect and control of the infection whereas a response at a later time, at which widespread infection in the lung is present, would result in extensive immunologically mediated pathology and disruption of normal pulmonary physiology. Similar views have been put forth by Zaia (15) and others and finds some support in the work of Shanley showing that continuous immunosuppression with cyclophosphamide can ameliorate CMV pneumonia despite increased viral replication in the lung in a mouse model (16). To explain the timing of CMV IP, we have also postulated that CMV may have enhanced replication in early myeloid cells and travel to the lung post-transplant by infected monocytes that then differentiate into alveolar macrophages and spread infection throughout the lung. Replication of CMV in human alveolar macrophages has been reported (17) but there has been no comparison of the CMV replicative capacity of alveolar macrophages from normal and immunosuppressed subjects.

In conclusion, CMV IP at our institution has diminished in importance from causing the death of approximately 15% of allogeneic patients to less than 1%. There is a significant correlation of the allogeneic setting and development of acute GVHD with the presence of this syndrome but the pathogenetic mechanism is unclear. Acute GVHD does not appear to cause activation of CMV in our patient population. The mode of virus acquisition is important with very few pre-BMT seronegative patients developing the syndrome, whether or not they seroconvert or excrete CMV post-transplant. Currently, the provision of seronegative blood products to seronegative recipients is feasible and at our institution prevents exposure to the virus in 95% of BMT patients so maintained. Although this has little influence on the development of CMV IP (since seronegative recipients seldom develop CMV IP), it may decrease the morbidity associated with CMV infection. The use of high dose ACV in seropositive patients may have a beneficial effect in lowering the incidence of CMV IP, but more effective control and prevention of acute GVHD and the use of cyclosporine may be more important factors.

VARICELLA-ZOSTER VIRUS

Reports from Seattle (18,19) and Stockholm (20) indicate that 30 to 40% of allogeneic patients develop zoster during the first year after transplant. This is consistent with our experience in which 65 of 188 (35%) of allogeneic patients transplanted from 1983 through mid-1986 developed reactivated zoster during the first year after BMT. Interestingly, only 7 of 124 (6%) autologous patients during that period developed zoster. Although prompt intravenous ACV treatment has been shown to be effective in zoster infections in the immunocompromised host (21), many of our patients develop zoster after returning home where it is sometimes not immediately recognized, resulting in delayed treatment. Despite marked decrease in virus isolation and shortening of the period to healing in ACV treated patients, relapses within two months often occurs (16%) in BMT patients and considerable morbidity may remain post-infection despite the treatment (19).

For these reasons a prophylaxis approach seems warranted. The use of oral ACV on a chronic basis to prevent VZV infection has several potential problems including the low serum concentrations achieved by oral ACV administration. Even so, during the six months of oral ACV administration to prevent HSV infections in BMT patients in Sweden, zoster was also prevented in these patients but not in the placebo-controlled patients (20). However, after ACV was discontinued these patients developed zoster at the expected rate so that overall the prophylaxed and untreated patients developed zoster with similar incidences although it was delayed in the former. A longer treatment period may be more effective in preventing zoster, but this approach may lead to an immunologically naive state for VZV and possibly more serious infection on later reactivation.

Hope-Simpson has hypothesized that the immune state following VZV infection is characterized by recurrent immune stimulation due to repeated subclinical reactivations of the virus from its latent state in dorsal root ganglia (22). Meyers suggested that the recovery of lymphocyte proliferation responses to VZV antigen after BMT in patients without zoster is due to subclinical virus reactivation (23). Strong support for the occurrence of subclinical reactivation of VZV following BMT and the role it plays in achieving effective immunity against VZV comes from the Swedish study (20). None of 19 BMT patients with evidence of subclinical reactivation (5-fold IgG titer rise to VZV and/or significant VZV antigen-induced lymphocyte proliferation) subsequently developed zoster whereas 26 of 54 patients without evidence of subclinical reactivation developed zoster. Although the number of patients was too small to draw firm conclusions, ACV prophylaxis appeared to reduce the occurrence of subclinical reactivation during its administration and resulted in diminished subsequent protection. Other studies have shown decreased humoral responses to HSV in patients treated with ACV for primary infection (24,25), and decreased cell-mediated responses to HSV following ACV prophylaxis for HSV in BMT patients (26).

These studies provide a basis for caution in considering longterm ACV administration to prevent VZV post-BMT. Without viral antigen stimulation, the VZV-specific memory lymphocytes adoptively transferred to the recipient from a seropositive host may diminish in number and leave the recipient in an immunologically naive state for VZV. In adults this may result in a "primary" infection from an exogenous source or after reactivation of the virus with serious consequences or mortality. An immunoprophylaxis approach may therefore be desirable and the use of an appropriate vaccine considered. The Oka live vaccine has been used safely in children undergoing chemotherapy for leukemia (27), but the use of a live vaccine in the BMT setting, particularly near the time of transplant, has not previously been recommended. In this case untoward replication and dissemination of the vaccine virus could be treated with ACV, but subunit vaccines using appropriate antigens produced through DNA recombinant techniques should also be considered.

EPSTEIN-BARR VIRUS

Over the past few years we have determined the serological status of 205 BMT patients and found 80% to be seropositive for prior Epstein-Barr virus (EBV) infection. Lymphocyte transformation assays or DNA hybridization techniques (28) were employed and 60% of 200 patients had at least one positive saliva sample positive for EBV and 42% had more than one weekly sample positive. No clinical correlations with demographic factors, hepatitis, pneumonitis, neurological complications or GVHD have been made, although the analysis has not been completed. Thus, although EBV infection is a common post-transplant event, clinical sequelae have not been associated with it except under special circumstances in which immunoblastic lymphomas have occurred.

HUMAN B LYMPHOTROPIC VIRUS

In 1986 a new herpesvirus joined the ranks of known human herpesviruses (29). During their search for human retroviruses in fresh peripheral blood mononuclear cell cultures from six patients with various lymphoproliferative disorders, investigators at the NIH noted the appearance of large, refractile cells in the primary cultures. A transmissible agent producing this cytopathic effect was isolated from these cultures and antibody from certain patients was found that could neutralize this agent and by immunofluorescence could be used to detect infection of freshly isolated B lymphocytes. A double stranded DNA virus was isolated and found to have characteristic herpesvirus morphology by electron microscopy and to be immunologically (29) and genetically (30) distinct from the four previously known human herpesviruses. Furthermore, sera against herpesviruses of Old World and New World primates failed to react with the virus. The virus therefore does not appear to be a newly acquired infection from lower primates. In a preliminary screening, sera from 4 of 220 healthy individuals were positive for antibody to the virus. With the high incidence of serious herpesvirus infections already documented post-BMT, an apparent 2% incidence of previous HBLV infection in the general population, and the large number of BMT patients being transplanted for lymphoproliferative malignancies, it is probable that there will be a significant incidence of HBLV infections of patients post-BMT.

In a preliminary survey in collaboration with Dr. R. Gallo's laboratory at the NIH, we found 5 of 22 selected patient pre-BMT sera were strongly positive for antibody to HBLV. This indicates that a significant number of BMT patients have had previous exposure to this virus prior to transplant. A comprehensive investigation of infection of these patients by HBLV is underway.

REFERENCES

1. Saral R, Burns WH, Prentice HG (1984) Herpes virus infections: clinical manifestations and therapeutic strategies in immunocompromised patients. Clin Haematol 13:645-59

2. Saral R, Burns WH, Laskin OL, Santos GW, Lietman PS (1981) Acyclovir prophylaxis of herpes-simplex-virus infections A randomized, double-blind, controlled trial in bone marrow transplant recipients. N Engl J Med 305:63-7

3. Wade JC, Newton B, Flournoy N, Meyers JD (1982) Oral acyclovir prophylaxis of herpes simplex virus infecitons after marrow transplant. Intersci Conf Antimicrob Ag Chemother 98

4. Ambinder RF, Burns WH, Lietman PS, Saral R (1984) Prophylaxis: A strategem to minimize antiviral resistance. Lancet i:1154-55

5. Burns WH, Saral R, Santos GW, Laskin OL, Lietman PS, McLaren C, Barry DW (1982) Isolation and characterization of resistant herpes simplex virus following acyclovir therapy. Lancet i:421-3

6. McLaren C, Chen MS, Ghazzouli I, Saral R, Burns WH (1985) Drug resistance patterns of herpex simplex virus isolates from patients treated with acyclovir. Antimicrob Ag Chemother 28:740-4

7. Hayward GS, Ambinder R, Ciufo D, Hayward SD, LaFemina RL (1984) Structural organization of human herpesvirus DNA molecules. J Invest Dermatol 83:29s-41s

8. Meyers JD, Flournoy N, Wade JC, Hackman RC, McDougall JK, Thomas ED (1983) Biology of interstitial pneumonia after marrow transplantation. In: Recent Advances in Bone Marrow Transplantation, pp 405-23

9. Weiner RS, Bortin MM, Gale RP, Gluckman E, Kay HEM, Kolb H-J, Hartz AJ, Rimm AA (1986) Interstitial pneumonitis after bone marrow transplantation. Ann Int Med 104:168-75

10. Pecego R, Hill R, Appelbaum FR, Amso D, Buckner CD, Fefer A, Thomas ED (1986) Interstitial pneumonitis following autologous bone marrow transplantation. Transplantation 42:515-7

11. Quinnan GV, Kirmani N, Rook A, Manischewitz JF, Jackson L, Moreschi G, Santos GW, Saral R, Burns WH (1982) Cytotoxic T cells in cytomegalovirus infection HLA-restricted T-lymphocyte and non-T lymphocyte cytoxic responses correlate with recovery from cytomegalovirus infection in bone marrow transplant recipients. N Engl J Med 307:6-13

12. Quinnan GV, Burns WH, Kirmani N, Rook AH, Manischewitz J, Jackson L, Santos GW, Saral R (1984) HLA-restricted cytotoxic T-lymphocytes are an early immune response and important defense mechanism in cytomegalovirus infections. Rev Infec Dis 6:156-63

13. Allison AC (1965) Genetic factors in resistance against virus infections. Arch Ges Virusforsch 17:280-94

14. Burns WH, Saral R (1985) Opportunistic viral infections Br Med Bull 41:46-9

15. Zaia JA (1986) The biology of human cytomegalovirus infection after bone marrow transpsantation Int J Cell Clon 4:135-54

16. Shanley JD, Pesanti EL, Nugent KM (1982) The pathogenesis of pneumonitis due to murine cytomegalovirus. J Infect Dis 146:388-96

17. Drew WL, Mintz L, Hoo R, Finley TN (1979) Growth of herpes simplex and cytomegalovirus in cultured human alveolar macrophages. Ann Rev Respir Dis 119:287-91

18. Atkinson K, Meyers JD, Storb R, Prentice RL, Thomas ED (1980) Varicella zoster virus infection after marrow transplantation for aplastic anemia or leukemia. Transplantation 29:47-50

19. Locksley RM, Flournoy N, Sullivan KM, Meyers JM (1985) Infection with varicella-zoster virus after marrow transplantation. J Infec Dis 152:1172-81

20. Ljungman P, Lonnqvist B, Gahrton G, Ringden O, Sundqvist V-A, Wahren B (1986) Clinical and sub-clinicial reactivations of varicella-zoster virus in immuno-compromised patients. J Infec Dis 153:840-7

21. Meyers JD, Wade JC, Shepp DH, Newton B (1984) Acyclovir treatment of varicella-zoster virus infection in the immunocompromised host. Transplantation 37:571-4

22. Hope-Simpson RE (1965) The nature of herpes zoster: a long term study and a new hypothesis. Proceedings of the Royal Society of Medicine 58:9-20

23. Meyers JD, Flournoy N, Thomas ED (1980) Cell-mediated immunity to varicella-zoster virus after allogeneic marrow transplant. J Infect Dis 141:479-87

24. Bernstein DJ, Lovett MA, Bryson YJ (1984) The effects of acyclovir on antibody response to herpes simplex virus in primary genital herpetic infections. J Infec Dis 150:7-13

25. Ashley RL, Corey L (1984) Effect of acyclovir treatment of primary genital herpes on the antibody response to herpes simplex virus. J Clin Invest 73:681-8

26. Wade JC, Day LM, Crowley JJ, Meyers JD (1984) Recurrent infection with herpes simplex virus after marrow transplantation: role of the specific immune response and acyclovir treatment. J Infect Dis 149:750-6

27. Gershon AA (1985) Perspective: Live attenuated varicella zoster. J Infec Dis 152:859-75

28. Ambinder RF, Wingard JR, Burns WH, Hayward SD, Saral R, Chin G, Perry HR, Santos GW, Hayward GS (1985) Detection of Epstein-Barr virus DNA in mouthwashes by hybridization. J Clin Microbiol 21:353-6

29. Salahuddin SZ, Ablashi DV, Markham PD, Josephs SF, Sturzenegger S, Kaplan M, Halligan G, Biberfeld P, Wong-Staal F, Kramarsky B, Gallo RC (1986) Isolation of a new virus, HBLV, in patients with lymphoproliferative disorders. Science 234:595-601

30. Josephs SF, Salahuddin SZ, Ablashi DV, Schachter F, Wong-Staal F, Gallo RC (1986) Genomic analysis of the human B-lymphotropic virus (HBLV). Science 234:601-3

28: Bacterial, Fungal, and Protozoan Infection After Marrow Transplantation

Joel Meyers, Finn B. Petersen, George W. Counts, Elizabeth C. Reed, Shawn J. Skerrett, Raleigh A. Bowden, Keith Sullivan, and C. Dean Buckner

INTRODUCTION

Bacterial, fungal, and occasionally protozoal infection continue to be important complications of marrow transplantation. Although bacterial infection as a primary cause of death is rare, such infection may add substantially to the morbidity and cost of transplantation. Moreover, bacterial infection is an important concomitant of both the treatment and outcome of acute graft versus host disease (GVHD). Fungal infection occurs less commonly than bacterial infection, but with a higher case fatality rate. Some fungi such as Aspergillus have emerged as frequent causes of death in individual transplant units [1]. The incidence of both bacterial and fungal infection is likely to increase in the future due to the increasing use of marrow purging (i.e. T-cell depletion) or autologous marrow storage, with a longer duration of neutropenia in some patients, and use of 2- or 3-antigen mismatched donors with an increased likelihood of acute GVHD.

Empiric and directed therapy of bacterial infection continues to evolve, with availability over the last few years of new antibacterial agents with a sufficiently broad spectrum of activity to be useful in "monotherapy" regimens. Despite the availability of these more potent antibiotics, prevention of infection remains a major goal, both to reduce morbidity and the occasional fatality due to infection and because of the putative relationship between bacterial colonization or infection and GVHD. Previous studies have established the efficacy of both the total protective environment and prophylactic granulocyte transfusions for infection prevention after marrow transplant [2,3], although not all studies of prophylactic granulocytes showed such benefit [4]. Among the newer approaches to infection prevention is selective decontamination. Orally administered quinolone antibiotics are being used for selective decontamination in some centers [5]. Passive immunoprophylaxis with immunoglobulins is another newer (or newly rediscovered) modality for infection prevention. This may have particular relevance to infections occurring among patients with chronic GVHD, in whom immunoglobulin levels are low and who become infected with organisms against which opsonization is an important host defense [6,7].

The risk of bacterial and fungal infection after marrow transplant can be divided into 3 phases: 1) The early neutropenic period extending to approximately 20 days after transplant except in patients with delayed engraftment (e.g. autologous or T-depleted transplants) or with graft failure or rejection. 2) The period of acute GVHD extending to approximately 90 days after transplant during which bacterial and fungal infections occur both as a concomitant of GVHD and associated with other iatrogenic risk factors such as the long-term intravenous catheter. 3) Infection in long-term survivors associated almost universally with chronic GVHD and its treatment. This review will focus on our recent experience with infection occurring in the first 2 time periods after marrow transplant.

BACTERIAL INFECTION

During the Neutropenic Period

Buckner et al. [8] and Navari et al. [9] summarized the experience with

Table 1. Comparison of the Protective Environment and Prophylactic Granulocyte Transfusions among Patients Transplanted for Acute Leukemia: Infection Before Engraftment*

	Protective Environment	Prophylactic Granulocytes
Patient Number	90	92
Local Infection	11 (.12)	6 (.07)
Bacteremia/Fungemia	14 (.16)	11 (.12)

*to a neutrophil count of 500/cu mm.
From Buckner et al. [8].

bacterial and fungal infections and the use of the protective environment and prophylactic granulocyte transfusions among patients transplanted for acute leukemia and aplastic anemia, respectively, during 1976 to 1980. The incidence of bacteremia or fungemia before engraftment averaged 14% (39 of 282) among patients transplanted for either aplastic anemia or leukemia. Among patients with leukemia, there was no difference between the protective environment and use of prophylactic granulocytes (Table 1). Among patients transplanted for aplastic anemia, less infection occurred among those transplanted in the protective environment whereas patients transplanted in conventional rooms without special infection prevention procedures developed both local major infections and bacteremia or fungemia more commonly (Table 2). In both studies, the most common blood isolate was coagulase-negative *Staphylococcus*, representing 10 of 27 (37%) isolates during the neutropenic period. Gram-positive organisms comprised 58% of all blood isolates, whereas aerobic Gram-negative organisms (31%) and *Pseudomonas* species (6%) in particular were less common.

Between 1981 and 1984, four methods of infection prevention were compared in 234 patients undergoing allogeneic transplant for hematologic malignancy [10,11]. In addition to the protective environment and use of prophylactic granulocyte transfusions, some patients received "prophylactic systemic antibiotics" (PSA) which were broad-spectrum intravenous antibiotics (usually an antipseudomonal penicillin and an aminoglycoside with or without vancomycin) given from the time the absolute neutrophil count decreased to less than 500/cu mm until the time that the neutrophil was again greater than 500. PSA was given both in conventional rooms and in the protective environment in these studies. The combination of the protective environment and PSA was associated with the lowest incidence of both local major infections and bacteremia, with only 4 episodes of bacteremia or fungemia among 54 patients receiving both modalities (Table 3). In contrast, patients receiving PSA in conventional rooms had slightly more bacteremia but fewer local major infections than patients receiving prophylactic granulocytes. There was a suggestion of more fungemia among patients receiving PSA in conventional rooms (5 of 45 patients, 11%) compared to all other groups (5 of 189, 3%). Otherwise, Gram-positive organisms again represented the most common isolates in all patients (27 of 45 isolates, 60%), with an even higher incidence of coagulase-negative *Staphylococcus* bacteremia (67% of isolates) among patients receiving prophylactic granulocyte transfusions.

The combination of the protective environment and PSA is the most effective approach to infection prevention studied in this unit. Prophylactic granulocytes appear to offer no advantage versus other methods of infection prevention and their prophylactic use has been discontinued for a variety of reasons including transmission of cytomegalovirus (CMV) infection and complications in the donor [11,12].

Table 2. Transplantation for Aplastic Anemia: Influence of the Protective Environment (PE), Prophylactic Granulocytes (PG) and Conventional Treatment (CT) on Infection Before Engraftment*

Infection Prevention Modality	Total Patient Number	Local Major Infection	Bacteremia/ Fungemia
PE	36	1 (.03)	2 (.06)
PG	33	5 (.15)	4 (.12)
CT	31	6 (.19)	8 (.26)

*to a neutrophil count of 500/cu mm.
From Navari et al. [9].

Table 3. Protective Environment (PE), Prophylactic Granulocytes (PG) and Prophylactic Systemic Antibiotics (PSA) for Infection Prevention Before Engraftment* Among Patients with Hematologic Malignancy

Infection Prevention Modality	Total Patient Number	Local Major Infection	Bacteremia/ Fungemia
PE + PSA	54	4 (.07)	3 (.06)
PE alone	68	13 (.19)	12 (.18)
PSA alone	45	9 (.20)	11 (.24)
PG	67	17 (.25)	13 (.19)

*to a neutrophil count of 500/cu mm.
Adapted from Petersen et al. [10,11].

Table 4. Influence of Infection Prevention Modalities on Infection after Engraftment*

Infection Prevention Modality	Total Patient Number	Local Major Infection	Bacteremia/ Fungemia
A. Patients with Acute Leukemia			
PE	86	9 (.10)	10 (.12)
PG	86	9 (.10)	10 (.12)
B. Patients with Aplastic Anemia			
PE	35	0	0
PG	32	5 (.16)	5 (.16)
CT	30	8 (.27)	5 (.17)

*from engraftment to day 100.
See Table 2 for abbreviations.
From Buckner et al. [8] and Navari et al. [9].

Infection After Engraftment

The risk of bacterial and fungal infection persists after initial engraftment. Moreover, the incidence of bacteremia and fungemia after engraftment is approximately equal to the incidence before engraftment, albeit over a longer time period (Table 4). Infection occurs commonly but not exclusively among patients with acute GVHD. Interestingly, patients transplanted for aplastic anemia in the protective environment had significantly fewer major local infections and less bacteremia or fungemia even after engraftment compared with patients who either received prophylactic granulocytes or who were treated in conventional rooms (Table 4) [9]. This apparent benefit of the protective environment after engraftment was not observed among patients transplanted for acute leukemia (Table 4) [8].

As in the pre-engraftment period, bacterial infection was most commonly due to Gram-positive organisms. In a review of complications associated with long-term Hickman catheters, Petersen et al. observed a constant probability of developing bacteremia during the first 100 days after transplant, with no change in risk at the time of engraftment. This may suggest that the catheter serves as a constant source of bacteremia for as long as it is in place. Alternatively, there may be a change in risk factors for infection (e.g. neutropenia initially versus GVHD later) which are coincidentally of equal magnitude. There are known defects in host defense after engraftment which may predispose to bacterial and fungal infection including defects in macrophage function and low antibody levels [13,14].

This continuing risk of infection after engraftment indicates the need for continuing efforts at infection prevent ion even after recovery of the circulating neutrophil count. One such approach would be selective decontamination with nonabsorbable or absorbable oral antibiotics. Another may be the use of immunoglobulin infusions to maintain levels of opsonizing antibody against some of these bacterial agents.

Prophylactic Immunoglobulin

Intravenous CMV immunoglobulin was compared to seronegative blood products for prevention of primary CMV infection among seronegative transplant recipients [15]. Although no protective effect of immunoglobulin against CMV infection or disease was observed, subsequent analysis of bacterial and fungal infection unexpectedly showed a lower probability of infection among the globulin recipients [16]. This effect was limited to the period after engraftment: 11 (26%) of 45 immunoglobulin recipients developed bacteremia or fungemia compared with 22 (42%) of 52 control patients (relative rate 2.1, $p = 0.039$ by Cox proportional hazards regression). The effect was further restricted to infections caused by organisms other than coagulase-negative *Staphylococcus* (relative rate of 2.4 among control patients versus immunoglobulin recipients, $p = 0.047$).

This apparent benefit will need reconfirmation in a study specifically designed to address bacterial infection. A recent study by Winston et al., also directed primarily at CMV infection, did not show a change in bacterial infection [17]. However, a previously available alkylated immunoglobulin (Gamimune, pH 6.8, Cutter Laboratories) was used in that trial and this preparation may have lesser opsonizing activity than native immunoglobulins. Passive immunoprophylaxis may be of even greater interest among patients with chronic GVHD.

Mortality

As noted, mortality from bacterial and fungal infection is fortunately low. In the studies summarized above, bacterial or fungal infection as a primary cause of death occurred in 17 of 516 (5%) patients before engraftment and in 29 of 503 (6%) patients after engraftment. At least 6 of the 29 patients dying after engraftment also had severe acute GVHD as a contributing cause of death.

Acute Graft versus Host Disease

Prevention of acute GVHD by total bacterial decontamination has received much attention. In a retrospective analysis of patients transplanted for severe aplastic anemia, Storb et al.

Table 5. Occurrence of Grade 2-4 Acute GVHD by Infection Prevention Modality

Study/ Modality	Total Number	With Acute GVHD: Number	Proportion
A. Acute Leukemics [8]			
PE	86	23	.27
PG	86	32	.37
B. Aplastic Anemia [9]			
PE	32	6	.19*
PG	31	11	.35
CT	22	11	.50*
C. Hematologic Malignancy [10,11]			
PE + PSA	54	21	.39
PE alone	68	32	.47
PSA alone	45	18	.39
PG	67	31	.46

*p = 0.08.
See Tables 2 and 3 for abbreviations.

observed that those transplanted in the protective environment had a significantly lower incidence of GVHD and better survival than patients transplanted in conventional rooms with or without the use of prophylactic granulocytes [18]. Use of prophylactic granulocytes had no independent effect. Although some patients were randomly assigned to the protective environment as part of other studies [2], this was not a randomized study. Although these results among patients with aplastic anemia have not been reconfirmed, all such patients in our center are transplanted in the protective environment.

This benefit has not been apparent in studies of patients transplanted for hematologic malignancy (Table 5). Patients transplanted for malignancy have more difficulty complying with the oral decontamination regimen and are rarely decontaminated for any substantial period of time [2,8,10]. It is possible that the lack of effect on GVHD among leukemia patients is due to inadequate decontamination.

FUNGAL INFECTION

Between 1969 and 1979 invasive fungal infection was discovered at autopsy in 22% of patients transplanted for hematologic malignancy and 44% of patients transplanted for aplastic anemia [19]. The higher incidence among patients with aplastic anemia was attributed to more common graft rejection and prolonged neutropenia. Invasive fungal infection, primarily candidal, was also associated with longer duration of neutropenia and with detectable colonization of multiple surveillance sites. This latter observation applied to both *albicans* and non-*albicans* *Candida*. Preliminary review of 1188 patients transplanted between 1980 and 1986 has identified 186 (15.6%) with *Candida* infection and 45 (3.8%) with *Aspergillus* infection.

Aspergillosis

Among the first 40 cases that have been reviewed, 25 (63%) had *Aspergillus* pneumonia only, 7 (18%) had multiple organ involvement and 8 (20%) had *Aspergillus* recovered from various culture sites without further documentation of invasive infection. Thirty of 32 (94%) with proven invasive infection died. Among the 32 with invasive infection, 12 (38%) had concomitant CMV pneumonia and 5 (16%) also had invasive *Candida* infection. Finally, 8 patients (25%) with invasive infection had *Aspergillus* cultured from sputum, 7 after and only 1 before clinical onset.

Candidal Infection

Review of 561 of the 1188 patients mentioned above identified 32 (5.7%) with fungemia within the first 100 days after transplant. This approximates the incidence observed in the infection prevention studies reviewed above. Eighteen of 32 episodes were due to *C. albicans*, 7 to *C. tropicalis*, 4 to other candidal species, and 3 to other fungi. The median day of first positive blood culture was 15 days after transplant. Nineteen of 32 patients had concomitant bacterial infections. The fatality rate was high, with 22 (69%) dying with fungal infection and 6 (19%) ultimately dying of other non-infectious causes. Only 4 patients survived.

Prevention of Fungal Infection

Although we found oral ketoconazole to be statistically superior to oral nystatin for prevention of fungal colonization among patients treated in the protective environment, neither was effective in eradicating carriage in patients already colonized [20]. Empiric amphotericin B is given to approximately 50% of our patients in the setting of persistent fever not responsive to broad spectrum antibiotics. This practice has not been shown to be effective in the prevention of (or in the early treatment of) fungal infection after marrow transplant and the potential for renal toxicity among patients receiving both amphotericin B and cyclosporine is high. No routine antifungal prophylaxis is given except in the protective environment at this time.

PROTOZOAN INFECTION

Pneumocystis Carinii Pneumonia

Pneumocystis infection has become rare since the advent of trimethoprim-sulfamethoxazole (TMP-SMX) prophylaxis. In contrast to a peak incidence of 14% observed in 1976, we now see only 1-4 cases yearly which invariably occur among patients who receive no TMP-SMX after transplant because of allergy or other intolerance. The parallel observation is that patients taking almost any amount of TMP-SMX after transplant appear to be adequately protected against *Pneumocystis carinii*.

A variety of prophylactic regimens have been used successfully. The initial regimen of daily TMP-SMX given at a TMP dose of 5 mg/kg (as one-half the dose every 12 hours) is clearly effective, but is also associated with gastrointestinal intolerance. Alternative regimens include a dose equivalent to 240 mg of TMP (3 tablets) given every 8 hours on 2 consecutive days of the week [21], and our present lower dose regimen of 2 tablets (or 1 double-strength tablet) given twice a day on 2 consecutive days of the week. This latter regimen is well tolerated and highly effective. The daily regimen continues to be used among patients with chronic GVHD in whom the goal is also prevention of bacterial infection.

Toxoxplasma gondii

We have observed 10 cases of toxoplasmosis after marrow transplant. The incidence is thus <1%. None were diagnosed during life, although 3 recent patients had pre-mortem blood cultures which became positive for toxoplasma after death [22]. All had involvement of both brain and heart and some also had toxoplasma pneumonia. All were seropositive before transplant, suggesting reactivation of infection, and none had a serological response to toxoplasma infection. Thus a high index of clinical suspicion and appropriate cultural and histologic studies must be performed to diagnose this treatable infection during life.

CONCLUSIONS

The risk of bacterial and fungal infection may be even greater in the future as newer methods of marrow manipulation and storage are introduced and as higher risk patients undergo marrow transplantation. More effective means of infection prevention will be needed to keep pace with such changes in the technology of marrow transplantation. Among these, better regimens for complete bacterial decontamination within the protective environment and perhaps use of selective decontamination both during the neutropenic period and thereafter may improve infection prevention. Adjunctive measures to restore host defenses, such as periodic immunoglobulin infusions, may also be of importance. Moreover, successful treatment or prevention of acute GVHD and CMV pneumonia and more effective regimens for prevention of leukemic relapse may increase the relative importance of mortality from bacterial and fungal infection, necessitating even greater focus on infection prevention.

This work was suported by grants CA 18029, HL 36444, CA 15704, CA 18221 and CA 18579 from the National Institutes of Health, DHHS.

REFERENCES

1. Peterson PK, McGlave P, Ramsay NKC, Rhame F, Cohen E, Perry GS, Goldman AI, Kersey (1983) A prospective study of infectious diseases following bone marrow transplantation: emergence of aspergillus and cytomegalovirus as the major causes of mortality. Infect Control 4:81-89

2. Buckner CD, Clift RA, Sanders JE, Meyers JD, Counts GW, Farewell CT, Thomas ED and the Seattle Marrow Transplant Team (1978) Protective environment for marrow transplant recipients. A prospective study. Ann Intern Med 89:893-901

3. Clift RA, Sanders JE, Thomas ED, Williams B, Buckner CD (1978) Granulocyte transfusions for the prevention of infection in patients receiving bone-marrow transplants. N Engl J Med 298:1052-1057

4. Winston DJ, Ho WG, Young LS, Gale RP (1980) Prophylactic granulocyte transfusions during human bone marrow transplantation. Am J Med 68:893-897.

5. Winston DJ, Ho WG, Nakao SL, Gale RP, Champlin RE (1986) Norfloxacin versus vancomycin/polymyxin for prevention of infections in granulocytopenic patients. Am J Med 80:884-890

6. Witherspoon RP, Storb, R, Ochs HD, Flournoy N, Kopecky KJ, Sullivan KM, Deeg HJ, Sosa R, Noel DR, Atkinson K, Thomas ED (1981) Recovery of antibody production in human allogeneic marrow graft recipients: Influence of time posttransplantation, the presence or absence of chronic graft-versus-host disease, and antithymocyte globulin treatment. Blood 58:360-368

7. Winston DJ, Schiffman G, Wang DC, Feig SA, Lin CH, Marso EL, Ho WG, Young LS, Gale RP (1979) Pneumococcal infections after human bone-marrow transplantation. Ann Intern Med 91:835-841.

8. Buckner CD, Clift RA, Thomas ED, Hersman J, Sanders JE, Stewart PS, Wade JC, Murphy M, Counts G, Meyers JD (1983) Early infectious complications in allogeneic marrow transplant recipients with acute leukemia: Effects of prophylactic measures. Infection 11:243-250

9. Navari RM, Buckner CD, Clift RA, Storb R, Sanders JE, Stewart P, Sullivan KM, Williams B, Counts GW, Meyers JD, Thomas ED (1984) Prophylaxis of infection in patients with aplastic anemia receiving allogeneic marrow transplants. Am J Med 76:564-572

10. Petersen FB, Buckner CD, Clift RA, Lee S, Nelson N, Counts GW, Meyers JD, Sanders JE, Stewart PS, Bensinger WI, Navari R, Thomas ED (1986) Laminar air flow isolation and decontamination: A prospective randomized study of the effects of prophylactic systemic antibiotics in bone marrow transplant patients. Infection 14:115-121

11. Petersen FB, Buckner CD, Clift RA, Nelson N, Counts GW, Meyers JD, Thomas ED (1986) Prevention of nosocomial infections in marrow transplant patients: A prospective randomized comparison of systemic antibiotics versus granulocyte transfusions. Infect Control 7:586-592

12. Hersman J, Meyers JD, Thomas ED, Buckner CD, Clift R (1982) The effect of granulocyte transfusions upon the incidence of cytomegalovirus infection after allogeneic marrow transplantation. Ann Intern Med 96:149-152

13. Clark RA, Johnson FL, Klebanoff SJ, Thomas ED (1976) Defective neutrophil chemotaxis in bone marrow transplant patients. J Clin Invest 58:22-31

14. Atkinson K, Farewell V, Storb R, Tsoi MS, Sullivan KM, Witherspoon RP, Fefer A, Clift R, Goodell B, Thomas ED (1982) Analysis of late infections after human bone marrow transplantation: Role of genotypic nonidentity between marrow donor and recipient and of nonspecific suppressor cells in patients with chronic graft-versus-host disease. Blood 60:714-720

15. Bowden RA, Sayers M, Flournoy N, Newton B, Banaji M, Thomas ED, Meyers JD (1986) Cytomegalovirus immune globulin and seronegative blood products to prevent primary cytomegalovirus infection after marrow transplantation. N Engl J Med 314:1006-1010

16. Petersen FB, Bowden RA, Thornquist M, Meyers JD, Buckner CD, Counts GW, Nelson MT, Newton BA, Sullivan KM, McIver J, Thomas ED (1987) The effect of prophylactic intravenous immune globulin on the incidence of septicemia in marrow transplant recipients. Bone Marrow Transplantation, in press

17. Winston DJ, Ho WG, Lin C-H, Bartoni K, Budinger MD, Gale RB, Champlin R (1987) Intravenous immune globulin for prevention of cytomegalovirus infection and interstitial pneumonia after bone marrow transplantation. Ann Intern Med 106:12-18

18. Storb R, Prentice RL, Buckner CD, Clift RA, Appelbaum F, Deeg J, Doney K, Hansen JA, Mason M, Sanders JE, Singer J, Sullivan KM, Witherspoon RP, Thomas ED (1983) Graft-versus-host disease and survival in patients with aplastic anemia treated by marrow grafts from HLA-identical siblings. Beneficial effect of a protective environment. N Engl J Med 302-307

19. Meyers JD, Thomas ED (1981) Infection complicating bone marrow transplantation. In: Rubin RH, Young LS (ed) Clinical Approach to infection in the immunocompromised host. New York: Plenum Press

20. Shepp DH, Klosterman A, Siegel MS, Meyers JD (1985) Comparative trial of ketoconazole and nystatin for prevention of fungal infection in neutropenic patients treated in the protective environment. J Infect Dis 152:1257-1263

21. Winston DJ, Gale RP, Meyer DV, Young LS, and the UCLA Bone Marrow Transplantation Group (1979) Infectious complications of human bone marrow transplantation. Medicine 58:1-31

22. Shepp DH, Hackman RC, Conley FK, Anderson JB, Meyers JD (1985) Toxoplasma gondii reactivation identified by detection of parasitemia in tissue culture. Ann Intern Med 103:218-221

29: Prevention and Treatment of Infections After Bone Marrow Transplantation

Drew J. Winston, Winston G. Ho, Robert Peter Gale, and Richard E. Champlin

Patients undergoing bone marrow transplantation are susceptible to many different types of infection caused by bacteria, fungi, viruses, and parasites [1,2]. Factors that cause immunosuppression and predispose to infection include pretransplant radiation and chemotherapy, transient granulocytopenia before marrow engraftment, and the post-transplant administration of immunosuppressive agents for the prevention and treatment of graft-versus-host disease (GVHD). It is the purpose of this review to summarize current and new approaches to the prevention and treatment of infections after bone marrow transplantation.

PREVENTION OF INFECTIONS DURING GRANULOCYTOPENIA

The most elaborate means for prophylaxis of bacterial and fungal infections in granulocytopenic marrow transplants is isolation in a laminar-air-flow room with concomitant administration of sterile food and oral antimicrobial agents for gastrointestinal decontamination. Several studies have demonstrated the efficacy of laminar-air-flow isolation for prevention of infection and possibly GVHD [3-5]. However, it does not significantly improve survival, is not cost-effective, and is thus not recommended except for institutions where Aspergillus infections are endemic [6,7].

A more practical approach for prevention of bacterial infections in granulocytopenic patients is the use of oral chemoprophylactic agents in patients who are managed in a private hospital room and are given a low bacterial diet devoid of fresh fruits, vegetables, and salads [8,9]. Decontamination of the gastrointestinal tract with oral nonabsorbable antibiotics (such as polymyxin and vancomycin) can effectively decrease infection but is limited by gastrointestinal side-effects and poor patient compliance [10]. Recently, the concept of selective decontamination or colonization resistance with oral trimethoprim-sulfamethoxazole has been popularized [11]. The routine use of prophylactic trimethoprim-sulfamethoxazole has not achieved widespread acceptance, however, due to reports of more prolonged periods of granulcoytopenia, a higher incidence of fungal colonization and superinfections, and the selection of trimethoprim-sulfamethoxazole resistant gram-negative organisms [12-15].

Another approach to oral chemoprophylaxis is the use of the new oral fluorinated quinolones. The fluorinated quinolones are especially active against the Enterobacteriaceae and Pseudomonas aeruginosa [16]. Their oral administration appears to preserve the anaerobic gastrointestinal flora and thereby maintain colonization resistance against the acquisition of new aerobic bacteria [17]. In a series of clinical trials, norfloxacin (400mg po bid), ciprofloxacin (500mg po bid), and ofloxacin (300mg po bid) have been compared to placebo, trimethoprim-sulfamethoxazole, or vancomycine-polymyxin for prevention of infection in granulocytopenic patients (Table 1) [17-22]. The quinolones reduced the incidence of microbiologically documented infections, especially gram-negative bacteremias. Only 3 of 163 patients (2%) given quinolone prophylaxis experienced gram-negative bacteremia compared to 26 of 155 patients (17%) receiving placebo, trimethoprim-sulfamethoxazole, or vancomycin-polymyxin. On the other hand, none of the quinolones or other chemoprophylactic regimens prevented gram-positive bacteremia. Isolation of quinolone-resistant organisms was infrequent. The quinolones were better tolerated than trimethoprim-sulfamethoxazole or vancomycin-polymyxin, which were commonly associated with either skin rashes or gastrointestinal side-effects.

In contrast to the effectiveness of oral antimicrobial agents for prevention of bacterial infections, oral antifungal prophylaxis with nystatin, ketoconazole, or amphotericin B has failed to produce consistently favorable results. Oral nystatin causes gastrointestinal irritability and is poorly tolerated by many patients. Oral ketoconazole (400-600mg per day) is better tolerated than nystatin but appears to be no more efficacious than nystatin in preventing serious invasive fungal infections [23,24]. Ketoconazole may also interfere with serum levels of cyclosporin and antagonize the activity of intravenous amphotericin B [25-27]. In a recent controlled prophylactic trial in granulocytopenic patients, oral amphotericin B suspension (1500mg per day) was compared to ketoconazole (600mg per day) or placebo [28]. A significant decrease in yeast colonization occurred in patients receiving amphotericin B or ketoconazole compared with patients receiving placebo, but there were no clinical benefits in terms of the number of febrile days, the initiation of intravenous amphotericin B, or the incidence of invasive fungal infections. These combined experiences suggest that the empiric use of intravenous amphotericin B in marrow transplants who remain persistently granulocytopenic and febrile on broad-spectrum intravenous antibiotics is the only reliable way to currently prevent fatal fungal infections [29]. A new formulation of amphotericin B (liposomal amphotericin B) is associated with less fever, chills, and nephrotoxicity and may improve the safety of empiric antifungal therapy [30].

Itraconazole and fluconazole are two new imidazoles that may also improve antifungal prophylaxis and therapy in the future. Itraconazole, which is administerd orally, may have some activity for Aspergillus as well as Candida [31,32]. Fluconazole can be given either orally or intravenously and has a unique pharmacokinetic profile that includes renal excretion and penetration into the central nervous system [33]. Fluconazole is currently being evaluated for treatment of cryptococcal meningitis in AIDS patients and for prophylaxis of fungal infections in granulocytopenic patients. Nasal sprays of amphotericin B for prevention of airborne aspergillus infections are also the subject of similar clinical trials [34].

Prophylactic granulocyte transfusions, intravenous immunoglobulin, and acyclovir have been used to prevent infections in granulocytopenic marrow transplants. The benefits of granulocyte transfusions in preventing bacteremia, however, are outweighed by the expense and potential complicatons (transfusion reactions, pulmonary infiltrates, and CMV infections) of these transfusions [35-38]. Consequently, prophylactic granulocyte transfusions are not recommended. In a recent trial of high-dose prophylactic intravenous immune globulin in marrow transplants, the intravenous immune globulin had no effect on the incidence or outcome of bacterial and fungal infections [39]. The intravenous immune globulin used in this trial was a preparation modified by reduction and alkylation [40]. An unmodified preparation might be more effective for prevention of bacterial and fungal infections. This issue is now being addressed in a controlled study. Both intravenous acyclovir (5mg/kg every 8 hours) and oral acyclovir (400mg five times daily) can prevent reactivation of herpes simplex viral infection in marrow transplants who are seropositive for herpes simplex viral antibody [41,42]. However, herpes simplex infection commonly occurs after the prophylactic acyclovir is stopped, and acyclovir-resistant strains of herpes simplex have occasionally been isolated [43]. Moreover, most of these herpes simplex infections are localized oral or genital infections that can be treated effectively when they occur. They are rarely fatal. Thus, we do not recommend the routine use of acyclovir for prophylaxis but reserve the drug for treatment of established herpes simplex or varicella-zoster infections. This approach is also more cost-effective.

TREATMENT OF INFECTIONS DURING GRANULOCYTOPENIA

The most important factor in the successful therapy of the febrile granulocytopenic patient with suspected or documented infection continues to be the prompt initiation of antibiotic therapy, usually with a combination of agents that are potentially synergistic and relatively nontoxic. Traditionally, a combination of an aminoglycoside plus an antipseudomonal beta-lactam has been used. In the granulocytopenic marrow transplant recipient, the frequent use of other nephrotoxic drugs (cyclosporine, amphotericin B) that may potentiate the nephrotoxicity of the aminoglycosides and the increasing incidence of gram-positive infections (Staphylococcus epidermidis, Staphylococcus aureus, Viridans Group Streptococcus, Corynebacterium) have led to the development of alternative antibiotic regimens [44]. One alternative approach is the use of a double beta-lactam regimen (a third generation cephalosproin and an antipseudomonal penicillin). Several controlled trials have recently evaluated the relative efficacy and safety of double beta-lactam antibiotic combinations which are synergistic in vitro and produce excellent serum bactericidal activity (Table 2) [45-50]. In general, the overall favorable response rates of proven infection in granulocytopenic patients to double beta-lactam therapy have been similar to those achieved with aminoglycoside-containing regimens (70% vs 70%). Furthermore, the incidence of nephrotoxicity is lower in patients treated with double beta-lactam combinations (1% vs 5%).

Another alternative approach to combination therapy with an aminoglycoside is single-agent therapy with a third-generation cephoalosporin. Monotherapy in the granulocytopenic patient has been most carefully evaluated in a controlled study at the National Cancer Institute in Bethesda, Maryland where ceftazidime alone was compared to a triple-drug regimen of cephalothin, gentamicin, and carbenicillin [51]. For patients with documented infection, the favorable response rates were 89% (82 of 92) for ceftazidime alone and 91% (58 of 64) for cephalothin, gentamicin, and carbenicillin. While these results with ceftazidime alone appear impressive, 50% of the patients initially given ceftazidime subsequently required additional antibiotics to achieve this "successful outcome with modification". Intravenous vancomycin or clindamycin was the antibiotic most commonly added due to the occurrence of gram-positive superinfections in patients given ceftazidime alone. We have also observed the emergence of ceftazidime-resistant Pseudomonas aeruginosa organisms during monotherapy of Pseudomonas infections with ceftazidime in nongranulocytopenic patients. Thus, we still recommend a two-drug regimen (an aminoglycoside plus an antipseudomonal beta-lactam or a double beta-lactam regimen) for the initial empirical therapy of the febrile granulocytopenic patient. On the other hand, imipenem, the first of a new class of beta-lactam antibiotics called the carbapenems, has the broadest antibacterial spectrum of any antibiotic yet developed and would appear to be the most promising agent for monotherapy [52]. Imipenem is very active against not ony gram-negative aerobic pathogens but also against many of the gram-positive aerobic pathogens now used in granulocytopenic patients. We are currently comparing monotherapy with imipenem with cefoperazone plus piperacillin or ceftazidime plus piperacillin in febrile granulocytopenic patients at UCLA. In a preliminary analysis, the overall clinical response to therapy was 86% (25 of 29) for cefoperazone plus piperacillin, 74% (20 of 27) for ceftazidime plus piperacillin, and 72% (21 of 29) for imipenem alone. The dosage of imipenem was 1.0 gram intravenously every 6 hours. Seizures occurred in 3 imipenem patients but in none of the patients given cefoperazone/piperacillin or ceftazidime/piperacillin. Thus, we are continuing the study but using a lower dosage of imipenem (500mg intravenously every 6 hours).

Due to the increasing number of gram-positive aerobic bacterial infections in cancer patients, especially those caused by Staphylococcus epidermidis [44], there has been concern that an initial two-drug regimen of an aminoglycoside plus a beta-lactam or of two beta-lactams may not be adequate therapy for many patients. Data showing the need to use empiric intravenous vancomycin with two other antibiotics in the initial therapy of the febrile granulocytopenic patient is conflicting [53,54]. We have found that most patients with a gram-positive bacterial infection initially improve or stabilize on the usual two-drug antibiotic regimens and that gram-positive bacterial infections are very rarely fatal. Thus, we currently do not recommend the routine use of an expensive antibiotic like vancomycin as part of the initial empirical therapy of a febrile granulocytopenic patient unless the patient has clinical evidence of a central intravenous catheter infection likely to be caused by Staphylococcus epidermidis or Corynebacterium. Similarly, we have found the routine administration of vancomycin to a patient who has persistent unexplained fever on other broad-spectrum antibiotics to be of no benefit and may only delay a more beneficial therapy like empiric intravenous amphotericin B. Indeed, we have seen an occasional patient given empiric intravenous vancomycin for persistent fever that was actually caused by fungal superinfection. There also is no need to use expensive and potentially hazardous granulocyte transfusions for treatment of suspected or documented infections complicating persistent granulocytopenia as long as appropriate antimicrobial therapy is given [55].

TREATMENT OF INTERSTITIAL PNEUMONIA

Since most cases of interstitial pneumonia after marrow transplantation are associated with CMV infections, treatment of interstitial pneumonia has focused on CMV infection [57,58]. Table 3 summarizes the results of several trials of antiviral therapy of CMV pneumonia. Earlier studies used vidarabine (adenine arabinoside), human leukocyte interferon, acyclovir, recombinant leukocyte interferon, lymphoblastoid interferon, foscarnet (trisodinm phosphonoformate hexahydrate), or combinations of these agents [58-65]. The responses with these agents were unfavorable in most cases (Table 3). Recently, a new acyclic nucleoside, 9-[1,3-dihydroxy-2-propoxymethyl] guanine (DHPG; ganciclovir) has been shown to have increased potency against CMV in vitro. Nevertheless, despite the elimination of CMV from cultures of respiratory secretions and other body fluids, only 3 of 19 patients with CMV interstitial pneumonia treated with DHPG at Seattle or UCLA survived [67,68]. Combining the anti-inflammatory effect of high doses of corticosteroids with the antiviral effect of DHPG also did not improve the outcome of CMV pneumonia (only 1 of 6 patients survived) [69]. The results of using CMV immune globulin for treatment of CMV pneumonia have been conflicting. Six of 9 marrow transplants with CMV pneumonia treated with a CMV immune globulin by Blacklock and colleagues in London survived [70]. In contrast, only 2 of 10 patients treated with a CMV immune globulin by Reed and colleagues in Seattle survived [71]. Recently, more favorable results and improved survival from CMV pneumonia have been reported by using a combination of DHPG plus high doses of intravenous immune globulin given daily.

For patients with idiopathic interstitial pneumonia presumably related to the pulmonary toxicity of radiation or chemotherapy, there is no therapy of proven value. Both controlled and uncontrolled studies suggest that cortocosteroids and other anti-inflammatory agents have no benefit [72]. Trimethoprim-sulfamethoxazole is still the drug of choice for treatment of Pneumoncystis carinii penumonia [73].

PREVENTION OF INTERSTITIAL PNEUMONIA

The ineffectiveness of antiviral therapy of CMV pneumonia in marrow transplants led to attempts to prevent or modify CMV infection by passive immunization with CMV immune plasma or globulin. These attempts were also prompted by animal studies demonstrating that passive immunization modified CMV infection and by earlier observations that CMV antibody synthesis may be associated with less severe CMV infection [74,75]. Table 4 summarizes the results of six controlled trials of CMV immune plasma, CMV hyperimmune globulin, or a polyvalent intravenous immune globulin containing CMV antibody (Gamimune) [78-81]. The polyvalent intravenous immune globulin was given at high doses (1000mg/kg once every week for four months), but was well tolerated [81]. More than 300 patients, most of whom were seronegative for CMV antibody, were evaluated in these trials. The incidence of CMV infection was 35% in the recipients of immune plasma or globulin versus 51% in control subjects. CMV pneumonia was reduced from 23% to 8%. These combined results suggest that immune globulin or plasma, although not necessarily preventing CMV infection, modifies the severity of infection and prevents CMV interstitial pneumonia in bone marrow transplants who are seronegative for CMV antibody. Similar results have been obtained in CMV-seronegative renal transplant patients [82].

Another approach for prevention of CMV infection in CMV-seronegative marrow transplants is the exclusive use of CMV-seronegative blood products [57,80]. The benefits of CMV-seronegative blood products appear limited to CMV-seronegative patients who have a CMV-seronegative marrow donor. A protective effect was not observed when the marrow donor was CMV-seropositive [80]. Moreover, this practice is limited by the ability of blood donor centers to provide large numbers of CMV-seronegative blood products in emergent situations and by the relative insensitivity of serological techniques for excluding latent viral infection. Indeed, we have observed occasional CMV infections in CMV-seronegative patients who had CMV-seronegative marrow donors and received only CMV-seronegative blood products. Although these patients were CMV-seronegative at the time of their marrow transplants, they had received many unscreened blood products before transplantation and presumably acquired latent CMV infection that was not detected by serological testing. Similarly, in patients who develop a major bleeding diathesis requiring immediate red cell and platelet transfusions, it is not always possible to provide only CMV-seronegative blood products. Thus, there may be a role for combined use of CMV-seronegataive blood products and intravenous immune globulin in CMV-seronegative patients. The intravenous immune globulin may have additional benefits such as the modification of GVHD and the prevention of bacterial and fungal infectious complications [81].

In patients who are seropositive for CMV antibody before transplantation, effective prophylaxis for CMV infection and pneumonia has not yet been established. Previously, prophylactic vidarabine (adenine arabinoside), human leukocyte interferon, and acyclovir have had no significant effect on the incidence of CMV infection [58,41,42,83]. Recently, patients seropositive for both CMV and herpes simplex virus were given high doses of prophylactic intravenous acyclovir (500mg/m^2 intravenously every 8 hours from 5 days before to 30 days after marrow transplantation) and compared to patients who were seropositive for CMV but seronegative for herpes simplex and who did not receive acyclovir [84]. The probability of CMV infection (68% vs 90%) and CMV pneumonia (19% vs 35%) was significantly lower in the recipients of the high doses of prophylactic acyclovir. Additional studies using high doses of intravenous and then oral prophylactic acyclovir for several months after transplantation are now being performed to confirm these results.

In contrast to the poor results of DHPG therapy of CMV pneumonia after marrow transplantation, all 6 UCLA marrow transplants who received DHPG for CMV viremia associated with high fever and generalized wasting survived. None developed pneumonia [68]. These results suggest that DHPG is more likely to be effective when given prophylactically or earlier in the course of CMV infection before the onset of CMV pneumonia. Accordingly, we have initiated a placebo-controlled, double-blinded trial of prophylactic DHPG in UCLA marrow transplants seropositive for CMV. The DHPG (2.5mg/kg intravenously every 8 hours) is given for one week before the transplant and then stopped the day before the transplant. When the post-transplant granulocyte count reaches 500/mm^3, the DHPG (6mg/kg once per day, Monday through Friday) is resumed until day 120 after the transplant. All patients entered into the study have had marrow engraftment, but the study code has not yet been broken.

Trimethoprim-sulfamethoxazole is effective for prevention of interstitial pneumonia due to <u>Pneumocystis carinii</u> and has reduced the incidence of <u>Pneumocystis carinii</u> pneumonia from 12.5% to less than 1% in allogeneic marrow transplants at UCLA [57]. The prophylactic trimethoprim-sulfamethoxazole (240mg of trimethoprim and 1200mg of sulfamethoxazole every 8 hours) is started at admission of the patient to the hospital and continued until 24 hours before transplantation. After transplantation, the trimethoprim-sulfamethoxazole (240mg of trimethoprim and 1200mg of sulfamethoxazole every 8 hours on any two consecutive days of each week) is resumed when the absolute granulocyte count reaches 1000/mm^3 and is continued until day 150 after transplantation. The trimethoprim-sulfamethoxazole can be given either orally or intravenously. Folinic acid is given with the trimethoprim-sulfamethoxazole to prevent marrow toxicity. For patients continuing to receive immunosuppressive therapy for chronic graft-versus-host disease, it is recommended that the trimethoprim-sulfamethoxazole be continued beyond day 150 after transplantation for prevention of Pneumocystis as well as bacterial infections.

PREVENTION AND TREATMENT OF LATE INFECTIONS

Most serious infections occurring more than four months after marrow transplantation are associated with chronic GVHD and its treatment with immunosuppressive agents. Bacterial infections of the upper and lower respiratory tract, cutaneous bacterial infections, and localized herpes zoster predominate [85,86]. Encapsulated bacteria, such as <u>Streptococcus pneumoniae</u>, <u>Hemophilus influenzae</u> and <u>Neisseria meningitidis</u>, and <u>Staphylococcus aureus</u> are common pathogens [87]. Continued prophylaxis with trimethoprim-sulfamethoxazole may prevent some of these infections [88]. Since patients with chronic graft-versus-host disease have subnormal antibody responses to pneumococcal and other vaccines [89,90], passive immunization with intravenous immune globulin is being evaluated in these patients. Intravenous acyclovir is the drug of choice for treatment of herpes zoster [91].

ACKNOWLEDGMENT

Support by grant CA 23175 from the National Cancer Institute.

REFERENCES

1. Winston DJ, Gale RP, Meyers DV, Young LS, UCLA Bone Marrow Transplant Group (1979) Infectious complications of human bone marrow transplantation. Medicine (Baltimore) 58:1-31.
2. Winston DJ, Ho WG, Champlin RE, Gale RP (1984) Infectious complications of bone marrow transplantation. Exp Hematol 12:205-215.
3. Buckner CD, Clift RA, Sanders JE, et al (1978) Protective environment for marrow transplant recipients. A prospective study. Ann Intern Med 89:893-901.
4. Navari RM, Buckner CD, Clift RA, et al (1984) Prophylaxis of infection in patients with aplastic anemia receiving allogeneic marrow transplants. Am J Med 76:564-572.
5. Storb R, Prentice RL, Buckner CD, et al (1983) Graft-versus-host disease and survival in patients with aplastic anemia treated by marrow grafts from HLA-identical siblings. Beneficial effect of a protective environment. N Engl J Med 308:302-307.
6. Peterson PK, McGlave P, Ramsay NKC, et al (1983) A prospective study of infectious diseases following bone marrow transplantation: emergence of Aspergillus and cytomegalovirus as the major causes of mortality. Infect Control 4:81-89.
7. Rotstein C, Cummings M, Tidings J, et al (1985) An outbreak of invasive aspergillosis among allogeneic bone marrow transplants: a case-control study. Infect Control 6:347-355.
8. Schimpff SC (1980) Infection prevention during profound granulocytopenia: new approaches to alimentary canal microbial suppression. Ann Intern Med 93:358-361.
9. Remington JS, Schimpff SC (1981). Please don't eat the salads. N Engl J Med 304:433-435.
10. Schimpff SC, Greene WH, Young WM, et al (1975) Infection prevention in acute nonlymphocytic leukemia: laminar-air flow room isolation reverse isolation with oral nonabsorbable antibiotic prophylaxis. Ann Intern Med 82:351-358.
11. Wade JC, Schimpff SC, Hargadon MT, Fortner CL, Young VM, Wiernik PH (1981) A comparison of trimethoprim-sulfamethoxazole plus nystatin with gentamicin plus nystatin in the prevention of infections in acute leukemia. N Engl J Med 304:1057-1062.
12. Dekker AV, Rozenberg-Anska M, Sixma JJ, Verhoef J (1981) Prevention of infection by trimethoprim-sulfamethoxazole plus amphotericin B in patients with acute nonlymphocytic leukemia. Ann Intern Med 95:555-559.
13. Wade JC, DeJongh CA, Newman KA, Crowley J, Wiernik PH, Schimpff SC (1983) Selective antimicrobial modulation as prophylaxis against infection during granulocytopenia. Trimethoprim-sulfamethoxazole vs nalidixic acid. J Infect Dis 147:624-634.
14. EORTC International Antimicrobial Therapy Project Group (1984) Trimethoprim-sulfamethoxazole in the prevention of infection in neutropenic patients. J Infect Dis 150:372-379.
15. Wilson JM, Guiney DG (1982) Failure of oral trimethoprim-sulfamethoxazole prophylaxis in acute leukemia. Isolation of resistant plasmids from strains of Enterobacteriaceae causing bacteremia. N Engl J Med 306:16-20.
16. Wolfson JS, Hooper DC (1985) The fluorequinolones: structures, mechanisms of action and resistance, and spectra of activity in vitro. Antimicrob Agents Chemother 28:581-586.
17. Karp JE, Merz WG, Hendricksen C, et al (1987) Oral norfloxacin for prevention of gram-negative bacterial infections in patients with acute leukemia and granulocytopenia. A randomized, double-blind, placebo-controlled trial. Ann Intern Med 106:1-7.
18. Winston DJ, Ho WG, Champlin RE, et al (1987) Norfloxacin for prevention of bacterial infections in granulocytopenic patients. Am J Med 82(6B):40-46.
19. Bow EJ, Louie TJ, Rayner E, Pitsanuk J (1985) Norfloxacin versus trimethoprim-sulfamethoxazole for infection prevention in patients with acute leukemia. In: Program and Abstracts of the Twenty-Fifth Interscience Conference on Antimicrobial Agents and Chemotherapy, Washington, D.C., American Society for Microbiology, 117.
20. Winston DJ, Ho WG, Nakao S, Gale RP, Champlin RE (1986) Norfloxacin versus vancomycin/polymyxin for prevention of infection in granulocytopenic patients. Am J Med 80:884-890.
21. Dekker AW, Rozenberg-Arska M, Verhoef J (1987) Infection prophylaxis in acute leukemia: a comparison of ciprofloxacin with trimethoprim-sulfamethoxazole and colistin. Ann Intern Med 106:7-12.
22. Winston DJ, Ho WG, Bartoni K, Bruckner DA, Gale RP, Champlin RE (1987) Ofloxacin versus vancomycin/polymyxin for prevention of infections in granulocytopenic patients. In: Program and Abstracts of the Twenty-Seventh Interscience Conference on Antimicrobial Agents and Chemotherapy, Washington, D.C., American Society for Microbiology.
23. Acuna G, Winston DJ, Young LS (1981) Ketoconazole prophylaxis of fungal infection in the granulocytopenic patient. In: Program and Abstracts of the Twenty-First Interscience Conference on Antimicrobial Agents and Chemotherapy, Washington, D.C., American Society for Microbiology, 852.
24. Shepp DH, Klosterman A, Siegel MS, Meyers JD (1985) Comparative trials of ketoconazole and nystatin for prevention of fungal infection in neutropenic patients treated in a protective environment. J Infect Dis 152:1257-1263.
25. Ferguson RM, Sutherland DER, Simmons RL, Najarian JS (1982) Ketoconazole, cyclosporin metabolism and renal transplantation. Lancet 2:882-883.
26. Sud IJ, Feingold DS (1983) Effect of ketoconazole on the fungicidal action of

amphotericin B in Candida albicans. Antimicrob Agents Chemother 23:185-187.
27. Schaffner A, Frick PG (1985) The effect of ketoconazole on amphotericin B in a model of disseminated aspergillus. J Infect Dis 151:902-910.
28. Meunier F (1987) Prevention of mycoses in immunocompromised patients. Rev Infect Dis 9: 408-416.
29. Pizzo PA, Robichaud KJ, Gill FA, Witebsky FG (1982) Empirical antibiotic and antifungal therapy for cancer patients with prolonged fever and granulocytopenia. Am J Med 72:101-111.
30. Lopez-Berestein G, Fainstein V, Hopfer R, et al (1985) Liposomal amphotericin B for the treatment of systemic fungal infections in patients with cancer. J Infect Dis 151:704-710.
31. Espinel-Ingroft A, Shadomy S, Gobhart RJ (1984) In vitro studies with R51, 211 (itraconazole). Antimicrob Agents Chemother 26:5-9.
32. Van Cutsen J, Van Gervan F, Van de Ven MA, Burgers M, Janssen PAJ (1984) Itraconazole, a new triazole that is orally active in aspergillosis. Antimicrob Agents Chemother 26:527-534.
33. Humphrey MJ, Jevons S, Tarbit MH (1985) Pharmacokinetic evaluation of fluconazole (UK-49,858), a metabolically stable triazole antifungal drug. Antimicrob Agents Chemother 28:648-653.
34. Meunier-Carpentier F, Snoeck R, Gerain J, Muller C, Klastensky J (1984) Amphotericin B nasal spray as prophylaxis against aspergillosis in patients with neutropenia. N Engl J Med 311:1056.
35. Clift RA, Sanders JE, Thomas ED, Williams B, Bruckner CD (1978) Granulocyte transfusions for the prevention of infection in patients receiving bone marrow transplants. N Engl J Med 298:1052-1057.
36. Winston DJ, Ho WG, Young LS, Gale RP (1980) Prophylactic granulocyte transfusions during human bone marrow transplantation. 68:893-897.
37. Winston DJ, Ho WG, Howell CT, et al (1980) Cytomegalovirus infections associated with leukocyte transfusions. Ann Intern Med 93:671-675.
38. Hersmen J, Meyers JD, Thomas ED, et al (1982) The effect of granulocyte transfusions on the incidence of cytomegalovirus infection after allogeneic marrow transplantation. 96:149-152.
39. Ho WG, Winston DJ, Bartoni K, Champlin RE, Gale RP (1983) A controlled trial of intravenous immune globulin for prevention of bacterial and fungal infections in immunosuppressed patients. In: Program and Abstracts of the Twenty-Third Interscience Conference on Antimicrobial Agents and Chemotherapy, Washington, D.C., American Society for Microbiology, 166.
40. Winston DJ, Ho WG, Rasmussen LE, et al (1982) Use of intravenous immune globulin in patients receiving bone marrow transplants. J Clin Immunol 2(supplement):425-475.
41. Saral R, Burns WH, Laskin OL, Santos GW, Leitman PS (1981) Acyclovir prophylaxis of herpes simplex virus infections. N Engl J Med 305:63-67.
42. Wade JC, Newton B, Flournoy N, Meyers JD (1984) Oral acyclovir for prevention of herpes simplex virus reactivation after marrow transplantation. Ann Intern Med 100:823-828.
43. Burns WH, Saral R, Santos GW, et al (1982) Isolation and characterization of resistant herpes simplex virus after acyclovir therapy. Lancet 1:421-423.
44. Winston DJ, Dudnick DV, Chapin M, et al (1983) Coagulase-negative staphylococcal bacteremia in patients receiving immunosuppressive therapy. Arch Intern Med 143:32-36.
45. Winston DJ, Barnes RC, Ho WG, et al (1984) Moxalactam plus piperacillin versus moxalactam plus amikacin in febrile granulocytopenic patients. Am J Med 77:442-450.
46. DeJongh CA, Joshi JH, Thompson BW, et al (1986) A double beta-lactam combination versus an aminoglycoside-containing regimen as empiric antibiotic therapy for febrile granuloctyopenic cancer patients. Am J Med 80(5C):101-111.
47. Fainstein V, Bodey GP, Bolivar R, et al (1984) Moxalactam plus ticarcillin or tobramycin for treatment of febrile episodes in neutropenic cancer patients. Arch Intern Med 144:1766-1770.
48. Feld R, Louie TJ, Mandell L, et al (1985) A multicenter comparative trial of tobramycin and ticarcillin vs. moxalactam and ticarcillin in febrile neutropenic patients. Arch Intern Med 145:1083-1088.
49. Joshi JH, Ruxen R, Newman K, et al (1984) Double beta-lactam versus an aminoglyoside plus beta-lactam combination as empiric therapy for granulocytopenic cancer patients. In: Program and Abstracts of the Twenty-Fourth Interscience Conference on Antimicrobial Agents and Chemotherapy, Washington, D.C., American Society for Microbiology, 383.
50. Winston DJ, Ho WG, Perkins J, et al (1986) Double beta-lactam antibiotic therapy in febrile granulocytopenic patients: cefoperazone/piperacillin vs. moxalactam/ piperacillin. In: Program and Abstracts of the Twenty-Sixth Interscience Conference on Antimicrobial Agents and Chemotherapy, Washington, D.C., American Society for Microbiology, 678.
51. Pizzo PA, Hathorn JW, Hiemenz J, et al (1986) A randomized trial comparing ceftazidime alone with combination antibiotic therapy in cancer patients with fever and neutropenia. N Engl J Med 315:552-558.
52. Wade JC, Standiford HC, Drusano GL, et al (1985) Potential of imipenem as single-agent empiric antibiotic therapy of febrile neutropenic patients with cancer. Am J Med 78(6A):62-72.
53. Karp JE, Dick JD, Angelopulos C, et al (1986) Empiric use of vancomycin during prolonged treatment-induced granulocytopenia. Randomized, double-blind, placebo-controlled clinical trial in patients with acute leukemia. Am J Med 81:237-242.
54. Rubin M, Pizzo PA (1986) Should vancomycin be

included in initial empiric management of febrile neutropenic patients? Analysis of its use in 550 episodes. In: Program and Abstracts of the Twenty-Sixth Interscience Conference on Antimicrobial Agents and Chemotherapy, Washington, D.C., American Society for Microbiology, 676.
55. Winston DJ, Ho WG, Gale RP (1982) Therapeutic granulocyte transfusions for documented infections: a controlled trial in ninety-five infectious granulocytopenic episodes. Ann Intern Med 97:509-515.
56. Meyers JD, Flournoy N, Thomas ED (1982) Non-bacterial pneumonia after allogeneic marrow transplantation: a review of ten years' experience. Rev Infect Dis 4:119-132.
57. Winston DJ, Ho WG, Gale RP, Champlin RE (1987) Treatment and prevention of interstitial pneumonia after bone marrow transplantation. In: Gale RP, Champlin RE (eds). Recent Advances in Bone Marrow Transplantation, New York, Alan R. Liss, in press.
58. Kraemer KG, Neiman PE, Reeves WC, Thomas ED (1978) Prophylactic adenine arabinoside following marrow transplantation. Transplant Proc 10:237-240.
59. Meyers JD, McGuffin RW, Neiman PE, Singer JW, Thomas ED (1980) Toxicity and efficacy of human leukocyte interferon for treatment of cytomegalovirus pneumonia after marrow transplantation. J Infect Dis 141:555-562.
60. Meyers JD, McGuffin RW, Bryson YJ, Cantell K, Thomas ED (1982) Treatment of cytomegalovirus pneumonia after marrow transplant with combined vidarabine and human leukocyte interferon. J Infect Dis 146:80-84.
61. Wade JC, Hintz M, McGuffin RW, Springmeyer SL, Conner JD, Meyers JD (1982) Treatment of cytomegalovirus pneumonia with high-dose acyclovir. Am J Med 73(A):249-256.
62. Wade JC, McGuffin RW, Springmeyer SL, Newton B, Singer JW, Meyers JD (1983) Treatment of cytomegalovirus pneumonia with high-dose acyclovir and human leukocyte interferon. J Infect Dis 148:557-562.
63. Winston DJ, Ho WG, Schroff RW, Champlin RE, Gale RP (1983) Safety and tolerance of recombinant leukocyte A interferon in bone marrow transplant recipients. Antimicrob Agents Chemother 23:846-851.
64. Meyers JD, Day LM, Lunn LG, Sullivan KM (1983) Recombinant leukocyte interferon A for the treatment of serious viral infections after marrow transplant: a phase I study. J Infect Dis 148:551-556.
65. Shepp DH, Newton BA, Meyers JD (1984) Intravenous lymphoblastoid interferon and acyclovir for treatment of cytomegalovirus pneumonia. J Infect Dis 150:776-777.
66. Ringden O, Wilczek H, Lonngvist B, Gahrton G, Wahren B, Lernestedt JO (1985) Foscarnet for cytomegalovirus infections. Lancet 1:1503-1504.
67. Shepp DH, Dandliker PS, De Miranda P, et al (1985) Activity of 9-[2-hydroxy-1-(hydroxy-methyl)ethoxymethyl] guanine in the treatment of cytomegalovirus pneumonia. Ann Intern Med 103:368-373.
68. Winston DJ, Ho WG, Bartoni KB, et al (1986) 9-(1,3-dihydroxy-2-propoxymethyl) guanine (DHPG) treatment of cytomegalovirus (CMV) infections. In: Abstracts of the Fourth International Symposium on Infections in the Immunocompromised Host, Ronneby, Sweden, 161.
69. Reed EC, Dandliker PS, Meyers JD (1986) Treatment of cytomegalovirus pneumonia with 9-[2-hydroxy-1-(hydroxymethyl)ethoxymethyl] guanine and high dose corticosteroids. Ann Intern Med 105:214-215.
70. Blacklock HA, Griffiths P, Stirk P, Prentice HG (1985) Specific hyperimmune globulin for cytomegalovirus pneumonitis. Lancet 2:152-153.
71. Reed EC, Bowden RA, Dandliker PS, Meyers JD (1986) The efficacy of cytomegalovirus immune globulin in marrow transplant patients with CMV pneumonia. In: Program and Abstracts of the Twenty-Sixth Interscience Conference on Antimicrobial Agents and Chemotherapy, Washington, D.C., American Society for Microbiology, 731.
72. Meyers JD, Thomas ED (1982) Infection complicating bone marrow transplantation. In: Young LS, Rubin RH (eds). Clinical Approach to Infection in the Immunocompromsied Host, New York, Alenum Press, 507-551.
73. Winston DJ, Lau WK, Gale RP, Young LS (1980) Trimethoprim-sulfamethoxazole for treatment of _Pneumocystis carinii_ pneumonia. Ann Intern Med 92:762-769.
74. Shanley JD, Jordan MC, Stevens JG (1981) Modification by adoptive humoral immunity of murine cytomegalovirus infection. J Infect Dis 143:231-237.
75. Neiman PE, Reeves W, Ray G, et al (1977) A prospective analysis of interstitial pneumonia and opportunistic viral infections among recipients of allogeneic bone marrow grafts. J INfect Dis 136:754-767.
76. Winston DJ, Pollard RB, Ho WG, et al (1982) Cytomegalovirus immune plasma in bone marrow transplant recipients. Ann Intern Med 97:11-18.
77. Meyers JD, Leszczynski J, Zaia JA, et al (1983) Prevention of cytomeglovirus infection by cytomegalovirus immune globulin after marrow transplantation. Ann Intern Med 98:442-446.
78. O'Reilly RJ, Reich L, Gold J, et al (1983) A randomized trial of intravenous hyperimmune globulin for the prevention of cytomegalovirus infection following bone marrow transplantation: preliminary results. Transplant Proc 15:1405-1411.
79. Kubanek B, Ernst P, Ostendorff P, Schaffer U, Wolf H (1985) Preliminary data of controlled trial of intravenous hyperimmune globulin in the prevention of cytomegalovirus infection in bone marrow transplant recipients. Transplant Proc 17:468-469.
80. Bowden RA, Sayers m, Flournoy N, et al (1986) Cytomegalovirus immune globulin and seronegative blood products to prevent primary cytomegalovirus infection after marrow transplantation. N Engl J Med 314:1006-1010.
81. Winston DJ, Ho WG, Lin CH, et al (1987) Intravenous immunoglobulin for prevention of interstitial pneumonia after bone marrow transplantation. Ann Intern Med 106:12-18.
82. Syndman DR, Werner BG, Heinze-Lacey B, CMVIG-IV Renal Transplant Study Group (1985)

Prevention of kidney transplant associated primary cytomegalovirus disease with an intravenous cytomegalovirus immune globulin. A preliminary analysis. In: Program and Abstracts of the Twenty-Fifth Interscience Conference on Antimicrobial Agents and Chemotherapy, Washington, D.C., American Society for Microbiology, 248.

83. Meyers JD, McGuffin RW, Thomas ED (1982) Prophylactic human leukocyte interferon after allogeneic marrow transplant: immunological and virologic effects. In: Program and Abstracts of the Twenty-Second Interscience conference on Antimicrobial Agents and Chemotherapy, Washington, D.C., American Society for Microbiology, 190.
84. Meyers JD, Reed EC, Shepp DH, et al (1986) Prevention of cytomegalovirus infection after marrow transplant with high-dose intravenous acyclovir. In: Program and Abstracts of the Twenty-Sixth Interscience conference on Antimicrobial Agents and Chemotherapy, Washington, D.C., American Society for Microbiology, 231.
85. Atkinson K, Farewell V, Storb R, et al (1982) Analysis of late infections after human bone marrow transplantation: role of genotypic nonidentity between marrow donor and recipient and of nonspecific suppressor cells in patients with chronic graft-versus-host disease. Blood 60:714-720.
86. Locksley RM, Flournoy N, Sullivan KM, Meyers JD (1985) Varicella-zoster virus infection after marrow transplantation. J Infect Dis 152:1172-1181.
87. Winston DJ, Schiffman G, Wang DC, et al (1979) Pneumococcal infections after human bone marrow transplantation. Ann Intern Med 91:835-841.
88. Sullivan KM, Dahlberg S, Storb R, et al (1983) Infection acquisition and prophylaxis in chronic graft-versus-host disease (GVHD). Blood 62:230A.
89. Witherspoon RP, Storb R, Ochs H, et al (1981) Recovery of antibody production in human allogeneic marrow graft recipients: influence of time post-transplantation, the presence or absence of chronic graft-versus-host disease and antithymocyte globulin treatment. Blood 58:360-368.
90. Winston DJ, Ho WG, Schiffman G, Champlin RE, Feig SA, Gale RP (1983) Pneumococcal vaccination of recipients of bone marrow transplants. Arch Intern Med 143:1735-1737.
91. Balfour HH, Bean B, Laskin CL, et al (1983) Acyclovir halts progression of herpes zoster in immunocompromised patients. N Engl J Med 308:1443-1453.

Table 1 CONTROLLED TRIALS OF ORAL FLUORINATED QUINOLONES FOR PREVENTION OF BACTERIAL INFECTIONS IN GRANULOCYTOPENIC PAITENTS

Reference	Regimen	Underlying Disease	Microbiologically Documented Infections	Gram Negative Bacteremia	Gram Positive Bacteremia
John Hopkins (Karp, 17) 1987	Norfloxacin vs placebo	Acute leukemia and autologous marrow transplant	20/35 (57%) vs 26/35 (79%)	3/35 (9%) vs 11/33 (33%)	4/35 (11%) vs 3/33 (9%)
Maryland (Joshi, 18) 1987	Norfloxacin vs Trimethoprim-sulfamethoxazole	Hematologic malignancy	10/26 (38%) vs 14/28 (50%)	0/26 (0%) 1/28 (4%)	5/26 (19%) vs 4/28 (14%)
Manitoba (Bow, 19) 1985	Norfloxacin vs Trimethoprim-sulfamethoxazole	Acute leukemia	9/17 (53%) 6/14 (43%)	0/17 (0%) 1/14 (7%)	5/17 (29%) vs 0/14 (0%)
UCLA (Winston, 20) 1986	Norfloxacin vs Vancomycin-polymyxin	Hematologic malignancy	12/36 (33%)vs 16/30 (53%)	0/36 (0%) 5/30 (17%)	9/36 (25%) vs 4/30 (13%)
Utrecht (Dekker, 21) 1987	Ciprofloxacin vs Trimethoprim-sulfamethoxazole	Acute leukemia	5/28 (18%) vs 14/28 (50%)	3/28 (11%) vs 5/28 (18%)	3/28 (11%) vs 6/28 (21%)
UCLA (Winston, 22) 1987	Ofloxacin vs Vancomycin polymyxin	Hematologic malignancy	8/21 (30%) vs 11/22 (50%)	0/21 (0%) vs 3/22 (14%)	6/21 (29%) vs 4/22 (18%)
	TOTAL	Quinolones vs Controls	64/163 (39%) vs 87/155 (56%)	3/163 (2%) vs 26/155 (17%)	32/163 (19%) vs 21/155 (14%)

Table 2 CONTROLLED TRIALS OF DOUBLE BETA-LACTAM COMBINATIONS IN GRANULOCYTOPENIC PATIENTS WITH PROVEN INFECTION

References	Combination	Favorable Responses/ Total Infections (%)	Nephrotoxicity
Winston 1984 (45)	Moxalactam/piperacillin vs Moxalactam/amikacin	46/61 (74%) vs 41/50 (82%)	2/136 (1%) vs 6/136 (4%)
De Jongh 1986 (46)	Moxalactam/piperacillin vs Moxalactam/amikacin	65/95 (68%) vs 60/83 (72%)	2/145 (1%) vs 12/130 (9%)
Fainstein 1984 (47)	Moxalactam/ticarcillin vs Moxalactam/tobramycin	73/113 (65%) vs 76/118 (64%)	0/217 (0%) vs 6/228 (3%)
Feld 1985 (48)	Moxalactam/ticarcillin vs Ticarcillin/tobramycin	38/64 (59%) vs 38/60 (55%)	2/88 (2%) vs 2/85 (2%)
Joshi 1984 (49)	Ceftazidime/piperacillin vs Ceftazidime/tobramycin	46/50 (82%) vs 46/61 (75%)	2/99 (2%) vs 7/103 (7%)
Winston 1986 (50)	Cefoperazone/piperacillin vs Moxalactam/piperacillin	24/32 (75%) vs 20/25 (75%)	0/59 (0%) vs 0/65 (0%)
TOTAL	Double beta-lactam Aminoglycoside+beta-lactam	311/440 (70%) 261/372 (70%)	8/809 (1%) 33/682 (5%)

Table 3 ANTIVIRAL THERAPY OF CYTOMEGALOVIRUS PNEUMONIA IN BONE MARROW TRANSPLANTS

Reference	Therapy	Response
Kraemer 1978 (58)	Vidarabine	1/6*
Meyers 1980 (59)	Human Leukocyte Interferon	0/8
Meyers 1982 (60)	Human Leukocyte Interferon + Vidarabine	1/7
Wade 1982 (61)	Acyclovir	1/8
Wade 1983 (62)	Human Leukocyte Interferon + Vidarabine	3/13
Winston 1983 (63)	Recombinant Leukocyte Interferon	3/5
Meyers 1983 (64)	Recombinant Leukocyte Interferon	0/5
Shepp 1984 (65)	Lymphoblastoid Interferon + Acyclovir	1/8
Ringden 1985 (66)	Foscarnet	0/9
Shepp 1985 (67)	DHPG (Ganciclovir)	1/10
Winston 1986 (68)	DHPG (Ganciclovir)	2/9
Reed 1986 (69)	DHPG (Ganciclovir) + Corticosteroids	1/6
Blacklock 1985 (70)	CMV Immune Globulin	6/9
Reed 1986 (71)	CMV Immune Globulin	2/10
TOTAL	22/114 (19%)	

*Survivors/Total Patients Treated

Table 4 CONTROLLED TRIALS OF PROPHYLACTIC IMMUNE PLASMA OR GLOBULIN IN BONE MARROW TRANSPLANTS*

Reference	Regimen	CMV Infection	CMV Pneumonia
UCLA 1982 (Winston, 76)	CMV Immune Plasma vs No Prophylaxis	12/24 (50%) vs 15/24 (63%)	3/24 (13%) vs 8/24 (33%)+
Seattle 1983 (Meyers, 77)	CMV Immune Globulin vs No Prophylaxis	10/30 (33%) vs 14/32 (44%)	2/30 (7%) vs 3/32 (9%)+
Sloan-Kettering 1983 (O'Reilly, 78)	CMV Immune Globulin vs No Prophylaxis	0/17 (0%) vs 10/20 (50%)	0/17 (0%) vs 6/20 (30%)
Europe 1985 (Kubanek, 79)	CMV Immune Globulin vs Normal Immune Globulin		1/26 (4%) vs 6/23 (26%)
Seattle 1986 (Bowden, 80)	CMV Immune Globulin vs No Prophylaxis	5/21 (24%) vs 8/20 (40%)	1/21 (5%) vs 1/20 (5%)
UCLA 1986 (Winston, 81)	Gamimune vs No Prophylaxis	18/38 (48%) vs 21/37 (54%)	6/38 (16%) vs 12/37 (32%)
TOTAL	Immune Plasma/Globulin vs No Prophylaxis	45/130 (35%) vs 68/133 (51%)	13/156 (8%) vs 36/156 (23%)

*Adapted from reference (57) with permission.
+Greater benefit with no WBC transfusions

X. Metabolic and Genetic Disorders: H. Mizoguchi and W. Krivit, Chairpersons

30: Bone Marrow Transplantation for Thalassemia: 156 Cases Transplanted in Pesaro

G. Lucarelli, C. Giardini, M. Galimberti, P. Polchi, E. Angelucci,
D. Baronciani, F. Manenti, P. Politi, D. Marchionni, M. Donati, O. Paradisi,
C. Giorgi, M. Manna, and F. Agostinelli

Bone marrow transplantation can be used to radically cure homozygous thalassemia (1,2,3,4). We present here the results of marrow transplantation in 156 consecutive patients with beta-thalassemia aged between 1 and 15 years.

PATIENTS AND METHODS.

All transplants were carried out between June 1983 and June 1987. The follow-up ranges from 45 to 1480 days post-transplant. All patients were prepared for transplant with busulfan 3.5 mg/Kg given orally in three divided doses on each of four consecutive days, followed by cyclophosphamide 50 mg/Kg administered intravenously on each of four consecutive days (5).
For acute graft-versus-host disease prophylaxis, 48 patients received methotrexate as in the Seattle Protocol but modified by substituting cyclophosphamide 7.5 mg/Kg on day 1 post-transplant; 26 patients received a combination of cyclosporine plus "short methotrexate" as proposed by the Seattle Group (6); 10 patients received cyclosporine alone from day -9 pre-transplant, and 72 received cyclosporine alone from day -2 pre-transplant. In all instances cyclosporine was administered i.v. 5 mg/Kg until day +5 post-transplant, when the dosage was reduced to 3 mg/Kg followed by 12.5 mg/Kg given orally from day + 21 to day 180 or 365 post-transplant. Cytogenetic analyses, performed on unstimulated marrow and phytohemagglutinin-stimulated peripheral blood reticulocytes when donor and recipient were of opposite sex, and determination of the pattern of globin chain synthesis with column chromatography of marrow cells and peripheral reticulocytes, were used as markers for the engraftment and for the functioning graft every six months. Acute and chronic graft-versus-host disease were graded according to the Seattle criteria.

Table 1. Results of bone marrow transplantation in thalassemia

No. of patients	156	
Age (yrs., ave.)	8	
Dead	24	(15%)
Alive	132	(85%)
Alive with return of thalassemia	11	(7%)
Alive disease-free (60 - 1500 days)	121	(78%)
A-GVHD incidence (grade 2 - 4)	24%	
A-GVHD fatality	3%	
C-GVHD incidence (grade Moderate-Severe)	11%	
C-GVHD fatality	2%	
Kaplan-Meier Survival (Probability)	84%, 376 days	
Patients at risk	89	
Kaplan-Meier Disease-Free Survival (Probability)	78%, 340 days	
Patients at risk	86	

RESULTS

Table 1 summarizes the results obtained after bone marrow transplantation in 156 patients aged between 1 and 15 years and suffering from beta homozygous thalassemia. Applying the Kaplan - Meier calculation, the probability of survival is 84% while the probability of disease-free survival is 78%.

DISCUSSION

This study shows that long-term disease-free survival can be achieved in a high proportion of patients with homozygous beta thalassemia transplanted between 1 and 15 years of age. Thalassemia is a progressive disease: organ iron overload increases with time; likewise, the presence of chronic aggressive hepatitis, chronic persistent hepatitis and periportal fibrosclerosis in liver biopsies becomes ever more frequent with age. Consequently, bone marrow transplantation has fewer both early and late post-transplant complications in young thalassemic patients (aged 1 to 8 years) than in older patients (8 to 15 years). Considering that the death rate is 10% in the younger group of patients, whereas in the older group it reaches 20%, it would therefore appear preferable to perform the transplant early in thalassemia rather than late.

REFERENCES

1. Thomas ED, Buckner CD, Sanders J, Pavayannopoulos T, Borgna-Pignatti C, Stefano P, Sullivan KM, Clift RA, Storb R (1982) Marrow transplantation for thalassemia. Lancet ii:227-28
2. Lucarelli G, Izzi T, Polchi P, Agostinelli F, Manna M, Delfini C, Galimberti M, Porcellini A, Moretti L, Manna A, Talevi S, Debiagi M, Nesci S, Sparaventi G, Andreani M, Filippetti A, Stramigioli S (1983) Bone marrow transplantation in thalassemia. J Exp Clin Cancer Res 3:313
3. Lucarelli G, Galimberti M, Polchi P, Giardini C, Politi P, Baronciani D, Angelucci E, Manenti F, Delfini C, Aureli G, Muretto P (1987) Marrow transplantation in patients with advanced thalassemia. N Engl J Med 316:1050
4. Lucarelli G, Polchi P, Galimberti M, Izzi T, Delfini C, Manna M, Agostinelli F, Giorgi C, Baronciani D, Angelucci E, Giardini C, Politi P (1985) Marrow transplantation for thalassemia following busulphan and cyclophosphamide. Lancet i:1355
5. Santos GW, Tutscha PJ, Brookmeyer R, Saral R, Beschorner WE, Bias WB, Brain HG, Burns WH, Elfenbein GJ, Kaizer H, Mellits D, Stuart RK, Sensenbrenner LL, Yeager AM (1983) Marrow transplantation for acute nonlymphocytic leukemia after treatment with busulphan and cyclophosphamide. N Engl J Med 309: 1347
6. Storb R, Deeg JH, Whitehead J, Appelbaum F, Beatty P, Beuriger W, Buckner CD, Clift R, Doney K, Forewell V, Hansen J, Hill R, Lum L, Martin P, McGuffin R, Sanders J, Stewart P, Sullivan K, Witherspoon R, Yee G, Thomas ED (1986) Methotrexate and cyclosporine alone for prophylaxis of acute graft versus host disease after marrow transplantation for leukemia. N Engl J Med 314:729-36

31: Improvement of Clinical Expression of Central Nervous System Manifestation in Lysosomal Storage Diseases Treated by Bone Marrow Transplantation

William Krivit, Chester B. Whitley, Gunnar Lund, Norma K.C. Ramsay, and John H. Kersey

INTRODUCTION

Bone marrow transplantation has amply proven itself capable of sowing normal hematopoietic seeds. Subsequent growth of normal cells throughout the reticuloendothelial system has been well established. Use of BMT for hematopoietic diseases such as aplastic anemia, leukemia, neutrophil disorders, and thalassemia have been reviewed extensively and will not be addressed here.

Less well recognized has been the therapeutic responses resulting from BMT in lysosomal storage diseases.[1,2]

As a direct result of replacement of reticuloendothelial cells, the congenital lysosomal storage disorders have been effectively treated by bone marrow transplantation.[3,4,5]

This review will specifically address the efficacy of such BMT for the central nervous system manifestations of lysosomal storage disorders.

Improvement in clinical expression of central nervous system manifestations in patients treated by bone marrow transplantation is becoming apparent. The data accumulated to-date is indicative of changes in the central nervous system which are permitting the children to attain a sustained more normal life. Cognitive capability has been enhanced subsequent to BMT in several patients. Motor functions and skills have also returned. The children who have been followed for several years have demonstrated a clinical course disparate from their untreated siblings and from previous experience.

METACHROMATIC LEUKODYSTROPHY

The patient (L.B.) at the University of Minnesota is now $2\frac{1}{2}$ years subsequent to successful bone marrow transplant. L.B. is now over 7 years of age and is achieving normal milestones in school and at home. Her scholastic capabilities as measured by specific psychometric tests at the University of Minnesota and, as measured by school accomplishments, are commensurate with her age. This is to be contrasted with her sister (K.B.) who was decerebrate and comatose at $6\frac{1}{2}$ years of age. The sister's typical course ended in demise at 8 years.[6,7]

We have also chosen to follow our patients' clinical course with serial magnetic resonance imaging (MRI). The impressive sensitivity of MRI in detecting abnormalities involving primarily the white matter was again demonstrated in our study. Over the period of $2\frac{1}{2}$ years subsequent to BMT, there is evidence of reversal and/or stabilization of demyelinating process.

This is the first radiological report of improvement of white matter disease in Metachromatic Leukodystrophy. We are reporting our observations in order to encourage BMT early in other patients with late infantile MLD before signs and symptoms appear.

MRI was performed using a super conductive magnet (Siemens Corporation). Prior to January, 1986 the unit was operated at .35 Tesla and after that date at 1 Tesla. Multislice, multiecho, spinecho sequences were used, SE 1.5/35-70 prior to January, 1986 and SE 2.3 to 3.3/35-70 EKG triggered sequences after that date.

The magnetic resonance images were first obtained in our patient at 4 years 8 months of age (8 months post BMT engraftment). The high intensity confluent areas in the periventricular white matter were identified as being typical of MLD. At 5 years of age, however, normal signals from MRI are seen in areas previously noted to have high intensity. Improvement was again noted at 6 years of age. And, most recently, at 7 years there is overall considerably less extensive area of abnormality around frontal and occipital horns. (Figure).

The comparison to the older sister who was similarly affected by MLD is critical for appropriate analysis. The sister died before MRI

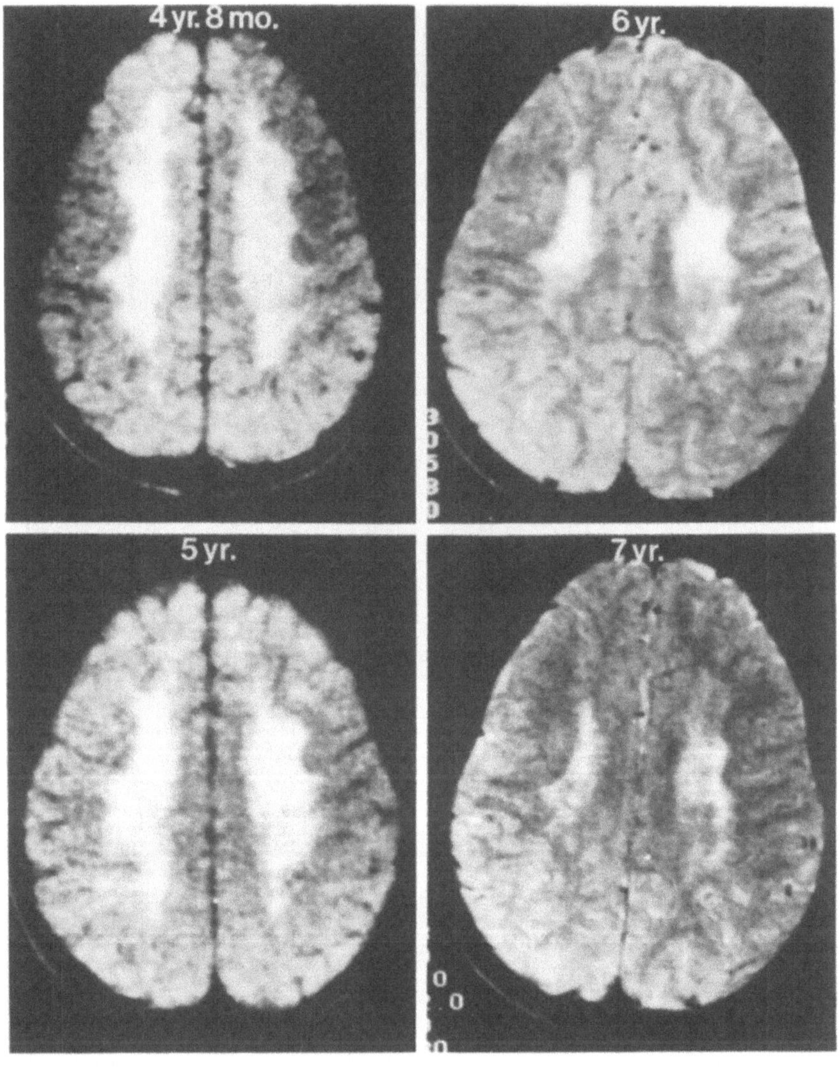

LEGEND
Figure 1

Sequential MRI were taken during the 2 years subsequent to BMT at age 4 years. The white densities are evidence of demyelination and represent significant amounts of water retained in these areas. The resolution of this demyelination is readily apparent.

was available at our facility. Her axial computerized tomographic examination was done at 8 years 11 months of age. Marked cerebral atrophy and ventricular dilatation are noted. In comparison, our patient does not have similar evidence of ventricular size change and/or cerebral atrophy.

We ascribe the beneficial effect of the BMT engraftment to the normal amount of Arylsulfatase A.

Therapeutic response has also been noted in two other patients with MLD subsequent to successful to BMT. Both are now sufficiently long past BMT (3½ years and 1 year) to indicate that the disease is not following the inexorable course that prior untreated siblings had. These untreated siblings had a course marked by the well documented rapid CNS decompensation and death.[8,9]

Concordance of clinical events in siblings in a family with MLD has been the dominant theme of previous literature review and experience.[10] The discordance between our BMT treated patients who are alive and their sibs who have died is striking. Central nervous system pathophysiology has been positively affected in MLD post BMT. The most striking demonstration of the efficacy of BMT has been the continued improvement in MRI in which areas of demyelination now have decreased and some are now demonstrating normal myelination.

The MRI alterations may be in keeping with remyelination in the brain. The data on interpeak latency (BAEP) and radiologic evidence from CT and MRI of the brain also suggest remyelination. However, peripheral motor nerve conduction velocities provide no evidence of improvement. The frequency distribution of myelinated fibers of sural nerve has shown a change from the nearly normal bimodal (before BMT) toward a unimodal (28 months after BMT) distribution. This finding implies worsening. The inhibition of CNS degeneration, and possibly even of improvement, is noticeably different than in peripheral nerve in which deterioration appears to be continuing. We have insufficient data to assess whether peripheral nerve impairment has been retarded. The difference in reconstitution in the central and peripheral nervous systems may reflect differences in enzyme concentrations.

HURLER SYNDROME

Hurler syndrome was the first lysosomal storage disease treated with bone marrow transplantation. The longest living post BMT Hurler patients are now 6 and 7 years of age. These patients now are attending school and have intelligence measurements consistent with their age attainments[11] (and personal observations of the London patients by Dr. W. Krivit).

CNS improvement in the patients with Hurler syndrome may be subsequent to reduction of apnea (hypoxia and anoxia) secondary to decrease in visceral disease and amelioration of cardiothoracic pharyngeal pathology. We have documented that sleep apnea resolves within days of beginning cytoreduction preparative regimen.[12] Obviously, prevention of recurrent otitis media, sleep apnea, and cardiac failure will help CNS development.[12]

The incontrovertible data concerning the glycosaminoglycan (GAG) levels in CSF, as developed by Whitley et al at Minnesota, must also be noted.[13] The cerebrospinal fluid GAG levels had been previously measured by Dekabon and Constantopulos and found to correlate very well with both progression of disease and with degrees of mental retardation.[14] CSF GAG levels in our patients have returned to normal levels.

The magnetic resonance imaging that we have obtained in our patients with Hurler syndrome subsequent to bone marrow transplantation at the University of Minnesota is confirmatory of that previously reported from London.[15] Although there have been episodes of change occurring immediately post bone marrow transplant period, the eventual resultant over the period of several months post BMT has been stabilization and return to a non progressive status.

The present authors are well aware of the several different types of disease within the family of mucopolysaccharidoses. Furthermore, there is a broad spectrum of clinical manifestations associated with the absence and/or deficiency of the L-iduronidase enzyme in Hurler syndrome[16,17,18]. Although we must await final results of periods of several years, we observe that the initial results are encouraging.

SANFILIPPO SYNDROME

The data from Westminster Children's Hospital on the twins who had BMT treatment for Sanfilippo disease (type B) is now quite interesting. These two children are now stable and are not deteriorating and attend school. This salient effect of attending school must be contrasted with their siblings who did not receive BMT. The untreated siblings had a decrement in clinical competency leading to demise quite characteristic of Sanfilippo.[19] We, at the University of Minnesota, also have had the opportunity to study 2 patients with Sanfilippo (III-A and III-B) who are post-BMT 2 months and 18 months. Although both continue to show no decline in cognitive or motor skills, there is no data to support improvement as yet.

ANIMAL EXPERIMENTS

Successful replacement of deficient enzyme activity by bone marrow transplantation has been done in several animal experiments. Furthermore, there has been demonstration by enzyme penetration into neuronal tissue. Appropriate changes of CNS abnormality include improvement ot status and prevention of CNS deterioration. These include animal models of human disease characterized by deficiencies of alpha L-iduronidase, arylsulfatase B, ^{B}-glucuronidase and B galactosyl cerebrosidase.

1) The canine model of mucopolysaccharide storage disease results from alpha L-iduronidase deficiency.[20] The characteristics of the canine disease are quite similar to that of human

counterpart of Hurler-Schie disease. The extensive work done by Shull and colleagues has included a definition of CNS pathology before and after bone marrow transplantation. The neuronal pathology includes the formation of lesions typical for the accumulation of lysosomal substrates. These are typical lysosomal inclusions before transplant. These and other abnormalities disappear afterwards. The enzyme also has been observed to penetrate and is at a level, which although quite low, may be sufficient to provide clearing of mucopolysaccharide material.

2) Correction of the CNS clinical abnormalities secondary to sulfatide accumulation in the brain of feline models due to abnormal arysulfatase B deficiency has been documented subsequent to bone marrow transplantation.[21] The abnormal morphologic characteristics of the neuronal cells disappear. Wenger and colleagues, however, have been unable to demonstrate enzymatic activity in the brain despite clearing of substrate and amelioration of symptoms. Whether or not this enzyme is membrane bound and cannot be measured has not been reviewed. Furthermore, the enzyme could potentially be effective at exceedingly limited amounts of exerting influence at a specific cellular site of focus. Antibody labeled studies could conceivably help provide data on this latter point.

3) The glucuronidase model studied so extensively by Hoogerbrugge and Associates demonstrate the presence of enzymes in the brain subsequent to bone marrow transplant but in very small amounts. The level of enzyme indicated in these articles is that of 4%. This too is being analyzed further to see if enzyme activity can increase.[22]

4) Yeager and coworkers have repeated their original observations on the "Twitcher mouse" model of "globoid cell" leukodystrophy. By completing the BMT at 7 days which was earlier than had been done before, these investigators have noted that CNS symptoms and signs and pathology are significantly delayed in onset and decreased in severity. The reduction and differences of psychosine and galactocerebroside substrate have been quite carefully documented in neuronal tissue subsequent to BMT as compared to control animals.[23]

Furthermore, there is specific monoclonal antibody staining data to indicate that globoid cells in globoid cell leukodystrophy (Krabbe disease) are macrophage derived cells and not a neuronal cell.[24] This data would indicate that globoid cell leukodystrophy (Krabbe disease) would be worthwhile for a BMT to be undertaken in appropriate circumstances in human disease counterpart. We at the University of Minnesota have treated two patients with Krabbe disease but it is too early to document results.

5) The established chimera in the cattle with mannosidosis (i.e. "snorter cattle") frequently has been mentioned as an example of failure to change or alter the clinical characteristics which resemble the human mannosidosis disease. The enzymatic activity in this model has not been quantitatively or qualitatively ascertained. Perhaps this in utero cross placental process of developing chimerism also offers alternative immunologic rationale for inhibition of lymphocyte and monocyte migration and replacement of r.e.s. fixed macrophage activity.[25]

6) Another animal model concerns development of normalcy subsequent to BMT in fucosidase deficiency.[26] In this model, the enzyme has clearly penetrated into CNS.

V. IN VITRO, EX VIVO EXPERIMENTS

Whereas, the replacement of recipients visceral r.e.s. macrophage by new monocyte from donor transplanted marrow can be readily documented in liver, spleen, peritoneum, osteoclast and pulmonary system, there has been considerable difficulty in fully establishing the origin of glial cells in the brain.

Monocytes labeled with H3 thymidine when injected into an experimental animal do migrate into CNS after either infection or trauma. The label from monocyte is now specifically found in the glial cell in the rabbit studies. This does require artifically induced exogeneous trauma or infection to be present.[27-30]

In humans several investigators have attempted to document the change of female to male chromosomes by fluorescent staining. This has not been demonstrable in the brain mainly because three specific technicalities have not been critically analyzed, 1) appropriate male-female donor recipient pair; 2) ability to stain and identify fluorescence; 3) documentative of specific glial cells. We have also tried specific X-Y fluorescent antibody stain in our catalase BMT model and were unable to distinguish because of high background activity.[31]

Glial cell cultures have been attempted and failed. This research will need to be pursued in the future with more vigor.

SUMMARY

There is every reason to believe that bone marrow transplantation will be effective in lysosomal storage diseases in correcting not only visceral lesions, but in prevention of damage to CNS and some degree of amelioration may also be anticipated post BMT.

Bone marrow transplantation for lysosomal storage diseases has now been accomplished in over 100 patients. The toxicities as measured by failure to engraft, loss of graft, infection, graft versus host disease and death have been enumerated. The data accumulated in these studies is generally considered acceptable as a Phase I beginning.

We now need to proceed to carefully construct Phase II studies. Individual diseases are considered in their own categories relative to therapeutic success. The degree of remission and eventual outcomes will need to be ascertained. This will require a concerted effort to combine data from all services throughout the world.

Finally, in the next several years, larger Phase III studies will be necessary to measure relative degrees of safety and effectiveness of different methods of preparation, age at which BMT should be done, use of additional lymphokines to aid in furthering enzyme production will need to be considered.

The number of diseases of inborn errors of metabolism which will be amenable to bone marrow transplantation has only been touched upon. To fully measure the potential will take many years and will require an enlargement of services and focus. Again, if there is to be a future in the use of "Gene Therapy", these studies now included in BMT protocols for inborn errors of metabolism will serve as forerunner and hallmark for the future. If gene therapy and molecular biological interventions are to be successful, this must first show merit in our present studies.

REFERENCES

1. Krivit W and Whitley CB (1987) Bone Marrow Transplantation for Genetic Diseases. NEJM 316:1085-1087

2. Editorial (1986) Bone Marrow Transplantation for Neurovisceral Storage Diseases. Lancet 2:788-789

3. Hobbs JR, Hugh-Jones K, Barrett AJ, Bryom N, Chambers D, Henry K and James DCO (1981) Reversal of clinical features of Hurler's disease and biochemical improvement after treatment by bone marrow transplantation. Lancet ii:709-712

4. Krivit W, Pierpont ME, Ayaz K, Tsai M, Ramsay NKC, Kersey JH, Weisdorf S, Sibley R, Snover D, McGovern M, Schwartz MF and Desnick RJ (1984) Bone marrow transplantation in the Maroteaux-Lamy Syndrome (Mucopolysaccharidoses Type VI). NEJM 311:1606-1611

5. Whitley CB, Ramsay NKC, Kersey JH and Krivit W (1986) Bone Marrow Transplantation for Hurler Syndrome: Assessment of Metabolic Correction. Birth Defects: Original Article Series. 22:7-24 Krivit W (Ed). Alan Liss, New York

6. Lipton ME, Lockman LA, Ramsay NKC, Kersey JH, Jacobsen RI, Krivit W. BMT in MLD. 56-68 (ibid)

7. Krivit W, Lipton ME, Lockman LA, Tsai M, Dyck PJ, Smith S, Ramsay NKC, and Kersey J (1987) Prevention of Deterioration in Metachromatic Leukodystrophy by Bone Marrow Transplantation. Accepted, Am J Med Sci

8. Ladisch S, Bayever E, Phillippart M, and Feig S (1986) Biochemical Findings After Bone Marrow Transplantation for Metachromatic Leukodystrophy. Birth Defects: March of Dimes. Original Article Series 22:165-176 Krivit W (Ed), Alan Liss, New York

9. Yeager A (Personal Communication)

10. MacFaul R, Cavanaugh N, Lake BD, Stephens R, and Whitfield AE (1982) Metachromatic Leukodystrophy: Review of 38 Cases. Arch of Dis of Child 57:168-175

11. Hugh-Jones K (1986) Psychomotor Development of Children with Mucopolysaccharidoses I-H Following Bone Marrow Transplantation. Birth Defects: Original Article Series 22:25-29 Krivit W (Ed), Alan Liss, New York

12. Malone BM, Whitley CB, Duvall AJ, Belani KG, Sibley RK, Ramsay NKC, Kersey JH, Krivit W, Berlinger N Resolution of Sleep Apnea in Hurler Disease After BMT. Am J Otolaryngology (submitted)

13. Whitley CB, Lockman LA, Lipton ME, Ramsay NKC, Kersey JH, and Krivit W (1986) A Blood-Brain Gateway: Access to the Central Nervous System After Bone Marrow Transplantation for Lysosomal Storage Diseases. Clin Res 34:984A

14. Dekabon AS, Constantopoulos G (1973) Mucopolysaccharidoses Relation of Elevated Cerebral Spinal Fluid Glycosaminoglycans to Mental Retardation. Arch Neurol 28:385-388

15. Johnson MA, Desai S, Hugh-Jones K, and Starer F (1984) Magnetic Resonance Imaging of the Brain in Hurler Syndrome. Am J Nuc Rad 5: 816-819

16. Roubicek M, Gehler J, Springer J (1985) The Clinical Spectrum of Alpha-1-iduronidase Deficiency. Am J Med Genet 20:471-481

17. Whitley CB, Gorlin RJ, Krivit W (1987) A Nonpathological Allele (I^W) for Low Alpha L-iduronidase deficiency. Am J Med Genet, in press

18. Stevenson RE, Howell RR, McKusick VA, Suskind R, Hanson JW, Elliott DE and Neufield EF (1976) The Iduronidase Deficient Mucopolysaccharidoses: Clinical and Roentgenographic Features. Pediatrics 57:111-122

19. Hugh-Jones K, Kendra J, James DCO, Hobbs JR (1983) Treatment of Sanfilippo Disease (MPS IIIB) by Bone Marrow Transplantation. Exp Haematol 19(10):50-51

20. Shull RM, Hasting NE, Selcer RR, Jones JB, Smith JR, Cullen WC, Constantopoulous G (1987) Bone Marrow Transplantation in Canine Mucopolysaccharidoses I. J Clin Invest 79: 435-443

21. Wenger DA, Gasper PE, Thrall MA (1984) Feline Arylsulfatase B Deficiency (mucopolysaccharidoses VI): correction by bone marrow transplantation. Am J Hu Genet 36:(suppl 1):80S

22. Hoogerbrugge PM, Poorthius BJHM, Wagemaker G and Bekkum DW Van (1987) Corection of Lysosomal Enzyme Deficiency in Various Organs of β-Glucuronidase-Deficient Mice By Allogeneic Bone Marrow Transplantation (1987) Transplantation 43(5):609-614

23. Toyoshima E, Yeager AM, Brennan S, Santos GW, Moser HW, Mayer RF (1986) Nerve Conduction studies in the Twitcher Mouse (murine globoid cell leukodystrophy). J Neurol Sci 74(2-3):307-318

24. Kobayashi S, Katayama M, Bourque E, Suzuki K and Suzuki K (1985) The Twitcher Mouse: Positive Immunohistochemical Staining of Globoid Cells with Monoclonal Antibody Against Mac-1 Antigen. Developmental Brain Research 29:49-54

25. Jolly RD, Thompson KG, Murphy CE, Mankelow BW, Brvere AN, Winchester BC (1976) Enzyme Replacement Therapy: An Experiment of Nature in a Chimeric Mannosidosis Calf. Ped Res 224:10219

26. Taylor RM, Farrow BRH, Stewart GJ, Healy PJ (1986) Enzyme Replacement in Nervous Tissue After Allogeneic Bone-Marrow Transplantation for Fucosidosis in Dogs. Lancet 772-774

27. Kronigsmark BW and Sidman RL (1983) Origin of Brain Macrophage in the Mouse. J Neuropathol Exp Neurol 22:643

28. Kosunen TV, Wahsman BH and Samuelson IK (1963) Radioautograph Study of Cellular Mechanisms in Delayed Hypersensitivity. J Neuropathol Exp Neurol 22:367-374

29. Ting JPL, Nixon DF, Weiner LP and Ferlinger JA (1983) Brain 1a antigen have a bone marrow origin. Immunogenetics 17:295

30. Perry VH, Hume DA and Gordon S (1985) Immunohistochemical Localization of Macrophages and Microglia in the Adult and Developing Mouse Brain. Neuroscience 15:313-326

31. Tuchman M, Blazar B, Krivit W (1986) Brain Catalase Activity Following Syngeneic Bone Marrow Transplantation in Acatalesemic Mice. Original Article Series: March of Dimes BMT for Lysosomal Storage. Krivit W (Ed) Alan Liss, New York, pp. 165-176

32: Bone Marrow Transplantation Following Nuclear Accidents

Robert Peter Gale

The medical response to nuclear accidents is complex and involves assessment of the source-term, containment, evacuation of individuals at risk, dose determination and medical interventions. For purposes of this review I will assume that the whole body dose of radiation have been determined either by physical simulation, or by physical or biologic dosimetry. Data regarding biologic dosimetry have been recently reviewed (1-4).

Several factors determine the nature of the medical response to nuclear accidents including the dose of radiation and the tissues affected. In the setting of a major radiation release, the primary target organs are the skin, bone marrow, gastrointestinal tract, liver and lungs. Depending upon the setting, these toxicities may be discrete or overlapping and are illustrated schematically in Figure 1. At one extreme,

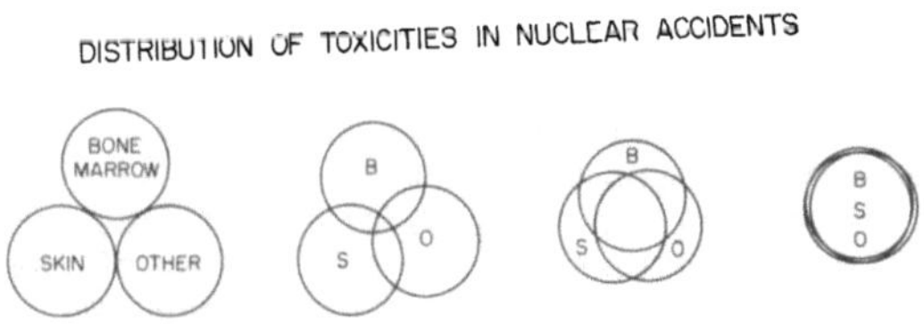

individuals with radiation induced skin damage are completely distinct from those with bone marrow damage as well as from other toxicities. The opposite extreme predicts completely overlapping toxicities. These relationships are complex and not completely understood. They are, however, of major importance in determining the medical response since each requires different interventions. For example, all individuals with irreversible bone marrow failure might also have ulitmately fatal skin or lung damage. In this case a bone marrow transplant can potentially prevent death from myelosuppression but cannot save lives since these individuals will utlimately die of other toxicities. If we consider the opposite case, then bone marrow transplants can potentially save lives since these other toxicities will not compromise transplant outcome.

This situation is even more complex since some toxicities are synergistic (Figure 2). For example a whole body dose of 2 Gy results in 100% survival in irradiated rats. Likewise a 1 cm skin burn has no immediate mortality. If, however, one combines these injuries, the mortality rate rises to 50%. This can be reduced by 20% (but not to zero) by surgical excision of the burn.

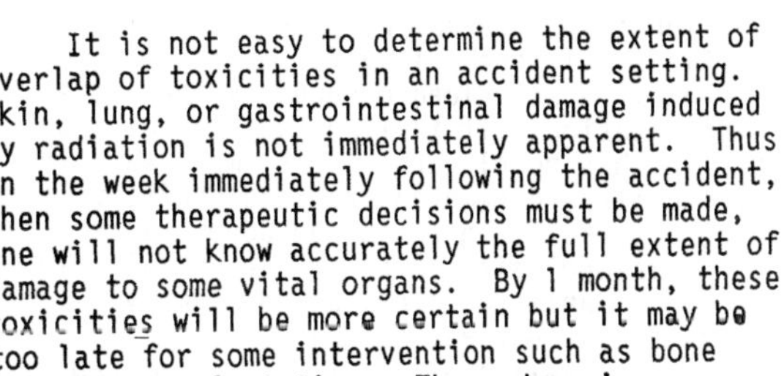

It is not easy to determine the extent of overlap of toxicities in an accident setting. Skin, lung, or gastrointestinal damage induced by radiation is not immediately apparent. Thus in the week immediately following the accident, when some therapeutic decisions must be made, one will not know accurately the full extent of damage to some vital organs. By 1 month, these toxicities will be more certain but it may be too late for some intervention such as bone marrow transplantation. These dynamic relationships are illustrated in Figure 3. In this situation the physician faces two possibilities, either intervene in all instances in which there is any possibility of survival or withhold therapy until the situation is resolved. This is not a simple decision. In the former instance, it means that many

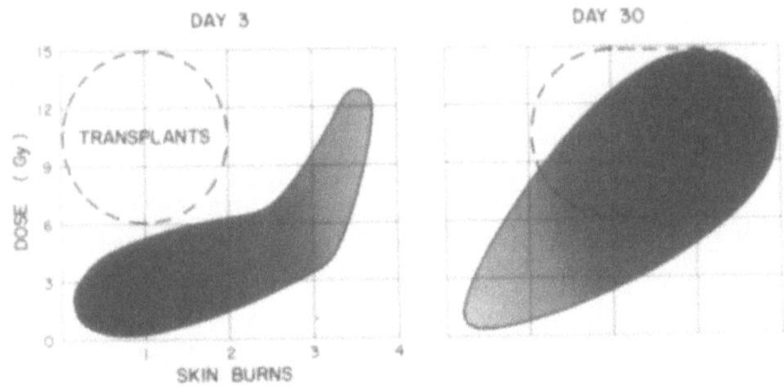

procedures which, while themselves successful, will not save lives because other toxicities will ultimately supervene. This is less a problem when the planned intervention is without inherent risk then when a risk is involved. At the other extreme, failure to intervene because of the possibility of other toxicities may lose lives if the efficacy of the intervention is compromised by waiting.

The recent accident at Cheronbyl has been reported in detail (5-8). This accident raised interesting questions regarding the potential role of transplantation in the medical response to nuclear accidents. Although a detailed discussion of this subject is beyond the objective of this review, it may be instructive to consider some of the major factors.

Transplantation of hematopoietic stem cells can unquestionably rescue animals and humans from otherwise bone marrow lethal doses of radiation. This rescue can occur by several mechanisms. In one instance, hematopoietic stem cells in the graft reconstitute hematopoiesis in the recipient. This reconstitution may be temporary or permanent. If reconsitution is temporary, survival of the recipient depends on recovery of endogenous hematopoiesis. Other possible mechanisms by which bone marrow transplantation can improve survival following high-dose radiation have also been described. For example, irradiated mice who receive transplants of histoincompatible, H-2 mismatched, T-cell depleted bone marrow transplants have a high rate of survival. However, blood cells in survivors are clearly of recipient and not donor origin (9,10). Thus, by an as yet unexplained mechanism, this type of transplant either stimulates recovery of recipient hematopoiesis or a temporarily functioning transplant permits the animal to survive sufficiently long for host hematopoietic recovery. Most evidence supports the latter interpretation. It is important to point out that in this model survival is improved only if the T-cells are removed from the graft; failure to do so results in sustained donor rather than host hematopoiesis. Also, these animals die rapidly of another complication, namely graft-vs-host disease (GvHD).

The potential efficacy of bone marrow transplant also depends on the dose of radiation. Mice that receive relatively lower doses of radiation (2-4 Gy) followed by transplantation of H-2 incompatible bone marrow cells have decreased survival compared to controls (11). This effect is referred to as a mid-lethal range effect. Studies using parental and F1-hybrid combination suggest that this decrease in survival is related to graft-rejection. It appears that rejection of incompatible bone marrow cells somehow decreased the likelihood or rate of endogensous hematopoietic recovery. This effect is illustrated schematically in Figure 4. Whether the same observations would pertain to T-cell depleted transplants is unknown. More importantly, most studies in large animals such as dogs and monkeys fail to show this mid-lethal range effect (12,13). Clinically this is not an important principle since transplants are not likely to be performed in individuals receiving radiation doses in this range.

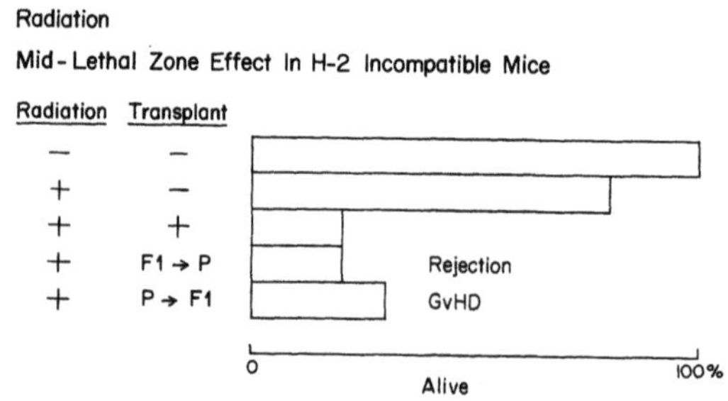

Major concepts regarding the use of bone marrow transplants include the notion that radiation induced bone marrow failure is a likely cause of death at high-doses of radiation, that other toxicities are not likely to be an important factor, that transplants may be beneficial but are unlikely to be harmful even if unsuccessful, and that sustained hematopoietic engraftment is not a requisite beneficial effect. Are these concepts correct? First, as I discussed, the likelihood of death from bone marrow failure alone without complicating toxicities, depends on the nature of the accident and will differ between accidents. Also, it may not be possible to make this determination at the time when a decision regarding bone marrow transplantation must be made. What of the absence of any potential negative effect of bone marrow transplants? Clearly this is an oversimplification. I have already discussed two potential adverse outcomes, the mid-lethal range effect (if it exists in man) and the possibility of inducing graft-vs-host disease. The probability of these potentailly adverse outcomes will depend on several factors including the dose of radiation, the histocompatibility relationship between donor and recipient, the efficacy of measures designed to prevent or modify GvHD such as T-cell depletion or cyclosporine and others. For example T-cell depletion clearly increases the risk of graft rejection while decreasing the likelihood of GvHD (14,15). The age and sex of the recipient and donor are also important since these are determinants of the likelihood and severity of GvHD in most instances (16). Clearly other factors may also be important in determining the likelihood of a negative consequence of bone marrow transplantation. It should be pointed out that some of these variables can be manipulated. For example, it is possible to change the dose of radiation received by an accident victim by administering additional radiation or immune suppression such as cyclophosphamide or antithymocyte globulin (ATG). In a practical sense, this approach is not likely to be useful for this purpose since individuals at risk of the mid-lethal range effect do not require bone marrow transplantation. Additional radiation might, however, be useful in the setting where an individual receives a dose of radiation with a high risk of death from bone marrow suppression, such as 8-10 Gy, but which is insufficient to permit sustained engraftment of genetically non-identical hematopoietic stem cells. In this instance, increasing the cumulative dose of radiation to 12-14 Gy or giving additional immune suppression might be useful therapeutically.

Is sustained engraftment necessary for a beneficial response to transplantation? Although this question cannot be answered definitively in man, considerable data from animal models including mice and dogs suggest that sustained engraftment is not required (10,13). This is not surprising since even extremely high doses of radiation are unlikely to eliminate all recipient hematopoietic stem cells. Furthermore data from transplants in the W/WV mouse indicate that hematopoietic repopulation can occur from a single pluripotent stem cell (17). For this to succeed, reconstitution must be extremely slow otherwise differentiation will predominate over stem cell self-renewal. It is also clear that a proportion of human transplant recipients with initial donor engraftment convert to recipient hematopoiesis after 1 to 2 years (18).

Presumably the correlation between transient engraftment, recovery of recipient hematopoiesis and improved survival relates to temporary function of the graft. This is more likely to occur in mice than man because of the considerably more rapid engraftment in the former, less than 1 week versus greater than 2-3 weeks. It is also possible that transient engraftment is beneficial for other reasons such as by providing accessory cells that stimulate hematopoiesis or by releasing hematopoietic growth factors. Whatever the mechanism, temporary engraftment followed by recovery of recipient hematopoiesis is an optimal outcome of bone marrow transplantation in this setting; it is preferred to sustained chimerism for obvious reasons.

The dose of whole body radiation thought to be lethal to 50 percent of normal individuals (LD_{50}) was 4.5 Gy (19,20). This calculation is based on studies in other species and limited data in atomic bomb survivors. The correct definition of the LD_{50} assumes that radiation is the sole cause of death, that the recipient population is relatively homogenous, that each individual receives an identical dose and that no supportive care, such as antibiotics or transfusions, are given. Clearly this concept has limited applicability to humans following a radiation accident. For example, it is difficult to calculate an effective dose when dealing with non-uniform radiation by different energies and by different routes. Although in theory this can be done, in practice it is difficult or impossible. Also, the LD_{50} for children is likely to be higher than for adults. Finally, supportive measures are likely to be utilized. Thus, the LD_{50} although of considerable biologic interest is, in my opinion, of limited importance in determining therapeutic strategy. Other measurements may be more useful; for example the $LD_{10/20}$ or the $LD_{80/90}$; these represent the 10% lethal doses respectively. The physician faces a range of therapeutic options. Some, such as red blood cell transfusions are of relatively low risk and might be given to any individual with severe anemia. Other interventions, such as prophylactic platelet transfusions or systemic antibiotics involve higher but still quite acceptable risks and might be given to individuals receiving an estimated LD_{10}. Finally some procedures, such as bone marrow transplantation, are associated with substantial risk; these might be used in individuals receiving an LD_{90} dose but not an LD_{10}.

Two other concepts merit consideration. First, the relationship between the mode of death at any lethal dose and the anticipated outcome of the therapeutic intervention should be clear. If, in a specific accident, most deaths occur from skin damage, an individual who receives an LD_{90} dose is unlikely to benefit from platelet transfusions since this can only decrease the chance of death from hemorrhage, not burns. Thus, the lethal dose must be operationally defined for each accident. This leads us to the concept of expressing the lethal dose in the context of a specific outcome. For example, if we knew an individual received a dose of radiation associated with a 90% probability of death from bone marrow failure, we are likely to consider a transplant unless it is certain that he will die of other causes. In contrast, an individual who receives a radiation dose associated with a 90% probability of death from skin damage may (in theory) have a 90% chance of recovery of bone marrow function should he survive his burns. One is unlikely to consider a bone marrow transplant in this instance.

The second factor which must be considered is the relative efficacy (or risk) of a planned intervention in a specific setting. As an example, transplantation of genetically identical bone marrow from a twin is associated with little if any risk. If a radiation victim had an identical twin one might consider a bone marrow transplant whether he received an LD_{10} or LD_{90} bone marrow dose. In contrast, an HLA-mismatched transplant in an older recipient is associated with substantial risks; it might be considered in someone receiving an LD_{90} but an and LD_{10}.

Although these considerations appear complex, they reflect a common decision making process in which one weighs the potential adverse outcomes associated with a disease process in a specific patient with the potential benefits and risks of a specific intervention in that individual. Thus, it is difficult to reach general conclusions regarding the applicability of different internventions; each individual must be considered specifically.

A final caution relates to the interpretation of the results of specific interventions. For example, an individual who receives a bone marrow transplant may survive a high dose of radiation. As I discussed, the origin of the hematopoietic cell post-transplant is not useful in determining if the transplant was successful in rescuing the recipient. Nor does the fact that a proportion of individuals who received what is estimated to be a similar dose of radiation permit us to define if a specific individual is alive because of the transplant. Under usual circumstances we would perform a randomized trial in which individuals receiving a certain dose would be randomly assigned to receive or not to receive a bone marrow transplant. Clearly this is not possible in the context of a radiation accident.

In summary, analysis of the potential role of bone marrow transplantation in nuclear accidents is complex. It is not possible to reach firm conclusions since the answer will vary from accident to accident and from patient to patient. In accidents which cause substantial, overlapping toxicities, such as with a graphite moderated reactor transplants probably play a minor role and the success rate is unlikely to exceed 25%. In other accidents, such as those more likley to occur with light water reactors which are most common in the United States, Europe and Soviet Union, the extent of overlappiing toxicities is likely to be less. Transplants may play a greater role and the anticipated success rate may exceed 50%.

Clearly additional studies are needed to precisely define the role of bone marrow transplantation in the range of nuclear reactor accidents which may occur. Areas of particular interest include determination of the uniformity of dose, the concept of additional immune suppression, and technics aimed at achieving temporary engraftment while avoiding GvHD. Some of these studies are in progress. Also of interest is the potentail use of fetal liver cells (21,22), of HLA-matched unrelated donors selected from volunteer donor poos (23), and the use of molecularly cloned hematopoietic growth factors (24).

ACKNOWLEDGEMENT

I would like to thank my Soviet and American colleagues for thoughtful discussion of several issues raised in this review. Special thanks are due to Drs. Angelina Guskova, Alexander Baranov, Andrei Vorobiev, Leonid ILyan of the USSR, Richard Champlin, Richard Jacobs, Paul Teraski, and Marvin Goldman of the USA, and Yair Reisner from Israel. Linda Rodman kindly typed the manuscript. My special thanks to Dr. Armand Hammer for his medical and humanitarian efforts.

Supported in part by Grant CA23175 NCI, NIH, USPHS, DHHS.

REFERENCES

1. Eisert WG, Mendelsohn ML (eds) (1984) Biological Dosimetery. Springer-Verlag: Berlin
2. Wald N (1986) Status of cytogenetic screening. In: Underhill DW, Radford EP (eds) New and Sensitive Indicators of Health Impacts of Environmental Agents. Pittsburg: University of Pittsburgh Press, pp 187-1999
3. IAEA Techinical Report 260 (1986) Biological Dosimetry: Chromosomal Aberration Analysis for Dose Assessment. Vienna
4. Barabanova AB, Baranov AE, Guskova AK, et al (1986) Acute radiation effects in man. National Committee Radiation Protection, Moscow
5. USSR (1986) <u>The Accident at Chernobyl Nuclear Power Plant and its Consequences</u>. Information compiled by the USSR State Committee on the Utilization of Atomic Energy for the IAEA Experts' Meeting, August 25-29, 1986, Vienna
6. IAEA (1986) Summary Report on the Post Accident Review Meeting on the Chernobyl Accident. International Atomic Energy Agency. International Safety Group (INSAG), Vienna
7. Goldman M, Catlin RJ, Anspaugh L, et al. Health and environmental consequences of the Chernobyl nuclear power plant accident. Department of Energy (To Be Released)
8. Ahearne JF (1987) Nuclear power after Chernobyl. Science 236:673-679
9. Ferrara J, Lipton J, Hellman S, Burakoff S, Mauch P (1987) Engraftment following T-cell depleted marrow transplantation. I. The role of major and minor histocompatibility barriers. Transplantation 43:461-467
10. Reisner Y, Lapidot J. Personal Communication
11. Trentin JJ (1959) Grafted-marrow-rejection mortality contrasted to homologous disease in irradiated mice receiving homologous bone marrow. J Natl CAncer Inst 22:219-228
12. Thomas ED, Leblond R, Graham T, Storb R (1970) Marrow infusions in dogs given mid-lethal and lethal irradiation. Radiat Res 41:113-124
13. Monroy RL, Vriesendorp HM, MacVittie TJ. Improved survival of dogs exposed to fission neutron irradiation and transplanted with DLA identical bone marrow. Bone Marrow Transplantation (In Press)
14. Gale RP (1987) T-cells, bone marrow transplantation and immunotherapy: Use of monoclonal antibodies. In: Fahey JL (moderator) Immune Interventions in disease. Ann Intern Med 106:257-274
15. Butturini A, Franchechini F, Gale RP (1987) Critical analysis of T-cell depleted bone marrow transplantation. In: Gale RP, Champlin RE (eds) Progress in Bone Marrow Transplantation, New York: Alan R. Liss, pp 323-335
16. Gale RP, Bortin MM, van Bekum DW, et al Risk factors for acute graft-versus-host disease. Br J Haematol (In Press)
17. Abramson S, Miller RG, Phillips RA (1977) The identification in adult bone marrow of pluripotent and restricted stem cells of the myeloid and lymphoid systems. J Exp Med 145:1567-1579

18. Hill RS, Petersen FB, Storb R, et al (1986) Mixed hematologic chimerism after allogeneic marrow transplantation for severe aplastic anemia is associated with a higher risk of graft rejection and a lessened incidence of acute graft-versus-host disease. Blood 67:811
19. Medical Research Council Committee on Effects of Ionizing Radiation. A forum on lethality from acute and protracted radiation exposure in man. (1984) Int J Radiat Biol 46:209-217
20. UNSCEAR (1982) Ionizing Radiation: Sources and Biologic Effects. Report to the General Assembly
21. Gale RP, Touraine J-L, Lucarelli G (eds) (1985) Recent Advances in Fetal Liver Transplantation. New York: Alan R. Liss
22. Touraine JL, Kochupillae V, Gale RP (eds) (1987) Fetal Liver Transplantation. Amsterdam: Martinus Nijhoff
23. Gale RP (1986) Potential utilization of a national HLA-typed donor pool for bone marrow transplantation. Transplantation 42:54-58
24. Metacalf D (1985) The granulocyte-macrophage colony stimulating factors. Science 229: 16-22

Conclusions

G.W. Santos

Great progress has been made in the last 2 decades since the first successful allogeneic marrow transplants were performed in man. Cure rates approaching 40-60% are possible in acute leukemias and chronic myelogenous leukemia, 50-70% in severe aplastic anemia and 70-80% in beta thalassemia. Data in animal disease models and early clinical results indicate that allogeneic marrow transplantation may assume a role in the therapy of lysosomal storage diseases. It is in these genetic diseases that gene transfer therapy may eventually be tried. Marrow transplantation is now a world wide endeavor. The International Bone Marrow Transplantation Registry estimates that more than 2,500 allogeneic and 1,000 autologous transplants are performed annually.

A number of problems remain, however; before marrow transplantation is able to realize its full therapeutic potential. Partial solutions to some of these problems have been presented in this symposium.

The results of autologous marrow transplantation in lymphomas and the acute leukemias are encouraging and provide potential solutions to the problem of lack of sufficient donors. Whether marrow purging with monoclonal antibodies, chemicals or depletion of leukemic contamination by long term marrow culture is necessary is perhaps controversial but early therapeutic results are quite encouraging.

Graft-versus-host disease (GVHD) remains a serious problem in most centers. T cell depletion of marrow may lessen or prevent this complication but often this is at the expense of marrow rejection or increase in relapse of leukemia. Other approaches to this problem are presented in this symposium. The development of an in vitro predictive model of human GVHD and the further insights into the immunobiology of syngeneic, acute allogeneic, and chronic GVHD are exciting findings that hopefully will provide new information as to the prevention and control of this complication.

Leukemic relapses present a continuing problem particularly in allogeneic transplants after T cell depletion, in patients transplanted in second or subsequent remissions and in autologous transplants. New creative approaches with new preparative regimens are needed. A few of the reports in this symposium suggest that there may be very valid regimens such as busulfan and cyclophosphamide and monoclonal antibody directed radiation that do not involve conventional total body irradiation.

Deaths due to bacterial, fungal, and viral infections are being reduced in many centers using some of the studies outlined in this symposium.

Although there are many problems that remain in the therapeutic application of marrow transplantation in human disease, it should be realized that solutions to many of the problems will be of direct applicability to the medical management of victims of nuclear accidents. With the current world wide intensity in basic and clinical research as evidenced by this international symposium we should look to the future with renewed dedication and optimism.

MIX
Papier aus verantwortungsvollen Quellen
Paper from responsible sources
FSC® C105338

If you have any concerns about our products,
you can contact us on
ProductSafety@springernature.com

In case Publisher is established outside the EU,
the EU authorized representative is:
Springer Nature Customer Service Center GmbH
Europaplatz 3, 69115 Heidelberg, Germany

Printed by Libri Plureos GmbH
in Hamburg, Germany